D1551903

THE WILEY BICENTENNIAL–KNOWLEDGE FOR GENERATIONS

*E*ach generation has its unique needs and aspirations. When Charles Wiley first opened his small printing shop in lower Manhattan in 1807, it was a generation of boundless potential searching for an identity. And we were there, helping to define a new American literary tradition. Over half a century later, in the midst of the Second Industrial Revolution, it was a generation focused on building the future. Once again, we were there, supplying the critical scientific, technical, and engineering knowledge that helped frame the world. Throughout the 20th Century, and into the new millennium, nations began to reach out beyond their own borders and a new international community was born. Wiley was there, expanding its operations around the world to enable a global exchange of ideas, opinions, and know-how.

For 200 years, Wiley has been an integral part of each generation's journey, enabling the flow of information and understanding necessary to meet their needs and fulfill their aspirations. Today, bold new technologies are changing the way we live and learn. Wiley will be there, providing you the must-have knowledge you need to imagine new worlds, new possibilities, and new opportunities.

Generations come and go, but you can always count on Wiley to provide you the knowledge you need, when and where you need it!

WILLIAM J. PESCE
PRESIDENT AND CHIEF EXECUTIVE OFFICER

PETER BOOTH WILEY
CHAIRMAN OF THE BOARD

Introduction to U.S. Health Care

Dennis D. Pointer, Stephen J. Williams, Stephen L. Isaacs, and James R. Knickman

with Tracy Barr

BICENTENNIAL
BICENTENNIAL
1807
WILEY
2007
BICENTENNIAL
BICENTENNIAL

Credits

PUBLISHER
Anne Smith

PROJECT EDITOR
Beth Tripmacner

MARKETING MANAGER
Jennifer Slomack

EDITORIAL ASSISTANT
Tiara Kelly

PRODUCTION MANAGER
Kelly Tavares

PRODUCTION ASSISTANT
Courtney Leshko

CREATIVE DIRECTOR
Harry Nolan

COVER DESIGNER
Hope Miller

COVER PHOTO
Gary S. Chapman/Getty Images, Inc.

This book was set in Times New Roman, printed and bound by R. R. Donnelley.

The cover was printed by Phoenix Color.

To order books or for customer service please, call 1-800-CALL WILEY (225-5945).

Library of Congress Cataloging-in-Publication Data

Introduction to U.S. health care/Dennis D. Pointer . . . [et al.].
   p. cm.
  Includes index.
  ISBN-13: 978-0-471-79075-4 (pbk.)
  ISBN-10: 0-471-79075-3 (pbk.)
1. Medical care—United States. 2. Medical Policy—United States. 3. Health facilities-United States. I. Pointer, Dennis Dale.
  RA395.A31496 2007
  362.10973—dc22   2006031239

ISBN-13 978-0-471-79075-4

ISBN-10 0-471-79075-3

Printed in the United States of America

10 9 8 7 6 5 4 3 2

PREFACE

College classrooms bring together learners from many backgrounds with a variety of aspirations. Although the students are in the same course, they are not necessarily on the same path. This diversity, coupled with the reality that these learners often have jobs, families, and other commitments, requires a flexibility that our nation's higher education system is addressing. Distance learning, shorter course terms, new disciplines, evening courses, and certification programs are some of the approaches that colleges employ to reach as many students as possible and help them clarify and achieve their goals.

Wiley Pathways books, a new line of texts from John Wiley & Sons, Inc., are designed to help you address this diversity and the need for flexibility. These books focus on the fundamentals, identify core competencies and skills, and promote independent learning. The focus on the fundamentals helps students grasp the subject, bringing them all to the same basic understanding. These books use clear, everyday language, presented in an uncluttered format, making the reading experience more pleasurable. The core competencies and skills help students succeed in the classroom and beyond, whether in another course or in a professional setting. A variety of built-in learning resources promote independent learning and help instructors and students gauge students' understanding of the content. These resources enable students to think critically about their new knowledge, and apply their skills in any situation.

Our goal with *Wiley Pathways* books—with its brief, inviting format, clear language, and core competencies and skills focus—is to celebrate the many students in your courses, respect their needs, and help you guide them on their way.

CASE Learning System

To meet the needs of working college students, *Introduction to U.S. Health Care* uses a four-step process: The CASE Learning System. Based on Bloom's Taxonomy of Learning, CASE presents key health care topics in easy-to-follow chapters. The text then prompts analysis, synthesis, and evaluation with a variety of learning aids and assessment tools. Students move efficiently from reviewing what they have learned, to acquiring new information and skills, to applying their new knowledge and skills to real-life scenarios:

▲ Content

▲ Analysis

▲ Synthesis

▲ Evaluation

Using the CASE Learning System, students not only achieve academic mastery of health care *topics,* but they master real-world health care administration *skills.* The CASE Learning System also helps students become independent learners, giving them a distinct advantage whether they are starting out or seek to advance in their careers.

Organization, Depth and Breadth of the Text

Introduction to U.S. Health Care offers the following features:

▲ **Modular format.** Research on college students shows that they access information from textbooks in a non-linear way. Instructors also often wish to reorder textbook content to suit the needs of a particular class. Therefore, although *Introduction to U.S. Health Care* proceeds logically from the basics to increasingly more challenging material, chapters are further organized into sections (4 to 6 per chapter) that are self-contained for maximum teaching and learning flexibility.

▲ **Numeric system of headings.** *Introduction to U.S. Health Care* uses a numeric system for headings (for example, 2.3.4 identifies the fourth sub-section of Section 3 of Chapter 2). With this system, students and teachers can quickly and easily pinpoint topics in the table of contents and the text, keeping class time and study sessions focused.

▲ **Core content.** This volume is designed to introduce students to the vast health care industry of the United States. Understanding the basics of the industry, how it is organized, the various health care models are all keys to making sense of one of the industries that affects the lives of everyone living in the United States. This understanding is crucial for anyone working in the health care industry.

The health care system used to be simple. The players were the physician, the nurse, the patient, the hospital, and one type of insurance.

Most people had insurance because almost all companies offered free or low cost insurance to their employees. Today the system is much more complex and involves technology, pharmaceutical companies, specialists, and a wide range of types of insurance. To further complicate matters, employers are shifting a greater percentage of the cost burden of insurance to employees. *Introduction to U.S. Health Care* addresses all these topics and breaks down every segment of the U.S. Health Care system, which can be overwhelming and confusing, into clear basic concepts. Every concept is illustrated with a real-world example to further reinforce the concepts.

The U.S. health care system is the only one of the industrialized nations that is not a public system where all citizens are provided basic health care coverage. One out of five citizens does not have any insurance coverage. This staggering statistic presents challenges to the U.S. health care system and affects the care that all of us receive. In addition to serving the uninsured, the health care industry faces additional challenges. The strain of an aging population and the shortage of nurses are just two of the obstacles that are assessed in *Introduction to U.S. Health Care*.

The book is divided into five distinct sections. The first section is, "Foundations," and it gives the student a knowledge base on the health care industry as a jumping off point for deeper discussions. The second section, "Health Care Organizing and Finance," examines different models of health care and how each one is financed. The third section, "Health Care Resources," discusses the workforce, technology, and research that comprise the health care industry and the day-to-day health care decisions that are made. The fourth section, "The Health Care Delivery System," assesses the evolution of the hospitals, long-term care, and ambulatory care. In addition, caring for the underserved populations is also discussed. The fifth section, "Challenges of U.S. Health Care," looks at the future challenges and present ideas to overcome them.

Part I: The U.S. Health Care System

This text begins with an introductory chapter entitled, The U.S. Health Care System. This chapter provides an introduction and overview of the nation's largest service industry and all the sectors it encompasses.

Chapter 2, Boards and Governance, outlines the role of governing boards and the challenges they face.

Part II: Health Care Organizing and Finance

Chapter 3, Health Care Provision, compares and contrasts the primary-care model and the specialty-care model with an emphasis on the primary-care model. This chapter also discusses recent health care reforms that affect the primary-care model.

Chapter 4, Financing the U.S. Health Care System, examines how we pay for health care, whether it is through insurance, Medicare, or Medicaid. Private and public finance models are covered as well as an examination of who has insurance and who does not.

Part III: Health Care Resources

Chapter 5, The Health Care Workforce, discusses the enormous workforce that supports the health care industry. The health care workforce includes diverse players such as nurses, medical assistants, general practitioners, specialists, pharmacists, and physical therapists. Each player has a unique role that is essential to the ability of the health care system to meet patients' needs.

Chapter 6, Research and Technology, discusses medical research and how medical miracles are financed. This chapter also includes an assessment of how technology is used to diagnose medical conditions at earlier stages than was previously possible.

Part IV: The Health Care Delivery System

Chapter 7, Hospitals in the U.S., looks at the evolution of hospitals throughout the nation's history and through their current state. The components and costs of hospitals are examined. Also assessed is how hospitals are classified.

Chapter 8, Ambulatory Care, assesses the reasons behind the growing reliance on ambulatory care. The chapter also discusses the different choices of ambulatory care settings and providers.

Chapter 9, Long-Term Care, discusses who needs long-term care, why, and what the choices are.

Chapter 10, Caring for Special Populations, discusses the challenges of providing health services for society's most vulnerable groups. The chapter discusses delivering services to the mentally ill, the homeless, immigrants, victims of violence, and people with AIDS and HIV. A section devoted to providing health care for veterans is also included as veterans often have unique medical challenges.

Chapter 11, Caring for Uninsured Patients, assesses the obstacles in caring for the uninsured and effectively handling the bureaucracy one encounters when trying to deliver medical services to the uninsured.

Chapter 12, Managed Care, examines the evolution of the managed care system as a solution to high health care costs. The types of managed care organizations such as health maintenance organizations (HMOs), Preferred Provider Organizations (PPOs), and Point-of-Service (POS) plans are discussed. The performance and impact of managed care organizations on the health care industry is also assessed.

Part V: Challenges of U.S. Health Care

Chapter 13, Promoting Health and Preventing Disease, discusses the current and future challenges for the health care industry. These challenges include: the growing complexity of the health care system, the strain on the system from the aging population, the needs of the underserved, incorporating advancing technology, the shortage of nurses, evolving public threats, and the financial state of hospitals.

Chapter 14, Public Health Policy, assesses the laws, regulations, and initiatives that have recently been implemented or are under consideration and how they will affect the ever-changing health care industry.

Learning Aids

Each chapter of *Introduction to U.S. Health Care* features the following learning and study aids to activate students' prior knowledge of the topics and orient them to the material.

▲ **Pre-test.** This pre-reading assessment tool in multiple-choice format not only introduces chapter material, but it also helps students anticipate the chapter's learning outcomes. By focusing students' attention on what they do not know, the self-test provides students with a benchmark against which they can measure their own progress. The pre-test is available online at www.wiley.com/college/pointer.

▲ **What You'll Learn in This Chapter and After Studying This Chapter.** These bulleted lists tell students what they will be learning in the chapter and why it is significant for their careers. They also explain why the chapter is important and how it relates to other chapters in the text. "What You'll Learn. . ." lists focus on the *subject matter* that will be taught (e.g. what ambulatory care is). "After Studying This Chapter. . ." lists emphasize *capabilities and skills* students will learn (e.g. how to compare and contrast different types of ambulatory care settings).

▲ **Goals and Outcomes.** These lists identify specific student capabilities that will result from reading the chapter. They set students up to synthesize and evaluate the chapter material, and relate it to the real world.

▲ **Figures and Tables.** Line art and photos have been carefully chosen to be truly instructional rather than filler. Tables distill and present information in a way that is easy to identify, access, and understand, enhancing the focus of the text on essential ideas.

Within-text Learning Aids

The following learning aids are designed to encourage analysis and synthesis of the material, and to support the learning process and ensure success during the evaluation phase:

▲ **Introduction.** This section orients the student by introducing the chapter and explaining its practical value and relevance to the book as a whole. Short summaries of chapter sections preview the topics to follow.

▲ **"For Example" Boxes.** Found within each section, these boxes tie section content to real-world organizations, scenarios, and applications.

▲ **Self-Check.** Related to the "What You'll Learn" bullets and found at the end of each section, this battery of short answer questions emphasizes student understanding of concepts and mastery of section content. Though the questions may either be discussed in class or studied by students outside of class, students should not go on before they can answer all questions correctly. Each *Self-Check* question set includes a link to a section of the pre-test for further review and practice.

▲ **Summary.** Each chapter concludes with a summary paragraph that reviews the major concepts in the chapter and links back to the "What You'll Learn" list.

▲ **Key Terms and Glossary.** To help students develop a professional vocabulary, key terms are bolded in the introduction, summary and when they first appear in the chapter. A complete list of key terms with brief definitions appears at the end of each chapter and again in a glossary at the end of the book. Knowledge of key terms is assessed by all assessment tools (see below).

Evaluation and Assessment Tools

The evaluation phase of the CASE Learning System consists of a variety of within-chapter and end-of-chapter assessment tools that test how well students have learned the material. These tools also encourage students to extend their learning into different scenarios and higher levels of understanding and thinking. The following assessment tools appear in every chapter of *Introduction to U.S. Health Care*:

▲ **Summary Questions** help students summarize the chapter's main points by asking a series of multiple choice and true/false questions that emphasize student understanding of concepts and mastery of chapter content. Students should be able to answer all of the Summary Questions correctly before moving on.

▲ **Review Questions** in short answer format review the major points in each chapter, prompting analysis while reinforcing and confirming student understanding of concepts, and encouraging mastery of chapter content. They are somewhat more difficult than the *Self-Check* and *Summary Questions,* and students should be able to answer most of them correctly before moving on.

▲ **Applying This Chapter Questions** drive home key ideas by asking students to synthesize and apply chapter concepts to new, real-life situations and scenarios.

▲ **You Try It Questions** are designed to extend students' thinking, and so are ideal for discussion or writing assignments. Using an open-ended format and sometimes based on Web sources, they encourage students to draw conclusions using chapter material applied to real-world situations, which fosters both mastery and independent learning.

▲ **Post-test** should be taken after students have completed the chapter. It includes all of the questions in the pre-test, so that students can see how their learning has progressed and improved.

Instructor and Student Package

Introduction to U.S. Health Care is available with the following teaching and learning supplements. All supplements are available online at the text's Book Companion Website, located at *www.wiley.com/ college/pointer*.

▲ **Instructor's Resource Guide.** Provides the following aids and supplements for teaching:

- *Diagnostic Evaluation of Grammar, Mechanics, and Spelling.* A useful tool that instructors may administer to the class at the beginning of the course to determine each students' basic writing skills. The Evaluation is accompanied by an Answer Key and a Marking Key. Instructors are encouraged to use the Marking key when grading students' Evaluations, and to duplicate and distribute it to students with their graded evaluations.

- *Sample syllabus.* A convenient template that instructors may use for creating their own course syllabi.

- *Teaching suggestions.* For each chapter, these include a chapter summary, learning objectives, definitions of key terms, lecture notes, answers to select text question sets, and at least 3 suggestions for classroom activities, such as ideas for speakers to invite, videos to show, and other projects.

▲ **Test Bank.** One test per chapter, as well as a mid-term and a final. Each includes true/false, multiple choice, and open-ended questions. Answers and page references are provided for the true/false and multiple choice questions, and page references for the open-ended questions. Available in Microsoft Word and computerized formats.

▲ **PowerPoints.** Key information is summarized in 10 to 15 PowerPoints per chapter. Instructors may use these in class or choose to share them with students for class presentations or to provide additional study support.

ACKNOWLEDGMENTS

No book is solely the product of its authors. Books tend to be culminations of accumulated experience that grow from many influences. We would like to thank all of the reviewers for their feedback and suggestions during the text's development. Their advice on how to shape *Introduction to U.S. Health Care* into a solid learning tool that meets both their needs and those of their busy students is deeply appreciated. We would like to thank:

Danny C. Borton, University of Michigan, Flint
Andre L. Lee, DPA, FACHE
Donna J. Slovensky, University of Alabama at Birmingham

In addition, the editors would also like to gratefully acknowledge the following people for their extensive contributions to the book:

Mary Ann Keogh Hass, Ph.D., Eastern Washington University
Robin Pickering, Eastern Washington University
Michael W. Posey, Franklin University

BRIEF CONTENTS

CONTENTS

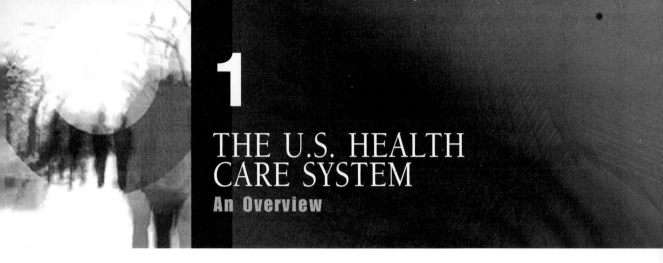

1

THE U.S. HEALTH CARE SYSTEM
An Overview

Starting Point

Go to www.wiley.com/college/pointer to assess your knowledge of health care industry basics.
Determine where you need to concentrate your effort.

What You'll Learn in This Chapter

▲ How large the U.S. health care industry is, based on expenditures
▲ The different types of health care organizations
▲ How health care organizations are structured into health systems
▲ The various industry sectors that comprise the U.S. health care system
▲ Triggers to health care utilization

After Studying This Chapter, You'll Be Able To

▲ Describe total health care expenditures and identify where the money goes
▲ Differentiate between the functions of private and public health organizations
▲ Identify differences between health systems
▲ Define health and disease
▲ Analyze factors affecting health care utilization
▲ Interpret the role of medical care research

Goals and Outcomes

▲ Understand the organization of the U.S. health industry
▲ Determine the role of health care organizations based on the organization's characteristics
▲ Explain the relationship between health sectors and health organizations
▲ Compare different health systems based on their affiliations with other health organizations
▲ Articulate how health care utilization factors impede or promote health care utilization

INTRODUCTION

The U.S. health care industry is vast. Understanding the basics of this industry—how large it is, how it's organized, what the various health sectors are—remains key to making sense of an industry that affects the lives of all people living in the United States. One of the largest enterprises in the United States, the health care industry represents over 15 percent of all goods and services produced in the country. The primary providers of health services are health care organizations (HCOs). HCOs seek to maximize the efficiency and cost-effectiveness of health care by combining organizations into coordinated units. The entire health care industry is intended to promote and protect the health and well-being of the U.S. population. However, how and when people access health care, as well as the factors influencing the availability of care, impact the overall health status of the nation.

The health care system in the United States is a combination of public and private services. It is the only health care system of the industrialized nations that is not a public system with all of its citizens provided basic health care coverage. The current estimates are that 1 of every 5 citizens does not have health insurance coverage. This lack of coverage challenges all aspects of the industry. Four main issues face health care today, driving one of the largest industries in the nation: cost, access, quality, and safety.

The "system" of health care used to be comprised of the physician, the nurse, the hospital, and the insurance plan, which was either private or public. Today the system is extremely complex and involves an ever-expanding continuum of care with new technology, new medications, new techniques, new sites for services. Some argue that with the lack of integration of services in the public sector, the private sector, and public/private sector, no true health care system exists in the United States.

1.1 Gauging the Size of the Health Care Industry

Today, health care is one of the U.S. economy's largest industries, employing more than 12 million people. This industry provides more than $1.8 trillion worth of **gross goods** (medications and medical supplies) and **services** (health care, public health initiatives, and so on). It is both an altruistic pursuit, enhancing citizens' well-being and quality of life, and a business enterprise, generating profits for private providers and suppliers.

Out-of-pocket expenses for a medical procedure or test, for a routine checkup or wellness exam, or for a prescription cost Americans quite a bit of money. The Office of the Actuary at the Centers for Medicare & Medicaid Services stated that Americans—individuals, insurers, and government agencies—spent nearly $1.9 trillion on health care in 2004. This amount is equal to 16 percent of the **gross domestic product (GDP)**—the total value of goods and services produced in the U.S.—which translates to $6,040 per capita, almost

Table 1-1: Projected National Health Care Expenditures, 2007

Good or Service	Amount in Billions*
Hospital care	$709.1
Professional Services	
Physician and clinical service	$496.5
Other professional services	$ 64.0
Dental	$101.3
Other private health care	$ 67.8
Nursing Home and Home Health Care	
Home health care	$ 57.3
Nursing home care	$134.8
Retail Sales of Medical Products	
Prescription drugs	$236.8
Other medical products	$ 61.1
Government Expenses	
For administration and net cost of private insurance	$236.8
Public health activities	$ 61.1
Investment	
Research	$ 48.9
Structures and equipment	$105.5

Source: Information is based on projections produced by the Office of the Actuary at the Centers for Medicare & Medicaid Services.

*Numbers may not add up due to rounding.

twice the median amount spent by other industrialized nations. Table 1-1 shows where the bulk of the money is expected to go.

Every year, the Office of the Actuary at the Centers for Medicare & Medicaid Services produces a report projecting health care expenditures for the coming decade. These projections describe how much money the United States spends on health care, show where that money comes from, and indicate what factors drive the increase (or decrease) in spending.

As Table 1-1 illustrates, the health care industry includes more than doctors, patients, and medical procedures and medications—the components that are often most obvious to consumers. To this list, add government health initiatives

---

FOR EXAMPLE

Impacting Health Expenditures

According to the most recent projections published by the Centers for Medicare and Medicaid Services, health care expenditures are expected to grow 7.1 percent annually. By 2014, the nation will spend $3.6 trillion on health care, comprising almost 20 percent of the GDP. One of the most significant events impacting these projections is the new prescription drug benefit plan passed by Congress and in effect January 2006.

---

and subsidies, ongoing medical research by both private and public organizations, and building and administrative costs, and you can understand how broad the health care industry is.

SELF-CHECK

- Define **goods** and **gross domestic product.**
- Cite the top expenditure in national health care for 2004.

1.2 Balancing Public and Private Health: Health Care Organizations

There are two types of health care organizations (HCOs): *private* and *public*.

▲ **Private HCOs** provide services that are consumed by, and affect, individuals, such as a physician office visit or an inpatient hospital stay. The goal of these organizations is to protect and enhance the health and well-being of individuals.

▲ **Public HCOs** provide services that targeted the health and well-being of populations or communities.

These distinctions, however, can become confusing because of the fluid nature of health services in the United States and the various entities—federal, state, and local government agencies and programs; commercial organizations (whether for-profit or nonprofit); philanthropic institutions; medical educational systems; and private individuals—that health care involves. Nevertheless, although fluid, the distinctions are helpful in understanding the complex U.S. health system.

1.2.1 Protecting Populations: Public Health Care Organizations

As previously stated, public health care involves the health and well-being of populations and communities. To that end, federal, state, and local government agencies create public policy affecting health-related issues. Examples of this aspect of public health care include the following:

▲ Federal and state funding for health programs.
▲ Public policies relating to infectious diseases.
▲ Antismoking legislation.
▲ Federal nutrition and exercise guidelines.
▲ State licensing procedures for medical professionals.
▲ Community sanitation laws.
▲ Government intervention in the control of infectious diseases.
▲ Pollution standards and controls.
▲ Government-sponsored and funded medical research.

These aspects of public health policy have an impact on personal health issues, but the primary goal of such policies and programs is to foster and support the health and well-being of an entire community, since health-related issues have a tremendous impact on society as a whole, both in terms of productivity and expense. (You can find out more about the role of the U.S. government in public health in Chapter 13.)

1.2.2 Serving Individuals: Private Health Care Organizations

Private health care focuses on the individual, usually in regard to a person's entry into, interaction with, and movement through the U.S. health care system. Even though this journey might include public health policy programs or support (a child whose medical expenses are paid for through Medicaid, for example, or an elderly person who uses his Medicare prescription drug benefit, or a veteran who goes to a VA hospital for treatment), it still falls within the realm of private health care because the primary goal is the health of the individual.

According to the U.S. Census Bureau, there are approximately 470,000 establishments that provide private health care services. Two-thirds are physicians' and dentists' offices; only 2 percent are hospitals, even though hospitals account for about 40 percent of the health care industry's employment. The distribution of health care establishments is contained in Table 1-2.

One distinctive characteristic of private HCOs is that they provide services, not products. Whereas products are tangible items that are first manufactured and then used (they make the car before you buy and use it, for example), **services** are intangibles that are produced and used simultaneously. The care a physician provides isn't needed, in other words, until a patient accesses it.

Table 1-2: Distribution of Private Health Care Organizations

Type of Organization	Percentage of All Establishments
Physicians' offices	41
Dentists' offices	25
Offices of other health care practitioners	19
Nursing homes	6
Medical and dental laboratories	4
Other	3
Hospitals	2

Karl Marx (in *Das Capital*), displaying unusual humor, described them as something you can buy but can't drop on your foot.

In terms of private HCOs, the same is true even for medical supplies (which you *can* drop on your foot) or capacity (the availability of both tangible and intangible resources). Although a defibrillator, for example, may be a product to the medical supply company that sells it and the hospital that buys it, it is not a product to the patient. Why? Because the patient doesn't buy it, even though he may have need of it. In that way, the defibrillator represents health care service that is available if needed.

Because health care services cannot be stored, capacity (such as an unused hospital bed) is lost forever. As a consequence, demand must be either accurately predicted or carefully controlled for an HCO's resources to be productively deployed.

Services (particularly health care) are also custom-designed while they are being produced; their form and content vary from patient to patient. One patient's aching wrist, for example, may indicate a fracture, whereas another patient's aching

---

FOR EXAMPLE

Planning for the Unpredictable

"Planning for need" is a key component of financial viability for organizations that provide services rather than products. For an HCO to use its resources productively and cost-efficiently, demand must be accurately predicted, or it must be carefully controlled. The managed care movement in the United States is a direct result of the burgeoning health care expenses of the last decades.

wrist is the result of arthritis. The service each patient receives is tailor-made to that patient's need.

Beyond being service based, private HCOs also share the following characteristics in order to address the essential needs of their patients:

▲ **Fulfill basic needs:** Health care services fulfill basic needs rather than peripheral wants and desires. For this reason, these services are critical. They have a huge impact on clients' quality of life (and often their survival); when needed, few offerings are as important.

▲ **Involve the emotional and physical:** Health care services and procedures, because they focus on the self, are often physically and psychologically invasive. They are also provided when a person is most threatened, frightened, and vulnerable. As a consequence, their use has a high emotional and spiritual charge.

▲ **Make services accessible to all:** Because of how crucial health care services are, access to basic health care services is an issue. It is faced by every HCO. Consumption is thought to be a right, although government has not guaranteed this. Currently, incarcerated individuals, mentally ill individuals, those 65 years of age and older, those disabled, those meeting federally established poverty requirements, and veterans may receive health care provided through government funded or provided programs. Some states such as Massachusetts and Vermont have developed basic health coverage for their citizens so that basic care is available. To date, health care is not a government-guaranteed right.

▲ **Are paid for by someone other than the patient:** For most goods, those who use the product are also the ones who pay for it. This is often not the case for health care services. Although individuals use these services, the services are often paid for (or "purchased"), in whole or in part, by employers and the government. In the past, because the use of most health care services is insured, patients make few if any out-of-pocket expenditures at the point where they consume care. The trend for out-of-pocket expenses paid by the patient has been changing, with a cost shifting occurring and patients paying more of these expenses.

  • Because those who purchase the services are often not the ones who receive the services, private HCOs must respond to two sets of potentially conflicting expectations and demands, one from purchasers and another from customers. Those who pay for the services want to keep down the costs. Those who receive the services want access to any resources that can satisfactorily address their health concerns. The tension between these two positions has had a dramatic impact on health care in the United States. (See Chapter 11 for more on this.)

▲ **Deal with the complexity of the human body:** The process of producing health care services is complex because the workings of the human body are incompletely understood and the store of knowledge regarding diagnostic and therapeutic technology is vast and building daily.

▲ **Rely on professional staff:** The health care workforce is highly professional; professionals are characterized by extensive, intensive, and lengthy training. Far more so than in other occupations, medical professionals are granted (through such mechanisms as licensing laws) and expect or demand a high degree of autonomy, discretion, and control over their work and the context in which they practice.

▲ **Relinquish control of key factors affecting the organization's operation:** Organizations typically employ the most critical personnel needed to produce their products and services. Airlines, for example, hire pilots, flight attendants, and mechanics; restaurants employ chefs. HCOs are a notable exception. Most do not employ physicians, even though the medical staff has tremendous influence over an organization's operation: specifically, who will be admitted; the course of treatment; the amount and type of resources employed; and as a consequence, costs, productivity, and margins.

▲ **Have a low tolerance of error:** Mistakes made in HCOs often have negative and irreversible consequences, jeopardizing well-being and causing death. Safety has become a major concern for all of health care. The Institute of Medicine Report, *To Err Is Human,* alerted the nation to the safety issues in health care. Since 2000, a major effort has been under way to make patient and worker safety the priority in health care.[1]

▲ **Operate full time:** Most HCOs operate 24 hours a day, 7 days per week, 365 days a year; they never close, must be continuously staffed, and have no downtime.

SELF-CHECK

- Differentiate between **private and public health care organizations.**
- Give three examples of public HCOs.
- Give three examples of private HCOs.
- Name four characteristics of private HCOs.

1.3 Identifying Health Systems

A health system combines into a single enterprise organizations that could function independently. Systems are typically defined or classified along two dimensions: the type of organizations that are combined and the way in which they are combined.

1.3.1 Types of Health Systems

There are two primary system types: *horizontal* and *vertical* (see Figure 1-1):

▲ **Horizontal systems** combine functionally similar organizations, such as groups of short-term general hospitals, physician practices, or nursing homes. Horizontal systems can be composed of similar organizations in a particular market (such as a city) or those spread across a number of markets (for example, hospitals located in various regions of the country).

Figure 1-1

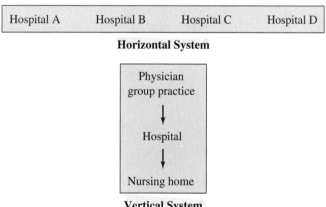

| Hospital A | Hospital B | Hospital C | Hospital D |

Horizontal System

Physician group practice
↓
Hospital
↓
Nursing home

Vertical System

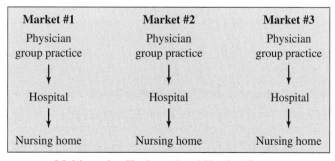

Market #1	**Market #2**	**Market #3**
Physician group practice	Physician group practice	Physician group practice
↓	↓	↓
Hospital	Hospital	Hospital
↓	↓	↓
Nursing home	Nursing home	Nursing home

Multi-market Horizontal and Vertical System

Types of health systems: A horizontal system *(top)*, a vertical system *(middle)*, and a multi-market horizontal and vertical system *(bottom)*.

▲ **Vertical systems** combine functionally different organizations, where patient outputs of one organization in the system (a physician group practice) are inputs of another (a hospital). Vertical systems always combine organizations within a given market. The reason is that patient flow among combined organizations requires geographic proximity.

These two system types can also be combined, as with several vertical systems operating in different markets.

From the mid-1980s through the 1990s, the private health care segment of the industry underwent significant consolidation. Horizontal combinations, particularly among hospitals, sought to achieve economies of scale (where fixed overhead costs were spread across organizations) and build share in local markets to increase bargaining power with health insurance plans. Vertical combinations were undertaken to create a continuum of services ("one-stop shopping") attractive to patients and managed care contractors. These systems, whether horizontal, vertical, or a combination, must be concerned with the consistent demonstration of quality and safety for the patients they serve.

1.3.2 Forming Health Systems

Health systems can be formed through a variety of mechanisms. These mechanisms can be employed alone or in combination:

▲ **Ownership:** Organizations are built or acquired through a purchase or merger.
▲ **Affiliation:** Organizations agree among themselves to cooperate with each other.
▲ **Contracts:** An arrangement is made in which one organization manages another.
▲ **Joint venture:** Two organizations cooperate to undertake a single, specific goal. For example, a hospital and collection of physicians working together to create a health plan.

FOR EXAMPLE

Building a Health System through Acquisition

Community Health Systems is a private health organization that operates general acute care hospitals throughout the United States. Based in Tennessee, the company currently owns, leases, or operates hospitals in 21 states. One of its recent planned acquisitions is the purchase of Newport Hospital and Clinic in Newport, Arkansas, whose assets Community intends to combine with that of another hospital, also in Newport, that the company already owns.

▲ **Lease:** One organization assumes control of another operation for a specified period of time. An example of such an arrangement would be when a hospital assumes control of a nursing home.

SELF-CHECK

- Differentiate between the two primary health system types.
- List the five mechanisms that form HCOs.

1.4 Classifying Health Care Industry Sectors

The health care industry is a complex mix of governmental organizations, non-profit and commercial organizations, and individuals. Each of these entities, or *sectors*, has a particular role in financing, providing, and regulating health care services. The following sections examine these sectors in more detail.

Keep in mind that these classifications are not exclusive: A particular agency may fall into two or more of the groups. A nursing home, for example, functions as an institutional provider (that is, it is an organization that provides health care services), but it also involves individual providers—the nurses, for instance, who actually care for the clients. Similarly, the federal Centers for Medicare and Medicaid Services (CMS) incorporates a financing function, a service provider function, and a regulatory function.

1.4.1 Financing

The *financing sector* reimburses health care providers. These can include any of the following:

▲ Federal agencies, such as the CMS.
▲ State programs, such as workers' compensation programs.
▲ Health insurance companies.
▲ Health maintenance organizations (HMOs).
▲ Employers both small (2–50 employees) and large (over 50 employees).
▲ Individuals.

Notice that, in the United States, those who reimburse health care providers are not necessarily the consumers of the goods or services (the patients). Although health care is, in the private sector, a business—that is, it sells products (medical services) for a profit—the person "buying" the product is often not the consumer, but an independent third party: the insurer. This insurer can be a for-profit organization, a nonprofit organization, or a government agency. (To learn more about the financial aspect of the U.S. health care system and the role of insurers, see Chapter 4.) Costs related to the provision and delivery of health care services continues to be a concern for all Americans. All projections show an upward trend for costs.[2]

1.4.2 Institutional providers

Institutional providers include organizations that provide private health care services and includes but is not limited to the following:

▲ Physicians' offices.
▲ Medical groups.
▲ Emergency care organizations.
▲ Hospitals.
▲ Mental health facilities.
▲ Nursing homes.
▲ Home health agencies (agencies that deliver medical services in the home).

Institutional providers, by their nature and design, are staffed by individual providers (see Section 1.4.3) and offer multiple services falling within their area of expertise or specialization. Mental health facilities, for example, can offer an array of mental health services, including inpatient treatment and outpatient counseling, and may specialize in emotional, psychiatric, or substance abuse issues. How broad the service offering is depends on the organization's stated mission, as well as its size and the resources (human and financial) available to it.

1.4.3 Individual Providers

Individual providers are the professionals who offer private health care services. Examples of individual providers include but are not limited to the following:

▲ Physicians.
▲ Dentists.
▲ Chiropractors.
▲ Nurses.
▲ Pharmacists.
▲ Psychologists.
▲ Licensed independent practitioners (LIPs).

Individual providers are often associated with one or more institutional providers. A pediatric dentist, for example, may have his or her own practice, in addition to serving as a staff member for a local pediatric hospital.

1.4.4 Public Health Agencies

Public health agencies are government agencies that promote health and prevent disease in populations, as opposed to dealing with the wellness of specific individuals. Examples of public health agencies include the Centers for Disease Control and Prevention, as well as state and local health departments.

1.4.5 Enablers

Enablers are organizations that support and facilitate the provision of health services. Enablers include the following:

▲ Trade and professional associations (for example, the American Hospital Association and the American Medical Association).
▲ Special-interest groups (for example, the American Heart Association).
▲ Research organizations (for example, the National Institutes of Health).
▲ Educational institutions (that is, medical and nursing schools).

Although the type of support these groups offer depends on the group's area of specialization and stated mission, these groups perform a variety of support functions, including participating in the development of public health policy, funding medical research and the study of public health status, training medical professionals, and promoting awareness of health issues.

1.4.6 Suppliers

Suppliers are organizations that provide products and services to the health care industry. Examples include pharmaceutical manufacturers, hospital supply and equipment companies, and medical consulting firms.

1.4.7 Regulators

Regulators are government agencies and private organizations that regulate health care institutions and professionals. Examples of such entities include the following:

▲ **State licensing boards:** Their primary responsibility is to ensure the proper licensing and regulation of physicians and, in some jurisdictions, other health care professionals.
▲ **State insurance departments:** Provide information on state statutes and regulations, as well as register complaints and take disciplinary action against insurance companies.
▲ **Federal agencies:** Include agencies such as the
  • *Food and Drug Administration (FDA)*, which, among other things, regulates the availability of medications.
  • *Department of Energy, Environment, Safety, and Health (ESH)*, which includes worker protection programs.

FOR EXAMPLE

The FDA

The Food and Drug Administration is a regulatory agency overseeing the introduction of health care products to the U.S. market. Comprising the FDA are five major centers: the Center for Biologics Evaluation and Research; the Center for Devices and Radiological Health; the Center for Drug Evaluation and Research (which you are probably most familiar with); the Center for Food Safety and Applied Nutrition; and the Center for Veterinary Medicine. In concert with to its regulatory function, the FDA also conducts research to test the products under its scrutiny.

- *Environmental Protection Agency (EPA),* which regulates environmental factors, such as pollution or the use of pesticides, that can impact human health.
- *Centers for Medicare and Medicaid Services (CMS)* that governs, regulates, and pays for services for citizens 65 years of age and older or disabled and those meeting federal poverty levels.

▲ **Medical specialty societies:** Include the American Academy of Neurology (AAN) and the American Psychiatric Association (APA), which are nonprofit professional organizations that set standards for membership, offer ongoing symposiums addressing issues and topics relating to their fields, and function as self-regulating entities for their members.

▲ **Nonprofit organizations:** Include the Joint Commission on Accreditation of Healthcare Organizations (JCAHO), a private, nonprofit association that evaluates medical organizations seeking accreditation.

Again, the agencies in the regulatory sector, like organizations in the financing and health care provider sectors, include both public agencies and private nonprofit groups.

SELF-CHECK

- Define **financing sector, institutional provider, individual provider, public health agencies, enablers,** and **regulators.**
- List examples of each of these sectors.

1.5 Defining Health and Disease

Who takes advantage of the 470,000 private HCOs (as outlined in Section 1.2)? Obviously, people who are not in good health—an obvious answer that leads to another question, this one with a not-so-obvious answer: What does it mean to be healthy? Is it simply a lack of illness?

Health is defined by the World Health Organization as complete physical, mental, and social well-being. This definition is notable because health, as define by the WHO, is not merely the absence of disease or infirmity.

The **World Health Organization (WHO)** is the United Nations agency whose function is to act as a coordinating authority on global health issues. The United States is a member state (as are all United Nations states, with the exception of one—Leichtenstein, if you're curious) and as such sends a delegate to the World Health Assembly, WHO's governing body. Although WHO standards and policies may occasionally differ from U.S. health standards and policies, the goals of both are essentially the same: to foster the health and well-being of people and communities. As such, WHO's definition of health, if not actually adopted by the United States, strongly informs U.S. health policies.

1.5.1 Causes of Disease

Disease impairs the functioning of a person. It can be caused by any of the following:

▲ Genetic flaws.
▲ The natural, preprogrammed, and progressive breakdown in biological systems that increases with age.
▲ External agents (chemical, biologic, radiological).
▲ Trauma (such as accidents).
▲ Personal behavioral habits.

Although any of these factors can cause disease, they are not always solely responsible for the actual development of disease, nor are they solely responsible for the path a disease may take once developed. A person may be exposed to an external agent, such as a virus, for example. He may not develop the disease at all, or he may develop a mild version or have a full-blown attack. Obviously, other factors come into play. These other factors include the following (listed here in decreasing order of importance):

▲ Genetic predisposition.
▲ Age.
▲ Context (including things such as income level, education level, housing, nutrition, sanitation, and environment).

FOR EXAMPLE

The U.S. Health Ranking

In its *World Health Report* 2000, WHO ranked the United States 37 out of 191 nations in ability to achieve vital health goals, even though it spends more per person than any other country on the list. This ranking generated a significant amount of press upon its publication, and affirmed for many Americans what they were already feeling: that they were paying more than ever for health care and getting less than they bargained for. This, in addition to projections showing significant increases in health expenditures during a time of economic slowdown, prompted Congress to address growing concerns about the accessibility and expense of health care in the United States.

▲ Race.

▲ The use of health care services.

Genetics, age, context, and race have a far greater impact on a person's health status than the amount and type of health care services consumed. The reason is that health care services primarily come into play only after the horse is out of the barn—when an illness or condition has already occurred. Meanwhile, other factors affect the probability that an illness or condition will appear in the first place.

1.5.2 Analyzing U.S. Health and Disease Status

Various mechanisms exist to test and represent the health status of the U.S. population. Researchers look at factors such as life expectancy at birth, infant mortality rates, cause of death, percentage of people with particular medical conditions or conditions that can negatively impact health, and so on. Generally, healthier societies have high life expectancy rates, low infant mortality rates, and low instances of chronic or debilitating health problems.

Infant Mortality Rate

In the United States, white and Hispanic infants have the lowest infant mortality rates, black infants the highest. Table 1-3 shows the statistics for the infant mortality rate.

In comparison with other selected countries, the infant mortality ranking of the United States is 27. Interestingly in 2002—and for the first time since 1958—the infant mortality rate increased in the United States. Upon further analysis of the data, the National Center for Health Statistics noted that of the ten most common causes for infant deaths, two causes showed a significant increase: low birthrate (up 5.3 percent) and maternal complications (up 14.2 percent).

Table 1-3: U.S. Infant Mortality Rate

Ethnicity	Deaths per 1,000 live births
White	6
Black	14
Hispanic	6
Other	9

Source: National Vital Statistics Report, Vol. 53, No. 5, October 12, 2004.

Life Expectancy and Cause of Death

In the United States, the average life expectancy is 74 for men and 79 years for women. Compared to other countries, America is number 20. What's killing Americans?

Table 1-4 lists the more common causes.

Table 1-4: Cause of Death

Cause of Death	Rate per 100,000 People
Heart disease	241.7
Cancer	193.2
Stroke	56.4
Chronic lower respiratory disease	43.3
Accidents	37.0
Diabetes	25.4
Pneumonia and influenza	22.8
Alzheimer's	20.4
Kidney disease	14.2
Homicide and firearms	16.6
Motor vehicle accidents	15.7
Suicide	11.0
Chronic liver disease and cirrhosis	9.5
HIV	4.9

Source: National Vital Statistics Report, Vol. 53, No. 5, October 12, 2004.

Table 1-5: Percentage of Chronic Health Conditions

Condition	Percentage
Adults (ages 20–74) with hypertension	24
Adults (ages 20–74) with an unhealthy weight	58
Children (ages 6–19) who are overweight	11

Population with Chronic Health Conditions

Another indicator of health status is the percentage of Americans who have a chronic or limiting health condition.

Consider these statistics shown in Tables 1-5 and 1-6.

Table 1-6: Population with Limitation of Activity Caused by Chronic Conditions

Age	Percentage
Under 18	6
18 to 44	6
45 to 54	12
55 to 64	20
65 to 74	26
Over 74	45

SELF-CHECK

- Give WHO's definition of **health**.
- Name the four causes of disease.
- Identify three of the five factors impacting a person's health status.
- Identify three common indicators of public health.

1.6 Accessing Health Services in the United States

Accessing health services is an ongoing issue. It can be a problem because of finances and availability or lack of knowledge and understanding of how this vast industry operates. The U.S. health care industry has the ability to meet the demands of all who need it. Staffed with professionals and stocked with advanced medical equipment, this industry has the technology and expertise that most U.S. inhabitants in medical crisis need. So how do people access the services they need?

1.6.1 Triggers to Utilizing the Health Care System

What affects the utilization of health care services? Simply feeling unwell isn't enough. Generally, before a patient steps foot in a medical facility, a sequence of events has occurred (see Figure 1-2):

1. **Need:** A person recognizes an underlying abnormal condition and judges it to warrant care and treatment. This condition can be physical, biological, or mental and it may be perceived or actual. The important thing is that the person *feels* that something is wrong and this feeling is disturbing enough to propel the person to the next stage.
2. **Demand:** Because of the depth of the discomfort caused by the underlying condition, the person is motivated to seek medical care and has the means to do so.
3. **Utilization:** Once believing that he or she has a need for medical care, the person then receives and uses the available medical services.

Figure 1-2

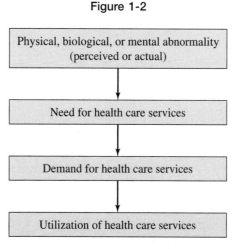

Key determinants in health care utilization.

Keep in mind, however, that the presence of a disease or condition does not necessarily cause need. Need may not precipitate demand, and demand may not result in utilization:

▲ **When condition doesn't lead to demand:** A person may have a condition that goes undetected because it is asymptomatic (that is, without symptoms). Or the underlying condition may not be defined as a disease (as was the case for many mental disorders in the early part of the last century).

▲ **When need doesn't lead to demand:** Individuals may need care yet not demand it because the condition is thought to be inconsequential. Conversely, a person can demand care without needing it (as in the case of a hypochondriac).

▲ **When demand doesn't lead to utilization:** The conversion of demand into consumption of health care services is most affected by the two-sided coin of access: individual wherewithal (knowledge, time, and money); and by how health services are organized, financed, and provided (industry structure and functioning).

Individuals also access services to prevent disease such as with immunizations. Public programs often emphasize preventive measures to ensure public and individual health.

1.6.2 Factors Affecting Utilization

A host of factors have been shown to affect the demand for and the utilization of health care services. Here are a few important ones:

▲ **Age:** Data show that the younger the person, the less likely he or she is to have a regular source of care. Keep in mind, however, that this could

FOR EXAMPLE

Addressing Disparities

Minorities in the United States (African Americans, Hispanic Americans, and others) have not benefited at the same level as their white counterparts in regard to health care. They are more likely to suffer from and die of cancer, heart disease, stroke, diabetes, and HIV/AIDS, and are less likely to get available immunizations. Infant mortality rates are also higher for minorities. The U.S. Department of Health and Human Services has launched programs to address these disparities. These efforts include engaging racial and ethnic minority communities in the fight against specific diseases and conditions that have a major impact on health, as well as finding ways to ensure that these populations get the necessary screening, diagnoses, and follow-up care.

be the result of a number of factors: The person may have fewer health problems, or may be less likely to have the financial means or insurance necessary to secure health care.

▲ **Insurance coverage:** People without insurance are more than four times as likely as people with insurance to forgo regular health care.

▲ **Race/ethnicity:** Hispanics are almost twice as likely as whites to be without regular health care, whereas the difference between white and black Americans is less pronounced.

▲ **Number and distribution of providers:** The Institute of Medicine's (IOM) promise of accessible care is meant to include all geographic regions of the country. But data suggest that inner cities and rural America aren't adequately served and a key reason is the dearth of physicians and facilities in those areas. This topic is one of the challenges facing the U.S. health care system. You can read more about it, and other challenges, in Chapter 13.

▲ **Education level:** People with lower levels of formal education are less likely to utilize or have access to medical services.

▲ **Provider referral patterns:** Given the relatively recent advent of managed care (which is discussed in detail in Chapter 11), whether a patient gets a referral to a specialist—and to which specialist—is often dependent upon the referral agreements stipulated by the health management organization (HMO) that the patient has.

▲ **Income level:** For reasons that are obvious, people in the lower socioeconomic brackets have less access to and utilize health care resources less than those in higher socioeconomic brackets.

▲ **Attitudes and beliefs:** The attitudes hampering adequate access and utilization of health care resources can be the individual's (a fear of doctors, for example, or a tendency to not follow the doctor's suggestions) or the physician's (who may, because of personal biases, be less aggressive with some populations than with others).

Table 1-7 lists the percentage of adults who have no regular source of medical care, categorized by age, gender, race, and insurance status.

1.6.3 The Role of Health Services Administration Research

Medical science does not make its contributions in a vacuum. Because the value of U.S. health care can be significantly affected by other factors, such as those listed in the preceding section, those factors can impede individuals from attaining better health. For that reason, health services administration research has an important role to play in assessing needs and evaluating how well medical services are delivered.

Table 1-7: Adults (18–64 Years of Age) with No Regular Source of Care

Category	Percentage
All	18
Age	
18 to 24	27
25 to 44	20
45 to 54	12
55 to 64	9
Gender	
Male	24
Female	12
Race	
White	17
Black	19
Hispanic	31
Insurance Status	
Insured	11
Uninsured	47

Health services administration research does not focus on diseases, but on the social, psychological, cultural, economic, informational, administrative, and organizational factors that impact both negatively and positively access to and delivery of health care to individuals and communities.

Health services administration research focuses on finding answers to questions such as these:

▲ What factors govern the patients' assumption or rejection of the "sick" role, or the "patient" role?

▲ What are the patients' sources of help in understanding and coping with their health problems?

▲ How do patients select their physicians, and conversely, how do physicians select their patients?

▲ Under what circumstances do physicians refer patients to other physicians and to medical centers?

▲ What kinds of patients, problems, and diseases are seen at different health facilities? Do the "right" patients get to the "right" facilities at the "right" time? What factors determine which person in every 1,000 adults will be referred to a university medical center each month? Are these processes in the best interests of all patients?

Health services administration research is as concerned with the health of those who do not use medical care resources as with the health of those who do. In essence, it is concerned with medicine as a social institution.

SELF-CHECK

- List the process by which people access the health system.
- Cite the factors affecting utilization of the health care system.
- Describe the role of health services administration research in health care.

SUMMARY

Understanding health care in the United States requires becoming familiar with the size and scope of the health care industry. The health care industry is one of the largest and represents over 15 percent of all goods and services produced in the nation. Health care organizations (HCOs) provide most of the primary care in the United States. In an effort to enhance the efficiency and cost-effectiveness of the health industry, HCOs are combined to create health systems. The entire health industry relies on health sectors to fulfill its mission. Still, U.S. health status is impacted by factors beyond the size and organization of the health care industry: How and when people access care, as well as the overall availability of care, determine to a large extent how successful the health system is.

KEY TERMS

Enablers	Organizations that support and facilitate the provision of health services, such as trade and professional organizations and public interest groups.
Gross domestic product (GDP)	The total value of goods and services produced in the U.S.
Gross goods	Medications and medical supplies.

Horizontal systems   Combine functionally similar organizations; can be composed of similar organizations in a particular market or those spread across a number of markets.

Individual providers   The professionals who offer private health care services such as physicians, dentists, chiropractors, and nurses.

Institutional providers Include organizations that provide private health care services, such as physician's offices, medical groups, hospitals and nursing homes.

Private HCOs   Provide services that are consumed by, and affect, individuals. The goal of these organizations is to protect and enhance the health and well-being of individuals.

Public HCOs   Provide services that targeted the health and well-being of populations or communities.

Public health agencies Government agencies that promote health and prevent disease in populations, such as the Centers for Disease Control and Prevention.

Regulators   Government agencies and private organizations that regulate health care institutions and professionals, such as state licensing boards, state insurance agencies, and federal agencies.

Services   Intangibles that are produced and used simultaneously.

Suppliers   Organizations that provide products and services to the health care industry, such as pharmaceutical manufacturers, hospital supply and equipment companies, and medical consulting firms.

Vertical systems   Combine functionally different organizations, where patient outputs of one organization in the system are inputs of another. Vertical systems always combine organizations within a given market.

World Health Organization (WHO)   United Nations agency whose function is to act as a coordinating authority on global health issues; established in 1948.

ASSESS YOUR UNDERSTANDING

Go to www.wiley.com/college/pointer to evaluate your knowledge of health care industry basics.

Measure your learning by comparing pre-test and post-test results.

Summary Questions

1. Indicate how large the U.S. health care industry is in terms of gross domestic product.
   (a) approximately 25 percent of GDP
   (b) approximately 15 percent of GDP
   (c) approximately 5 percent of GDP
   (d) as a service, health care isn't figured into GDP
2. The services that account for the top three health care expenditures are hospital care, professional and clinical care, and _____.
   (a) prescription drugs
   (b) medical research
   (c) nursing home care
   (d) public health activities
3. The goal of private HCOs is to use government programs to promote and protect the health and well-being of communities. True or false?
4. Public HCOs are government agencies that make health care policy and implement public health care initiatives. True or false?
5. Which of the following is *not* an example of a private HCO?
   (a) veteran's hospital
   (b) FDA
   (c) inner-city health clinic
   (d) all of the above
6. Which of the following accurately defines a health system?
   (a) a health system is one of the four major systems—respiratory, circulatory, and so on—in the human body
   (b) a health system is an organization that combines into one enterprise HCO that could otherwise function independently
   (c) an organization that includes health care professionals from various fields and offers a variety of treatment options for its patients
   (d) all of the above
7. Which of the following is *not* a mechanism for forming a health system?
   (a) joint venture
   (b) lease

    (c) association

    (d) ownership

  8. Health sectors are

    (a) health regions throughout the country, as defined by the DHHS.

    (b) specific roles that health care providers have in promoting and protecting health.

    (c) types of health care (geriatric care, pediatric care, oncology, and so on).

    (d) categories of disease as defined by the CDC.

  9. Which of the following are examples of institutional providers?

    (a) a nursing home specializing in Alzheimer's care

    (b) a physician providing care in a hospital

    (c) a government agency implementing public health policy

    (d) a and c

  10. The World Health Organization defines *health* as

    (a) absence of disease or infirmity.

    (b) complete physical well-being of both individuals and populations.

    (c) complete physical, mental, and social well-being.

    (d) the WHO doesn't define health, instead leaving the definition up to its member states.

  11. Apart from the physical causes of disease, which of the following factors can impact the course a disease may take once developed?

    (a) age

    (b) genetic predisposition

    (c) environment

    (d) education

    (e) all of the above

  12. A sequence of events generally occurs before a person seeks medical attention. Which of the following most accurately represents this sequence?

    (a) Demand => Need => Utilization

    (b) Utilization => Demand => Need

    (c) Need => Demand => Utilization

    (d) none of the above

  13. Which of the following factors affects utilization of health care?

    (a) age

    (b) insurance coverage

    (c) income level

    (d) education

    (e) all of the above

Review Questions

1. The health care industry provides both goods and services. Of the following, explain which are goods and which are services.

    (a) medication

    (b) follow-up care

    (c) stethoscopes

2. As the U.S. population ages, what will be the impact on health care expenditures?

    (a) expenditures will stay roughly the same

    (b) expenditures will increase

    (c) expenditures will decrease

3. Cite three characteristics of private HCOs.

4. Private HCOs address health issues of the individual; public HCOs address the health needs of the population as a whole. In the following scenarios, state whether the situation includes a private HCO, a public HCO, or both.

    (a) a general practitioner working in a clinic diagnoses an elderly woman with breast cancer and refers her to an oncologist working in a hospital setting

    (b) FDA officials pull a popular cholesterol drug from pharmacy shelves because additional studies indicate it isn't safe

    (c) as part of a statewide "Smile" program, local dentists volunteer their time to give elementary school children dental checks at school

5. Indicate whether the following are examples of vertical health systems or horizontal health systems.

    (a) an organization comprised of several nursing homes throughout a geographic region

    (b) an organization comprised of dental offices within a city

    (c) an organization comprised of hospitals and nursing homes

6. In the mechanisms used to form health systems, identify the main difference between organizations that are formed through ownership and those formed through affiliation.

7. Indicate whether each of the following is a health sector.

    (a) enablers

    (b) providers

    (c) regulators

    (d) users

8. Describe the role of regulator.

9. What are the contextual factors impacting the status of disease?

10. Explain why the use of health care services has less of an impact on a person's health status than the other factors.
11. In what situations does a health care need *not* lead to demand?
12. What factors affect health care utilization?

Applying This Chapter

1. Evaluate the data in Table 1-1 and determine which sectors spend the most money. Given the aging population and upcoming changes in health policy (such as federal prescription drug plan for seniors), identify which areas may be most affected and briefly explain why.
2. Identify the type of health system being described in each of the following:
   (a) a clinic specializing in geriatrics refers a patient to a hospital for immediate care; the hospital, after stabilizing the patient, refers the patient to local nursing home facility for recuperation
   (b) an organization operates hospitals in several cities across a particular region
   (c) a managed care organization that contracts with general physicians practices, specialty practices, hospitals, and nursing care facilities in various regions
3. Identify which sectors each of the following falls into. Note that some may fall into more than one sector:
   (a) doctors in a health clinic
   (b) the research department of a community hospital
   (c) a company that sells syringes and other medical supplies
   (d) a state health department
   (e) a national health insurance company
   (f) a pharmacist
4. Good Samaritan Children's Hospital is a research, training, and treatment center for children with cancer and catastrophic diseases. Physicians from around the country refer children to this facility, and it also has an outreach program that works in partnership with research facilities and medical centers around the world. Describe this hospital in terms of
   (a) the type of HCO it is.
   (b) the type of health system it represents.
   (c) the health sectors it falls into.
5. Create a profile of a person *least* likely to access health care; of a person *most* likely to access health care.

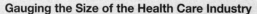

Gauging the Size of the Health Care Industry

You are responsible for identifying the source of health care expenditures. Indicate what components you would include in your report.

Balancing Public and Private Health: Health Care Organizations

Of all the HCOs, hospitals account for only 2 percent, yet they employ over 40 percent of the total HCO work-force. Explain why this seeming discrepancy exists and extrapolate what that means in terms of where hospitals stack up in terms of expenditures.

Identifying Health Systems

Draw up your own plan for a health system that provides services to elderly people. Indicate the services you intend to provide and identify the type of health system you've created.

Classifying Health Care Industry Sectors

As a director of a nursing home that employs registered nurses and provides services to patients with dementia (such as Alzheimer's), indicate what other type of health care sectors you would be involved with.

Defining Health and Disease

Based on the data regarding the health status of U.S. citizens, if you were charged with reducing preventable causes of death and improving the overall health of Americans, what issue(s) would you target? Explain why.

Accessing Health Services in the United States

Health care is available to all. Defend or refute this statement, using information from this chapter to support your position.

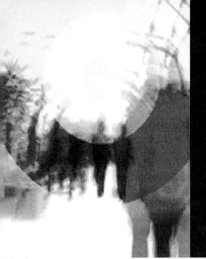

2

BOARDS AND GOVERNANCE
Hospital and Health System Decision Makers

Starting Point

Go to www.wiley.com/college/pointer to test your knowledge of boards and governance.
Determine where you need to concentrate your effort.

What You'll Learn in This Chapter

▲ What a governing board is
▲ The characteristics of governing board members
▲ The functions that a governing board performs
▲ The legal and ethical challenges that governing boards face

After Studying This Chapter, You'll Be Able To

▲ Identify organizational characteristics that make a governing board necessary
▲ List the four core functions governing boards perform
▲ Compare the duties of standing committees
▲ Analyze the challenges facing health system boards

Goals and Outcomes

▲ Discern the relationship between a health organization's governing board and the organization's chief executive officer
▲ Analyze the structure and composition of governing boards
▲ Identify important differences between hospital and health system governing boards
▲ Discuss potential ethical conflicts that may come from being the member of a health system board.

INTRODUCTION

Health systems, hospitals, and government health agencies are overseen by **governing boards.** In the United States, there are approximately 7500 hospital and health system boards, including subsidiary boards, and about 120,000 people serving on them. Three types of hospitals and health systems exist: for-profit, nonprofit, and government. The for-profit and nonprofit hospitals and health systems must have boards in order to maintain their legal status as a corporation. Board members are often called directors or trustees. Government hospitals and health systems often have elected officials, executive staff, and citizens on their boards. For-profit board members have one primary objective: to maximize profits. For-profit board members are generally paid for this service. Nonprofit board members serve to meet the needs of the community. Board members are not compensated other than for out-of-pocket expenses. They must be free of conflict regarding their duties as a board member and may not profit from any association with the organization. The decisions that boards make have a profound impact on the quality of care the organization provides and the environment in which that care is given. From a legal standpoint the board is responsible for actions taken by the organization.

2.1 Understanding the Role of Governing Boards

The fundamental obligation of all governing boards is to represent an organization's owners to ensure that resources and capacities are deployed in ways that benefit the organization.

Who the "owner" is depends on the type of organization: In for-profit health care organizations, the owners are stockholders; in nonprofits, they are stakeholders (such as the community); and in governmental facilities they are constituents (voters). Similarly, just as there are numerous types of owners, there are numerous types of organizations. Organizations can be independent institutions, such as small, privately owned hospitals; complex health systems including multiple health care organizations; and any configuration in between (refer to Section 1.3 for a discussion of types of health systems). Regardless of the type of organization, a board must perform four core responsibilities (described in detail in the following sections).

▲ Determine mission, vision, and values.
▲ Ensure a high level of management performance.
▲ Ensure the quality and safety of patient care.
▲ Ensure the organization's financial health.

Not all health care organizations have—or need—governing boards. Health care services that are solely owned, partnerships, or limited liability corporations are not legally required to have boards. The *Joint Commission on Accreditation of Healthcare Organizations (JCAHO)* has recommended that governance responsibilities be in writing for hospitals across the nation. Because of this, there is great conformity in terms of hospital board structure in the United States. For a board to be formed, there must be a charter or bylaws that dictate the operation and authority of the board.

2.1.1 Determining Mission, Vision, and Values

All health care organizations exist to fulfill a purpose, be it altruistic, economic, or a combination of the two. This **mission statement,** or *vision,* provides the context under which all decisions are made and the standard against which all strategies and outcomes are evaluated. The health organization governing board defines the organization's vision and creates a mission statement that embodies that vision and articulates the values.

Vision and Mission Statements

Consider the following example of a mission statement from Children's Hospital in Columbus, Ohio:

> *Children's believes that no child should be refused necessary care and attention for lack of ability to pay. Upon this fundamental belief, Children's is committed to providing the highest quality patient care including: Advocacy for children and their families, pediatric research, education of patients, families and future providers, and outstanding service to accommodate the needs of patients and families.*

Depending on how an organization wishes to structure its mission and what type of image it wants to build, a mission statement may include:

▲ The purpose, or why the organization exists.
▲ Characteristics and values of the organization that make it unique.
▲ Identification of target customers and markets.
▲ Organizational philosophy and values.
▲ The types of services the organization delivers.

The board determines the organization's mission by examining the organization's values, its philosophies, its core beliefs, and the characteristics that make the organization unique. It also identifies the needs of the community/market. Often the organization receives a mandate from the community and its stakeholders to provide specific services and resources or to move in a particular direction.

Taking all these things into consideration, the board formulates the organization's mission that serves all stakeholders, both customers and employees of an organization, whether they are shareholders or community residents.

In many ways, public and private organizations are very similar in terms of how they formulate their visions and mission statements. Although private health care organizations don't rely on the community for funding and in theory answer only to their shareholders, they still must be responsive to the community in their mission. Private institutions operate within the public sphere and within the public marketplace and therefore try to remain responsive to community concerns to be successful.

The Organization's Strategic Plan

The governing board also approves the organization's strategic plan to achieve the vision and carry out the mission (as embodied in the vision or mission statement). For example, whereas the mission statement for an urban hospital may include the mandate to provide high-quality health care to inner-city poor people, some specific goals to realize this mission may include:

▲ Decreasing the average wait-time of patient visits.
▲ Increasing the number of professional staff in clinical areas.
▲ Increasing the quality of medical equipment.
▲ Providing fee-free services for immunizations and preventive health care.

2.1.2 Ensuring Management Performance

Another key function of a health care organization's governing board is to ensure a high level of management performance. As mentioned previously, the board articulates the organization's mission and sets the overarching goals that lead to fulfillment of that mission. However, it must rely on the **chief executive officer (CEO)**—the management executive responsible for the day-to-day operation of the facility or health system—and the management team he or she puts in place to institute policies and strategies that support the mission. For this reason, ensuring CEO performance is a key function of the governing board. To that end, the board is responsible for the following:

▲ Recruiting and selecting the CEO.
▲ Specifying CEO performance expectations.
▲ Assessing the CEO's performance and contributions.
▲ Adjusting the CEO's compensation.
▲ If the need arises, terminating the CEO's employment.

Although the governing board establishes the organization's mission and its attendant goals, it is the CEO who formulates strategies that support these goals. For example, a CEO may develop the following strategies to accomplish the goal of meeting the prenatal needs of people who are economically disadvantaged:

instituting a visiting nurse program for women who lack transportation to the area health clinic, disseminating pamphlets on prenatal care in community centers, and so on. The board is responsible for ensuring that the management-developed strategies can achieve the board-developed goals and fulfill the organization's mission.

2.1.3 Ensuring Quality of Care

One of the other core obligations of a health organization's governing board is to ensure the quality of patient care. For that reason, the board is responsible for

▲ Appointing or reappointing members of the medical staff and determining their privileges.
▲ Making sure that necessary quality, utilization, and risk measurement and management systems are in place and functioning effectively.
▲ Assessing the quality and safety of care provided for patients, employees, and services delivered.

Boards carry out these functions through a committee structure. These committees deal with a specific area of organizational functioning, such as personnel, finance, planning, or even quality, performance, and process improvement. The committees usually have the authority to delegate tasks to others within the committee or the organization's administrative structure. These committees work on tasks such as developing assessment procedures or guidelines or developing strategic plans for the organization. The board also appoints the CEO of the organization with whom they work closely. It is through this committee structure combined with delegating duties that the board carries out many of its governing functions.

2.1.4 Ensuring Financial Health

The board is responsible for the financial health of the organization. As such, it performs the following functions:

▲ Specifying financial objectives.
▲ Approving the organization's annual budget.
▲ Determining whether management-devised budgets are aligned with financial objectives and to the organization's key strategic plan, vision, and mission.
▲ Monitoring and evaluating financial performance and outcomes in relation to approved budget.
▲ Ensuring that financial controls are in place and the organization's financial statements accurately reflect its financial status.
▲ Protect the assets of the organization.

FOR EXAMPLE

Sarbanes-Oxley and Health Care Governing Boards

The Sarbanes-Oxley Act, passed in 2002, was intended to protect investors by improving the accuracy and reliability of financial statements and by establishing harsher penalties for those who violate the law. Although directly applicable to publicly traded companies, this act is likely to impact the boards of nonprofit organizations as well. Key components of the act include mandates regarding board composition and financial and auditing responsibilities. In some hospitals and health systems, the financial committee is separate from the audit committee sharing perhaps one committee member to ensure the integrity of the audit function.

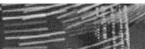

SELF-CHECK

- Describe who the owners of a hospital or health system can be.
- What must be in place for the board to operate?
- Define what a **mission statement** is.
- List the four core functions of a governing board.

2.2 Board Composition, Structure, and Infrastructure

A **board of directors,** of any organization, is a group of people who oversee the affairs of a corporation. To fulfill its myriad responsibilities, a board must have the right structure, composition, and infrastructure. This information is outlined in the charter or bylaws for the board.

- ▲ **Board structure:** How the is board divided and coordinates the governance work within the organization. It deals with such things as board size, the number and type of committees, and (in systems) the number of boards and their relationships.
- ▲ **Board composition:** Focuses on board members—their characteristics, knowledge, skills, perspectives, and experience.
- ▲ **Board infrastructure:** Includes the resources and systems that support the performance of governance work.

The following sections describe these components for both hospitals and health systems.

2.2.1 Health Systems

When multiple health care organizations that could function independently are combined into single enterprise organizations, a health system is created (see Chapter 1). Their structure can range from relatively simple (the combination of functionally similar organizations within a geographic area, for example) to highly complex (the combination of multiple health systems across a geographic area, for example).

Information about the composition, structure, and infrastructure of a typical health system board is presented in the following subsections.

Structure

Health systems, as previously explained, unite various organizations into a single enterprise. Typically, each individual organization within the system has its own governing board. As a result, a health system can have numerous functioning boards. The total number of boards in a health system and the relationship between them depend on the health system's mission, scope of service, strategic plan, and organizational realities.

Although a health system may have multiple functioning boards (called **subsidiary boards**) for each organization within its system, there is almost always one centralized (or corporate) board from which representatives of the smaller boards operate and to which they are responsible. For example, if a health system is made up of three hospitals and two small clinics, each individual institution may have a board for its own local organization, but a **parent board**—a systemwide board—ties them all together. The larger board serves as a big-picture-type board and reserves power to make sure the centralized mission, values, and philosophy are maintained and perpetuated across the various institutions. Again, the work of these boards is carried out through a committee structure.

To perform its core responsibilities (refer to Section 2.1), boards often form committees to address specific areas. The most common system **standing committees**—often permanent, but sometimes temporary, committees that address specific areas of needs—are

- ▲ **Executive:** The **executive committee** consists of senior-level board members and officers of the board.
- ▲ **Finance:** The **finance committee** deals with budgeting guidelines and performance, long-range financial planning, debt structure, and asset protection and is usually composed of the treasurer, chief financial officer (CFO), and others.
- ▲ **Planning or strategy:** The **planning** or **strategy committee** looks at long-range institutional planning and organizational strategic planning.
- ▲ **Quality credentialing:** The **quality credentialing committee** deals with ensuring that privileges, credentials, licensures, and certifications are appropriate, up-to-date, and in compliance.

▲ **Nominating:** The function of the **nominating committee** is the nominating of new board members and officers.

▲ **Audit:** The **audit committee's** responsibilities include ensuring that audits are conducted and reported to the board of directors.

▲ **Compensation:** The **compensation committee** looks at performance issues in regard to salary, benefits, and bonuses

▲ **Quality/performance/process improvement:** The **quality/performance/ process improvement committee** has ongoing responsibility in reviewing quality and safety initiatives regarding care and service delivery.

Board Composition

Boards must be able to fulfill their core responsibilities. Meeting these responsibilities determines the number of members and their skills, experience, and resources. Boards may be of any size, which determines the composition of the members. Some suggest that the "most effective boards have between 10 and 15 members and vary in effectiveness when they have 16 to 25 members"[1]. Boards have term limits. These are typically identified in the charter or bylaws. Health care organizations are encouraged to appoint a physician to the board, although in nonprofit organizations medical staff cannot make up the majority of the board. Board members are appointed as individuals, not as representatives of a certain entity, and act on behalf of the community as a whole.

Infrastructure

Most health care systems have a person assigned to provide staff support to the board; a fewer number have a designated board coordinator. In most health systems, staff support to the board comes from an executive assistant, who is typically attached to the office of the president or the CEO.

Some system boards meet monthly, others meet every other month, and some meet quarterly. The typical system board meeting lasts three and one-half hours.

2.2.2 Hospitals

In many respects, the board of a hospital functions in much the same way as does the board of a health system. Hospital boards may tend to be smaller than system boards.

Structure

As in health systems, the most common standing committees in hospital boards are executive, finance, planning or strategy, quality credentialing, nominating, and audit (see Section 2.2.1).

Fifty-six percent of hospital boards meet monthly, 19 percent meet every other month, and 8 percent meet quarterly. The average hospital board meeting lasts two hours.

Board Composition

The average hospital board is composed of 15 members: 1 insider, 3 medical staff directors, and 11 outsiders.

▲ Eighteen percent of hospital directors are female.

▲ Minorities compose 7 percent of hospital directors; 6 percent are black, 0.7 percent are Hispanic, and 0.3 percent are Asian.

▲ Fifty percent of hospital boards have no racial or ethnic minority members.

Fifty percent of hospitals have term limits (the median is three terms), and the typical hospital director spends about 17 hours per year involved in governance education.

Infrastructure

Ninety-four percent of hospitals have a person assigned to extend staff support to the board. In hospitals with governance staff support, 15 percent have a formally designated board coordinator; 80 percent use an executive or administrative assistant or secretary, and 5 percent assign a member of the management team.

FOR EXAMPLE

Governing Boards in Action

Nebraska's Health and Human Services System is responsible for overseeing health care and health policy throughout the state. To facilitate mental health services, for example, Nebraska is divided into six regions, each with its own regional governing board. These boards are responsible for planning, organizing, directing, and coordinating mental health care within the various regions. Each county within a region appoints a commissioner to sit on the board, and each board has a regional program administrator who hires support staff. Together, the program administrator, the board members, and the support staff work to devise and implement mental health services within their regions.

SELF-CHECK

- Define **structure, composition,** and **infrastructure** as they relate to governing boards.
- List the most common standing committees for health system and hospital boards.

> ## FOR EXAMPLE
>
> ### Coming Around to Quality of Care
>
> Even though one of the four core responsibilities of health care governing boards has been quality of care, many boards, following the example of boards in non–health care related corporations, have focused their attention on the board's fiduciary responsibilities. As health care quality of care and safety come under scrutiny, however, health care organizations are coming to realize that ensuring quality has implications on the financial health of an institution. In that way, the board's role in overseeing quality is as important as its role in overseeing the organization's finances. To highlight the role of health care boards in ensuring quality of care, the Joint Commission on Accreditation of Healthcare Organizations convened a Leadership Accountabilities Task Force. The task force concluded that the overall responsibility for quality of care lies with the health organization's governing board, but that the board must work in concert with the medical staff and health care management to achieve the quality of care target.

2.3 Challenges Facing Boards

As health care evolves, the challenges that governing boards face have evolved as well. More complex health systems, the rising costs of health care, and the changing regulations regarding board composition and accounting have all impacted how boards function. Although costs for health care have steadily been on the rise—102 percent over the past two decades[2]—the financial status of hospitals has been in a decline since the passing of the Balanced Budget Act of 1997. "In 2003, nearly one-third of hospitals lost money overall" according to the AHA[3]. Health care has been "pummeled by pressures to reduce costs, improve quality, assume economic risk and broker affiliations"[4]. These are serious issues that plague the industry that must be dealt with by these boards in their own communities.

2.3.1 Liability of Board Members

In today's litigious environment, any person who sits on a governing board of a health care organization faces possible legal and public scrutiny. All boards face this reality, and many take measures to structure the organization so that these risks are minimized. One way to reduce the risk is to put safeguards in place within the organization to distance board members from liability and undue scrutiny, while at the same time making sure that the board is still held accountable to all stakeholders. All board members have liability insurance coverage through the organization. Board members may choose to obtain additional coverage at their own expense.

In addition, the organization's **general counsel** (the chief attorney for a corporation) should be available to the board at any time. Board members can consult the general counsel when necessary.

To help minimize the legal liability of board members, Congress passed specific policies such as the **Health Care Quality Improvement Act of 1986 (HCQIA)**. The HCQIA was established primarily to protect individuals and hospitals conducting medical peer review against legal action by physicians whose practice privileges were revoked.

2.3.2 Reporting and Disclosure of Accounting Information

Congressional acts like the **Sarbanes-Oxley Act**, although not specific to health care, have profound legal implications in terms of the reporting and disclosure of accounting information. Boards must make sure they and their organizations are in compliance with all appropriate laws, regulations, and rules. The board member in today's health care organization must take into account the myriad legal issues that exist in today's business environment.

2.3.3 Conflict of Interest

Balancing conflict between making money for shareholders and providing care for patients is also a concern for boards. One way to address this issue is to construct organizational mission statements and strategic plans in such ways that value patient care and safety as most important. By making and publicly stating organizational values in such a way, an organization has a guidepost from which to operate when it comes to the conflict between patient care and monetary gain. Annually all board members sign a statement declaring that they are free of any conflicts of interest. Should an individual feel that an issue may be a conflict of interest, he or she can declare that to the board and abstain from voting on any related issue or ask the board for a determination on what his or her status should be regarding the issue.

To minimize any ethical conflicts, health care organizations can also take the following steps:

▲ Before appointing someone to the board or making certain decisions, research and address all possible conflicts of interest and document the rationale behind the decision or appointment.

▲ Ensure that no individual profits from a nonprofit corporation. Although a nonprofit organization can make a "profit," in that it can generate income in excess of its expenses, the profit must be used by the organization in achieving its philanthropic, educational, or scientific goals. The money *cannot* go to enrich individuals (as it can in a for-profit organization).

▲ Prohibit board members and the organizations to which they serve from negotiating the conversion of a nonprofit to for-profit ownership without regulatory and judiciary review.

2.3.4 Board Performance

Boards have a responsibility to evaluate their effectiveness on an annual basis. Evaluation must center on the core responsibilities. Unsatisfactory performance requires a course redirection by the board at the committee level or with CEO or board membership.

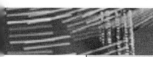

SELF-CHECK

- List the three main challenges facing governing boards.
- Define the **Health Care Quality Improvement Act of 1986.**

SUMMARY

Governing boards in general perform a vital function in the organizations they serve; the same is true of the governing boards of health care organizations. They represent the health organizations' stakeholders, ensure that resources are used in a way that benefits the organization, and perform the same core functions. How the board is organized and who its members are depends on the type of organization it serves, whether it is a single entity or a health system. In addition to performing their core functions, boards today must also be aware of the legal and ethical scrutiny they attract.

KEY TERMS

Audit committee	Standing committee responsible for ensuring that all necessary audits are conducted and reported to the board of directors.
Board composition	The characteristics, knowledge, skills, perspectives, and experience of board members.
Board infrastructure	The resources and systems that support the performance of the board's work.
Board of directors	A group of people who oversee the affairs of a corporation.
Board structure	How the board is divided and coordinates the governance work within the organization, specifically relating to board size, the number

	and type of committees, and the number of boards and their relationships.
Chief executive officer (CEO)	The management executive responsible for the day-to-day operation of the facility or health system, who formulates strategies that support the goals outlined in an organization's mission statement.
Compensation committee	Standing committee that looks at performance issues in regard to salary, benefits, and bonuses
Executive committee	Standing committee consisting of senior-level board members, which conducts the business of the board.
Finance committee	Standing committee that deals with budgeting guidelines and performance, long-range financial planning, and debt structure. Standing committee members typically include the treasurer, CFO (chief financial officer), and others.
General counsel	The chief attorney for a health care organization.
Governing board	The entity charged with overseeing the affairs of a corporation.
Health Care Quality Improvement Act (HCQIA) of 1986	Act established primarily to protect individuals and hospitals conducting medical peer review against legal action by physicians whose practice privileges were revoked.
Mission statement	The statement of purpose for an organization. It generally provides the context under which all decisions are made and the standard against which all strategies and outcomes are evaluated.
Nominating committee	Standing committee responsible for nominating new board members and officers.
Parent board	In a health system, the one centralized (or corporate) board comprised of representatives of the smaller boards. The parent board is responsible for ensuring that the health system's centralized mission, values, and philosophy are maintained and perpetuated across the various subsidiary institutions.
Planning or strategy committee	Standing committee responsible for long-range institutional planning and organizational strategic planning.

Quality credentialing committee	Standing committee that deals with ensuring that privileges, credentials, licensures, and certifications are appropriate, up-to-date, and in compliance.
Quality/performance/process improvement committee	This committee has ongoing responsibility in reviewing quality initiatives and performance regarding patient care, safety, and service delivery.
Sarbanes-Oxley Act	Act, passed in 2002, intended to protect investors by improving the accuracy and reliability of financial statements and by establishing harsher penalties for those who violate the law.
Standing committees	Often permanent (but sometimes temporary) committees that address specific areas of needs.
Subsidiary board	Functioning board for a health care organization that exists as part of a larger health system and that is accountable to the health system's parent board.

ASSESS YOUR UNDERSTANDING

Go to www.wiley.com/college/pointer to evaluate your knowledge of boards and governance.
Measure your learning by comparing pre-test and post-test results.

Summary Questions

1. Name one significant difference between health system and hospital boards.
2. Identify which of the following organizations do not require governing boards:

   (a) an independent group practice

   (b) Planned Parenthood Federation of America

   (c) Women's Hospital of Greater Indianapolis

   (d) Metropolitan Area Agency on Aging
3. The Sarbanes-Oxley Act requires that all health care organizations have a governing board. True or False?
4. According to the Joint Commission on Accreditation of Healthcare Organizations, all health care organizations must have a governing board. True or False?
5. A subsidiary board is the governing board of a health care organization that is part of a health system. True or False?
6. The Sarbanes-Oxley Act applies to all nonprofit and for-profit businesses, and therefore applies to health care organizations. True or False?
7. Board members cannot be sued individually for the actions of the board, although the board itself can be sued. True or False?
8. As long as board members of a nonprofit health care organization do not enrich themselves personally through the organization's profits, they can avoid charges of conflict of interest. True or False?

Review Questions

1. Identify the primary functions of a health care governing board.
2. Name the executive who works closely with the board on achieving the organization's mission.
3. What is the relationship between a hospital or health system governing board and CEO?
4. Name the most common standing committees on a health system board.
5. What steps can a health system board take to minimize ethical conflicts?

Applying This Chapter

1. Indicate what standing committee would be responsible for each of the following functions.
    (a) ensuring that organization accreditation is current
    (b) reporting the results of accounting audits to the board of directors
    (c) setting long-range planning goals
    (d) setting budgetary guidelines
    (e) evaluating salaries and bonuses
2. As a board member, what would you do to protect yourself from scrutiny and possible legal action?

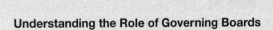

Understanding the Role of Governing Boards

As a member of a governing board, what areas would you expect the CEO to focus on in the execution of his or her duties?

Board Composition, Structure, and Infrastructure

Discuss one significant difference between health system and hospital boards.

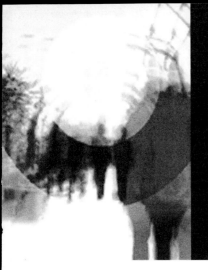

3

HEALTH CARE PROVISION
Organization and Dispersal of Health Care Providers

Starting Point

Go to www.wiley.com/college/pointer to assess your knowledge of the health provision.
Determine where you need to concentrate your effort.

What You'll Learn in This Chapter

▲ The definition of primary care and specialty care
▲ How well primary care addresses patient needs in terms of access, continuity, comprehensiveness of care, and more
▲ Primary innovations relating to how health care is provided
▲ The three types of primary care specialties
▲ Which health care providers other than primary care physicians perform primary care functions

After Studying This Chapter, You'll Be Able To

▲ Illustrate primary care and specialty care
▲ Distinguish the benefits of primary care and specialty care
▲ Evaluate the performance of primary care
▲ Analyze primary care innovations in health care
▲ Compare the types of primary care specialties
▲ Articulate why specialists and others perform primary care functions
▲ Examine what HPSAs are and which populations they most significantly affect

Goals and Outcomes

▲ Master the terminology of health care provision
▲ Understand the evolution of primary care in the United States
▲ Identify hurdles to the full implementation of primary care in this country
▲ Propose solutions to problems facing the full implementation of primary care
▲ Draw a connection between accessibility in primary care and health profession shortage areas (HPSAs)
▲ Predict the impact if the United States reverts to specialty care

INTRODUCTION

A key component of any health system is its organization and the location of health care providers. U.S. health care traditionally has been a system of specialty care rather than primary care. The requirements of modern health care and the advent of the managed care system, however, have generated a shift toward a system that is more primary care based. Managed care systems utilize primary care physicians (PCPs) as gatekeepers for access to specialty care. The success of a primary care based system in the United States depends on whether patients receive the continuity of care and comprehensiveness of care they expect. To address such expectations, primary care providers are innovating the way in which health care is dispensed. As the U.S. system remains in flux and specialty care and primary care exist side-by-side, however, primary care struggles to find its niche because both PCPs and specialists perform primary care functions. The current mix of physicians in the United States is about one-third generalists to two-thirds specialists."[1] Exacerbating the problem is that this nation has a shortage of PCPs, which is most keenly felt in health professional shortage areas (HPSAs).[2,3]

3.1 Health Provision at a Glance: Specialty Care vs. Primary Care

Traditionally, health care systems involve three types of care: primary care, secondary care, and tertiary care.

▲ **Primary care:** General preventive and curative care that is provided to a person over an extended period of time (not infrequently the course of that person's life). Another function of primary care is to coordinate all the care—primary, secondary, and tertiary—that the patient receives. All family physicians and most pediatricians and internists are in primary care.

▲ **Secondary care:** Care that is provided by medical specialists who generally don't have first contact with patients; instead, patients are referred to them through PCPs.

▲ **Tertiary care:** Specialized consultative care, usually on referral from primary or secondary health care providers. Tertiary care, generally delivered in teaching institutions that have the personnel and facilities for special investigation and treatment, handles rare and complicated illnesses.

The way in which people access the various types of health care, whether they must follow a referral process or seek out care individually, is determined by the type of insurance they have or their ability to gain access without insurance. Some systems are highly structured and hierarchical; that is, access to the various levels of care requires that patients begin at a certain level (usually the primary care level) and access other levels through a system of referrals. Other systems

FOR EXAMPLE

General practitioners in the United Kingdom

In the United Kingdom, general practitioners (GPs) take care of a defined group of patients (and families) who sign on with them. Although self-employed, they sign a contract with the U.K.'s National Health Service to be responsible for the health of the patients on their lists in return for a mixture of **capitation** and fee-for-service payments. In addition to palliative care (treating illnesses), GPs are also responsible for preventive care and receive incentives for meeting certain public health goals; for example, they're rewarded financially if they ensure that more than 90 percent of eligible children on their lists have been immunized. Their work includes social as well as medical care, such as decisions about eligibility for public housing.

are much more flexible, in that patients themselves determine at which level they seek treatment.

3.1.1 Primary Care Model

In some countries—the United Kingdom and Scandinavia are examples—health care systems are highly structured. Primary care is the foundation of this structure and manages the prevalent health problems and needs of the majority of the people. In the primary care model, systems require patients to consult with a primary care provider for all except emergency health problems; difficult problems are referred to secondary or tertiary levels of the system after an initial evaluation by the primary care gatekeeper. Secondary care, provided by specialists and general hospitals, involves the management of more complex problems. Tertiary care, generally delivered in teaching institutions, handles rare and complicated illnesses. Primary care clinicians play a role in coordinating secondary and tertiary care through referrals and the integration of specialty care provided in non–primary care settings.

3.1.2 Specialty Care Model

Historically most care in the United States has taken place within a more dispersed model, allowing patients access to the secondary and tertiary levels without their first seeing their primary care clinician. The **specialty care model,** a more dispersed model than the primary care model, doesn't require patients to consult with a primary care provider before seeking general or specialty care.

The development of such a model is easier to understand if one considers that, in the mid-1960s, for example, 45 percent of the population had no regular physician.[4] Without a regular physician to see about health care issues and concerns—or to promote preventive care—people pursued health care independently, without first consulting a general care practitioner.

But this system came at a price, literally. It became evident that the United States' specialist-centered system encouraged the overuse of diagnostic procedures, surgeries, and prescription drugs. Such overuse of health care resources contributed to the rising costs of health care. In the 1960s, the community medicine movement questioned this model and advocated a more central role for primary care. According to the March 2006 *Report to the Congress: Medicare Payment Policy* by the Medicare Payment Advisory Commission (MedPAC), "analysts believe that because of their training, specialists suspect serious pathology more frequently than generalists, and conduct or order more diagnostic workups to rule out their suspicions. Others note that specialists in the United States provide a larger share of visits for evaluation and management."[5] This continues to contribute to rising costs today.

SELF-CHECK

- Define **primary, secondary,** and **tertiary care.**
- Describe the primary care model.
- Describe the specialty care model.

3.2 Primary Care Reforms in the United States

A number of commissions and reports during the 1960s promoted primary care reforms. Their findings resulted in the establishment of the family medicine specialty in 1969. Creating such a specialty was a vital sign that generalist medicine is important to U.S. health care.[6] (To understand why such a designation confers status on family practice, see Section 5.2.)

Further bolstering the central role of the PCP was the advent to managed care in the 1980s. The rapid growth of managed care transformed much of our health care into a system based on primary care. In the **managed care model,** the health organizations control—manage—care and cost by funneling all medical necessities through a primary care provider: the PCP.

Read more about managed care in Chapter 12, and about HMOs (health maintenance organizations) in Section 4.7. With many of the 80 million patients enrolled in HMOs required to gain permission from their PCP to get to secondary and tertiary referrals, it is no wonder that the profile and status of PCPs rose.

FOR EXAMPLE

The Decline of the General Practitioner

The general practitioner of old—otherwise known as the family doctor—is largely disappearing. The reason for the declining number of GPs was the creation of the family practice specialty in 1969. Since 1969, obtaining certification in family practice medicine requires a three-year residency program, similar to many of other specialty fields. To emphasize that family practice was a new field—and different from the general practice—general practitioners were not grandfathered in to family practice, even though they performed many of the same functions.

3.2.1 Benefits of the Primary Care Model

Over the past two decades, research has demonstrated that the more structured primary care system has advantages over a dispersed system that emphasizes specialist care over generalist care.

▲ **Quality of care:** The primary care model offered these benefits in terms of quality of care:
  - Continuity of care and the coordination of care are more likely to exist when care is given by primary care providers rather than specialists.
  - Nations with strong primary care based systems tend to have better outcomes on such measures as infant mortality and life expectancy.[7]
  - The quality of care for a variety of common conditions such as low back pain, diabetes, and hypertension is similar between generalists and specialists.

▲ **Cost containment:** The primary care model offered these benefits in terms of cost containment:
  - The model has led to greater use of preventive services, reductions in hospitalization, and reductions in overall health care costs.
  - Generalists have been found to practice a less expensive style of medicine, and health care costs are higher in regions with higher specialist-to-generalist ratios.

▲ **Public sentiment:** The American public wants primary care. According to a recent survey
  - 94 percent of the patients enrolled in California physician groups valued having a PCP who knew about all their medical problems.
  - For common ailments, such as coughing, knee pain, and so on, most people prefer to seek care from their PCP rather than a specialist.

- 89 percent wanted their PCP to participate in the process of specialty referral.

3.2.2 Predicting Primary Care's Future in the United States

At the dawn of the twenty-first century, the influence of managed care is declining. As primary care based managed care recedes in importance, the health care pendulum may swing back toward the dispersed and specialty-centered model of care, even though research shows that a primary care based system is preferable and that the American public wants primary care. As a result, the United States faces a major choice: renewed support for primary care or reversion to the dispersed model of care.[8]

SELF-CHECK

- List the benefits of a primary care model.
- Define the **managed care model.**
- What recent event is jeopardizing the continuation of the primary care model in the United States?

3.3 Performance of the Primary Care Model in the United States

The waning of managed care has given rise to fears that the recently arrived primary care centered system will wither despite its proven advantages and remarkable popularity. To better understand the future prospects of primary care, one needs to understand the forces that have made it difficult to flourish in this country. To be maximally effective, primary care, as the first point of entry into the health system, must

▲ Be accessible.
▲ Be comprehensive, handling most health care needs.
▲ Provide continuity of care over time, as a sustained partnership with patients.
▲ Interact easily, in its coordinating role, with the secondary and tertiary rungs of the health system.
▲ Be held accountable to the entire population the health system serves rather than merely to individual patients.

Has primary care risen to these challenges? Thus far, not entirely—in part because of the many political and economic forces that inhibit primary care and in part because of primary care's own reluctance to innovate. Primary care faces major new tensions, outlined in the following sections, in achieving each of its cardinal tasks.

3.3.1 Accessibility

Accessibility refers to how easily a patient can obtain and make use of medical care from his or her physician, and how timely such access is. For the following reasons, primary care is not as accessible as it needs to be in order to flourish in the United States:

▲ This nation has a shortage of PCPs.
▲ Many rural and inner-city areas qualify as health professional shortage areas (see Section 3.6), meaning that these populations lack adequate access to health care.
▲ Recent studies indicate that even patients who have access to health providers often have difficulty obtaining timely appointments with any clinician in their primary care practice.[9]

3.3.2 Continuity

Continuity of care refers to the systematic ability to have relevant information about previous episodes of care move with the patient among providers. When a primary care provider is used as a gatekeeper for access to specialties, coordination of care is better served. Information on treatments, medications, and need for services can be tracked if the primary care approach is used. Oftentimes specialists are not able or equipped to facilitate or provide continuity regarding a patient's care.

FOR EXAMPLE

Primary Care Report Card

In 2004, the Commonwealth Fund, a philanthropic organization founded in 1918, conducted a series of international surveys focused on primary and ambulatory care in five countries: the United States, Australia, New Zealand, Canada, and the United Kingdom. In terms of accessibility, adults in the United States reported the following: 17 percent of U.S. adults in the have no regular doctor. Only 37 percent had a long-term relationship with their doctors (defined as being five years or longer). Sixty-three percent claimed getting access to care on nights, weekends, or holidays without having to go to an emergency room for treatment was "very or somewhat difficult."

3.3.3 Comprehensiveness

Over the past two decades, the management of many illnesses has become far more complicated, placing a great strain on primary care's ability to handle most health care needs. Thus comprehensiveness of care has grown broader, meaning that PCPs have to provide more services (preventive and curative) than in the past, without referral to specialists. **Comprehensiveness of care** refers to the breadth and depth of care that primary physicians provide directly to their patients (beyond the coordinating and referral function).

The scope of care provided in primary care without referral to specialists has increased, with one-quarter of PCPs feeling that they are doing more than they are comfortable doing. Consider the change in what constitutes preventive care: In years past, preventive care included DPT and polio immunization, Pap smears, and breast exams. Today, preventive care includes these as well as multiple periodic screenings for cancers, lipids, and coronary heart disease; treating numerous childhood and adult infections; and providing advice on healthy lifestyles. Primary care tasks in chronic illness management have multiplied geometrically. As the U.S. population ages, chronic disease management of multiple diseases will be a major challenge for all primary care providers.

3.3.4 Coordination

Modern health care creates complex coordination problems for primary care. To perform their functions as coordinators of health care (as well as providers of health care) PCPs must interact with a growing number of organizations and personnel involved in the care of many patients, such as home health agencies, public health nurses, mental health professionals, pharmacists, and physical therapists.

Primary physicians' relationship with these other health care providers doesn't end with the patient referral, however. These collaborating organizations and professionals generate more requests to PCPs for authorization of services and orders and additional information to incorporate into treatment plans.

3.3.5 Accountability to the Community

PCPs may have their clinical practice under constant surveillance—and at times made public through report cards and the Internet—by employers, Medicare, health plans, physician groups, and hospitals. This level of accountability requires primary care to concern itself not only with patients who make appointments to be seen but also with those who do not. The reason is a relatively new idea of the **population-based medicine,** a concept that requires PCPs be concerned with *every* patient on their panel, not only those who actively seek health care.

3.3.6 Its Effect on Primary Care Providers

Given the current design of primary care practice (refer to Section 3.3.5), it has become increasingly difficult to convert the definition of primary care into daily reality. Many PCPs are stressed out and overwhelmed with crammed schedules, inefficient work environments, and unrewarding administrative tasks.

Primary care visits last an average of 16 to 18 minutes and include a median of three patient problems, requiring the physician to make an average of 2.75 decisions per visit. At least half of these decisions are relatively complex.[10]

SELF-CHECK

- List the characteristics that ensure a maximally effective primary care system.
- Define **continuity** and explain the challenges primary care faces in this regard.
- Define **comprehensiveness** and explain the challenges primary care faces in this regard.

3.4 Primary Care Innovations

For the primary care model to make good on its promises (accessibility and continuity and comprehensiveness of care; for example, see Section 3.3), it needs to be redesigned in such a way as to

▲ Relieve the time stresses on physicians.
▲ Reconceptualize the meaning of continuity of care.
▲ Enable acute patients to be seen in a timely fashion.
▲ Provide optimal management to the entire panel of chronic patients.

Fortunately, medical innovators are initiating redesign projects in all four of these areas.

3.4.1 The Primary Care Team

One concept underlying the redesign efforts is the **primary care team.** At some primary care sites, a team of caregivers is being developed to relieve time pressures on the physician, to become the vehicle for continuity of care, and to allow a complementary division of labor. One model of a primary care team might bring together two family physicians, two nurse practitioners, a health educator, two medical assistants, and a receptionist. The physicians might directly care for 8 to 10 (rather than 25 to 30) patients a day, spending 30 to 45 minutes with more complex patients, thereby making the encounters more meaningful to both patient and physician. The physician would spend considerable time consulting with other team members and arranging referrals.

More routine visits would be handled by nonphysician clinicians. Medical assistants would be trained to perform routine tasks associated with preventive health care and chronic illness, thereby relieving the physician of time-consuming work that is easily handled by caregivers with far less training.

The issue of continuity of care in a team-based system is more complicated. Patients expecting to see their own doctor would need to be willing to be seen by the team instead. Given how often patients currently see clinicians other than their own PCP, they may find it an improvement to be guaranteed access to a stable team, even if they can't see the physician.

Such access would be enhanced by guaranteeing that patients could see the appropriate caregiver on the primary care team the same day that they call for an appointment. Some medical practices have already redesigned their scheduling systems along these lines. For example, the scheduling innovation known as open access emphasizes providing same-day appointments for all patients, irrespective of whether they have routine or urgent needs.

3.4.2 Chronic Care Model and Collaborative Care

Improved management of chronic illness may be achievable through a set of innovations known as the **chronic care model.** The chronic care model proactively addresses health concerns of people with chronic illnesses, such as diabetes and asthma, by using **evidence-based research** to overcome obstacles to care. Such obstacles include physicians who don't follow established guidelines, lack of coordinated care, lack of follow-up services, and patients inadequately educated on how to best manage their illnesses.

Components of this model, some of which have been adopted at a number of primary care sites, include the creation of disease registries to allow for population-based care of chronic illnesses; reminder systems and performance feedback for physicians; intensive case management of challenging patients; and planned chronic care visits with groups of patients.

Chronically ill patients may also benefit from a new model of providing health care variously called provider–patient partnerships, patient empowerment, and collaborative care. The essence of collaborative care is that the caregiver and the patient agree on a written plan to improve the patient's health. Collaborative care, which may be more effective than having physicians tell patients what they are supposed to do, takes more time than traditional care, but physicians do not need to do all the work involved; other team members can be trained to work with patients on their action plans.

FOR EXAMPLE

Problem Solving for Chronic Care

In 1995, about 99 million people in the United States had chronic conditions. By 2030, that number is expected to increase to 150 million. The direct costs for medical services for these people will grow as well, to nearly $800 billion by 2030. In 1997, Dorothy Rice, professor emeritus at the University of California, San Francisco, suggested integrating medical and social services to address the growing numbers because treating chronic conditions requires both medical and nonmedical services. The National Chronic Care Consortium, an allliance of 30 health care networks from across the country, has set up chronic-care networks in which providers would evaluate a patient's needs from every angle and address them accordingly. Such a system would require setting up an information system to help care providers share data and have a more global view of a patient's situation.

According to MedPAC *Report to Congress*, "As estimated from Medicare claims data, about 78% of the Medicare population had at least one chronic condition in 1999, and 63% had two or more."[11] With an increase in population longevity, there is an increase in chronic disease. The U.S. system of care has been based on an acute care approach and has not focused on long-term chronic disease management.

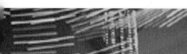

SELF-CHECK

- Define **collaborative care.**
- Identify three characteristics of the primary care team approach.
- Describe the chronic care model.

3.5 Identifying the PCP

Not only are their days hectic and their time with patients cut short by sheer volume and administrative tasks (refer to Section 3.3), but PCPs face another dilemma: identifying who is, in actuality, the primary care provider.

In European countries, the primary care provider is the PCP. In the United States, however, the answer is vastly more complicated because no single physician specialty has a monopoly on primary care.

In this country general practitioners (GPs) are virtually an extinct species, crowded out by the proliferation of specialists over the past century (refer to Section 5.2 to learn about the draw of specialty medicine and what this has meant for the generalist). The GP was reincarnated in the United States as the family physician with the advent of the board-certified specialty of family practice in 1969. But by then—after years of a lack of general practitioners available to provide primary care—the ecological niche of primary care was partly occupied by physicians in general internal medicine and general pediatrics. Currently, the United States has approximately equal numbers of the three types of generalist specialties: family physicians, general internists, and general pediatricians.

Collectively, these three generalist specialties account for one-third of all American physicians. All three specialties fulfill the essential primary care functions, although many observers consider family medicine the quintessential primary care specialty in the United States because, unlike physicians in internal medicine and pediatrics, those in family medicine care for patients irrespective of age. They also often perform services—obstetrical care and surgery—outside the scope of practice of the two other generalist specialties.

3.5.1 Permeable Boundaries between Generalist, Specialist, and Other Functions

As if having three primary care specialties instead of one (see Section 3.5) did not make for a confusing enough situation, the dispersed health care model complicates matters even more. In the U.S. system, there are no clear distinctions between who performs primary and secondary care. PCPs provide secondary care, specialists provide primary care, and hospitalists—a relatively new player in the U.S. health care arena—provide general care in hospital settings.

3.5.2 Specialists Providing Primary Care

Other specialties (beyond the three generalist specialties of family physician, general internist, and general pediatrician) lay claim to portions of the primary care turf. Many women, for example, consider their obstetrician-gynecologists to be their primary care doctors—even though studies have shown that specialties other than family medicine, general internal medicine, and general pediatrics do *not* fulfill the essential core functions of primary care in either practice or training. Obstetrician-gynecologists, for example, can provide first contact and continuity of care, but they don't provide truly comprehensive care because of their focus on reproductive-health-related problems.

3.5.3 Generalists Providing Secondary Care

The uncertain boundaries between primary, secondary, and tertiary care levels in the traditional health system have not only allowed specialists to perform some

> ## FOR EXAMPLE
>
> ### Nonprimary Primary Care Providers
>
> According to a 2004 study by the Robert Graham Center in Washington, DC, titled "Specialist Physicians Providing Primary Care Services in Colorado," in Colorado physicians outside primary care fields provide approximately a third of the primary care medical services. For the purposes of the study, primary care fields included physicians in family medicine, general practice, general internal medicine, or general pediatrics. The research found that specialists perform about a third of the primary care functions (preventive care, routine physicals, and treatment of common ailments) in the state and that the care is generally of lower quality than that provided by PCPs.

primary care functions, they've also forced PCPs into more of a secondary care role, particularly in comparison with PCPs in other nations.

Whereas general practitioners in most nations work only in ambulatory care settings, family physicians in the United States have traditionally served as inpatient attending physicians. This arrangement, at least according to the traditional American view, allowed better continuity of care. In addition, inpatient practice has had important political and financial benefits for PCPs: Insurance plans pay much higher fees for inpatient than ambulatory visits, and the acute hospital setting has conferred professional prestige in the specialty-oriented world of American medicine.

3.5.4 Hospitalists Dedicated to General Inpatient Care

Recent trends are forcing a reconsideration of the role of PCPs in inpatient medicine. Many health care organizations now have a dedicated staff of physicians who handle all general inpatient services. PCPs voluntarily, or in some cases compulsorily, hand over care of their inpatients to a dedicated staff of hospitalists, doctors employed by a hospital who handle all general inpatient services.

Although the term **hospitalist** is an American invention, the hospitalist arrangement is a long-standing one in most European nations. The role of general internists and general pediatricians in these nations is in fact largely that of hospitalists. Although hospitalists are well accepted in these nations, their advent in the United States is causing controversy. Many PCPs, particularly those in general internal medicine, are reluctant to relinquish hospital practice. On the other hand, research has indicated that many PCPs may welcome a reduced role in the hospital because the demands of inpatient service often detract from the ability of generalist physicians to concentrate their efforts on the most critical dimension of primary care—ambulatory care.

3.5.5 Nonphysician Primary Care Clinicians

In addition to the hospitalist movement explained in Section 3.5.4, PCPs in the United States face another major development that has implications for their future: The nation is in the midst of an explosion in the supply of nonphysician primary care clinicians. These clinicians—nurse practitioners and physician assistants—have considerable overlap in functions with those of PCPs, and research has demonstrated that they can perform most of the tasks usually undertaken by PCPs with comparable quality of care.

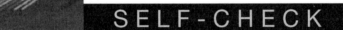

SELF-CHECK

- Define **hospitalist**.
- Name the three primary care specialties.
- Identify three health care providers other than PCPs who provide primary care services.

3.6 PCPs and the Populations They Serve

The previous sections describe the health care provided in the United States and its continuing evolution. In essence, the theme of the earlier sections is *how* Americans access health care: In other words, which organization, primary or secondary—impacts how people enter and move through the U.S. health care system. This section focus on another issue: *whether* people access the system.

Although this nation has a large number of physicians, not all people have access to health care. The question, then, becomes why not? The answer is threefold:

▲ Despite the overabundance of physicians in general, the United States has too few generalists and too many specialists. (You can find out about how many physicians America's medical schools are turning out and the distribution of specialists to generalists in Section 5.2.)

▲ Arguably the single most critical barrier to health access in the United States is the lack of health insurance and the inability of the nation to agree on some form of universal coverage so that all people can have the benefits of health care, including primary care. (Chapter 4 provides information on how the U.S. health care system is financed.)

▲ The maldistribution of PCPs leaves many regions in the United States without the doctors they need for adequate care. Called *health profession shortage areas* (HPSAs), these are the areas—most often rural and inner city—that lack access to medical care because they lack health care providers.

Interestingly, the preceding points qualify as three of the most pressing challenges facing the U.S. health care system. These challenges, and others, are discussed in detail in Chapter 12.

3.6.1 Health Profession Shortage Areas (HPSAs)

Tremendous geographic variation exists in the supply of PCPs. Physicians have tended to locate their practices in urban areas and, within cities, have gravitated toward more affluent neighborhoods. Although it is to be expected that many specialists will locate their practices in urban areas near tertiary care hospitals, PCPs are also disproportionately concentrated in urban areas. The result? About 2,500 communities in the United States qualify as primary care **health profession shortage areas (HPSAs).** HPSA is a federal designation meaning that the population lacks adequate access to health care. One of the major criteria for receiving such a designation is having fewer than one PCP for every 3,500 residents.

Despite the increase in the overall number of physicians (see Section 5.1), the number of HPSAs increased by 25 percent between 1980 and 2000. Places that lack adequate access to medical services are primarily rural and inner-city areas.

Rural regions have fewer physicians than urban areas do. Consider these statistics:

▲ Whereas 20 percent of the population resides in rural areas, only 9 percent of the nation's physicians have offices there.

▲ Two-thirds of all HPSAs are in rural regions. In many sparsely populated regions, even individuals with the best health insurance coverage often find their access to care compromised by an absence of physicians within a convenient distance.

FOR EXAMPLE

Mental Health Shortage Areas

PCPs aren't the only health care professionals in short supply in some areas. The federal government designates regions as mental health profession shortage areas, as well. As of December 2003, over 1,400 were designated mental health HPSAs, up from 900 in 2002. To qualify, in addition to a population-to-mental-health-professional ratio (which varies, depending on the mental health professional), the population within the area must be considered to have unusually high needs for mental health services, defined as followed: 20 percent below the poverty level, a high number of young people or a high number of elderly people, a high prevalence of alcoholism, or a high degree of substance abuse.

Rural communities face many challenges in recruiting and retaining PCPs. Some of these challenges stem from community characteristics that are difficult to modify, such as a lack of job opportunities for spouses of physicians; limited choices of schools; lack of cultural, recreation, and shopping opportunities; and an inhospitable climate. Other obstacles are related to the nature of primary care practice in rural areas.

▲ The higher rate of poverty in rural communities limits the number of persons with commercial health insurance coverage, making it difficult to financially sustain private primary care practices.
▲ The distance from specialists and hospitals poses obstacles to referrals and consultations and may compel primary care practitioners to provide a broader scope of care than they would in an urban setting.
▲ The lack of a critical mass of colleagues requires primary care practitioners to be on call more frequently and makes it difficult to leave town for professional conferences or vacation.

Although the shortage of physicians and medical facilities is most significant in rural areas, cities also have shortage areas. Neighborhoods with a high proportion of minority residents are most likely to have a low supply of PCPs and to be designated as HPSAs. The relationship between the supply of physicians and access to care is probably less clear cut in urban neighborhoods than in rural counties; most urban neighborhoods with few physicians are surrounded by communities with an abundant supply of physicians. However, inadequate public transportation and related factors may make it difficult for low-income people to avail themselves of health services outside their neighborhood. Such difficulty argues for the importance of local primary care.

3.6.2 Federal and State Strategies

Federal and state agencies have developed policies to improve the geographic distribution of physicians.

▲ **National Health Service Corps and Loan Repayment Program:** One of the most prominent programs administered by the federal Bureau of Primary Health Care, the **National Health Service Corps and Loan Repayment Program** provides scholarships to medical students and loan repayment to recent residency graduates in exchange for medical service in HPSAs. Several states operate similar loan repayment programs.
▲ **Grants:** The federal government provides grants to community health centers in underserved communities and to supplement Medicare fees for physicians practicing in HPSAs. Other federal and state programs have awarded grants to medical schools and residency training programs to encourage training opportunities that emphasize service to needy populations.

▲ **Focused recruiting of medical students:** Physicians who grew up in rural communities are much more likely than other physicians to locate their practice in rural communities when they complete their residency training. Similarly, physicians from minority racial and ethnic groups are much more likely to practice in underserved urban neighborhoods. A recent study demonstrated that four factors are highly predictive of which physicians care for underserved populations:

- Being a member of a minority group.
- Participating in the National Health Service Corps.
- Having a strong interest before medical school in practicing in an underserved area.
- Growing up in an underserved area.

Eighty-six percent of the physicians with all four characteristics worked in shortage areas or cared for substantial numbers of underserved patients, compared with only 22 percent with none of these characteristics. By working to recruit students who possess these characteristics, the medical education system can increase the number of physicians who are likely to practice in underserved areas.

SELF-CHECK

- Define **health profession shortage area (HPSA)**.
- List the two underserved areas.
- Explain the strategy of focused recruiting on addressing underserved areas.

SUMMARY

Providing health care involves not only diagnoses and treatment but also access to health care, continuity of care, coordination of care, and more. How a health system coordinates all these functions determines its health model. The primary care model, popular in Europe, is growing in popularity in the United States and challenging this country's reliance on a specialty care model. The success of a primary-based system in the United States depends on how well primary care can meet patient expectations regarding access to and quality of care. Certain primary care innovations, such as a chronic care model and creation of primary care teams, are intended to address these concerns. Because specialists and other health care providers often perform the same functions as PCPs, and because there are fewer PCPs than needed, the primary care model continues to struggle for a secure foothold in the United States.

KEY TERMS

Accessibility	How easily a patient can obtain and make use of medical care from his or her physician, and how timely such access is.
Capitation	A fixed amount of money paid in advance to a physician for the delivery of health care services.
Chronic care model	Health care model that uses evidence-based research to proactively address health concerns of people with chronic illnesses, such as diabetes and asthma.
Comprehensiveness of care	The breadth and depth of care that primary physicians provide directly to their patients (beyond the coordinating and referral function).
Continuity of care	The systematic ability to have relevant information about previous episodes of care move with the patient among providers.
Evidence-based medicine	A medical movement that bases care decisions for individual patients on evidence from clinical studies.
Hospitalists	Doctors, employed by a hospital, who handle all general inpatient services.
Health Profession Shortage Area (HPSA)	A federal designation meaning that that population lacks adequate access to health care.
Managed care model	Model in which health organizations manage care and cost by funneling all medical necessities through a primary care provider.
National Health Service Corps and Loan Repayment Program	Federal program providing scholarships to medical students and loan repayment to recent residency graduates in exchange for medical service in HPSAs.
Population-based medicine	A concept that requires PCPs to be concerned with every patient on their panel, not only those who actively seek health care.
Primary care	General preventive and curative care that is provided to a person over an extended period of time, including coordination of all primary, secondary, and tertiary care that the patient receives.

Primary care team

A team approach to primary care in which division of labor is shared among a group of primary caregivers.

Secondary care

Care that is typically provided in a hospital by medical specialists who generally don't have first contact with patients

Specialty care model

A health care model in which patients are not required to consult with a primary care provider before seeking general or specialty care; nor do patients have to have their care coordinated through a PCP.

Tertiary care

Specialized consultative care, usually on referral from primary or secondary health care providers. Tertiary care, generally delivered in teaching institutions that have the personnel and facilities for special investigation and treatment, handles rare and complicated illnesses.

ASSESS YOUR UNDERSTANDING

Go to www.wiley.com/college/pointer to evaluate your knowledge of health care models.

Measure your learning by comparing pre-test and post-test results.

Summary Questions

1. In a primary care system, a patient, as the primary decision maker, is free to seek medical care from any physician without first consulting a PCP. True or False?

2. The United States uses a highly structures primary care model. True or False?

3. Which of the following promoted the visibility of primary care in the United States?

    (a) the advent of managed care in the 1960s

    (b) the creation of a family medicine specialty in 1969

    (c) millions of patients enrolled in HMOs

    (d) all of the above

    (e) a and b

4. Which of the following explains why primary care is less expensive than specialty care?

    (a) PCPs offer more preventive services

    (b) primary care patients receive less comprehensive care

    (c) specialists offer greater continuity of care

    (d) none of the above

5. To flourish in the United States, primary care must be

    (a) accessible.

    (b) comprehensive.

    (c) accountable to the community.

    (d) all of the above.

6. Comprehensiveness of care refers to the scope of care that primary physicians provide directly to their patients. Identify why the PCPs struggle to provide comprehensive care.

    (a) because they often work in teams, PCPs have more patients to attend to than ever before

    (b) as specialists outnumber PCPs, PCPs find themselves competing with specialists in the services they must provide

(c) as managing illnesses grows more complex, PCPs have to provide more services than they have in the past

(d) all of the above

7. A primary care team reconceptualizes the meaning of continuity of care in the following way.

    (a) by freeing up the PCP to be available on a same-day basis for any patient who calls seeking an appointment

    (b) by relying on team members to provide follow-up care based on the primary physician's instructions

    (c) by altering the definition of continuity to mean the availability of any member of the practice rather a particular physician

    (d) by making it possible for patients to see the same doctor at every appointment, regardless of scheduling conflicts

8. What primary care innovations directly address the care of chronic patients?

    (a) the managed care model, which provides a series of services to patients with chronic conditions

    (b) the collaborative care model, which relies on proactive interaction between patient and physician

    (c) the secondary care model, which relies on a secondary care provider specializing in the condition to help the PCP develop a treatment plan

    (d) the chronic care model, which addresses specific obstacles impeding the delivery of adequate care for chronic conditions

9. Primary care is provided by

    (a) pediatricians and internists.

    (b) family practitioners.

    (c) specialists.

    (d) all of the above.

    (e) a and b.

10. Which of the following are primary care specialties?

    (a) gynecologists

    (b) family practice physicians

    (c) general internists

    (d) all of the above

    (e) b and c

11. A hospitalist is

    (a) a physician who provides inpatient care in hospitals.

    (b) a PCP whose practice is based in a hospital.

    (c) a physician assistant who provides primary care to hospitalized patients.

    (d) a researcher who studies the impact of primary care on hospitalization rates.

12. Explain why not all Americans have access to health care, even though the United States has an abundance of physicians.

    (a) lack of health insurance

    (b) shortage of general practitioners

    (c) poor distribution of health care providers

    (d) all of the above

13. Define HPSA.

    (a) health profession shortage area: an area that lacks adequate health care providers or access to health care providers

    (b) health profession study area: a geographic region featured in studies on health care trends in the United States

    (c) health profession service area: a geographic area identified by the type and number of both primary and secondary health care providers

    (d) none of the above

14. Identify the area most likely to be classified as an HPSA.

    (a) suburban area

    (b) business district

    (c) inner-city area

    (d) rural area

Review Questions

1. Health care is divided into primary, secondary, and tertiary care. Define *secondary care*.

    (a) general preventive and curative care that is provided to a person over an extended period of time

    (b) care that is typically provided in a hospital by medical specialists ho generally don't have first contact with patients

    (c) specialized consultative care, usually on referral from a primary health care provider

    (d) none of the above

2. Why is the U.S. system based on the specialty care model?

    (a) general preventive and curative care in the United States has traditionally been provided by specialists rather than generalists; hence, people have come to expect specialty care for general health concerns

(b) the specialty care model is more dispersed than the primary care model; hence, people in sparsely populated areas had few general practitioners and therefore had to rely on specialists

(c) nearly half of the U.S. population lacked a regular physician to function as a point of first contact; hence, they pursued health care independent of a referral from a PCP

(d) a and c

3. In what way does managed care foster a switch from the specialty care model to the primary care model?

(a) the advent of managed care plans coincided with the decreasing number of specialists in the United States; as more people turn from specialty care to general care, the role of the PCP becomes more vital and necessary

(b) managed care plans require that patients access health care through the PCP; as more people become members of managed care plans, the role of the PCP becomes more vital and necessary

(c) in the United States managed care isn't fostering a switch; currently both systems exist side-by-side, and no research suggests that primary care will become the dominant health model

(d) none of the above

4. In what way does the primary care model outperform the specialty care model?

(a) continuity of care and coordination of care

(b) infant mortality and life expectancy

(c) cost

(d) all of the above

5. PCPs are responsible for coordinating a patient's health care needs. Identify the purpose of this coordination.

(a) to facilitate medical services by interacting with other organizations and health providers and authorizing services and referrals

(b) to reduce costs and promote continuity of care by acting as a gatekeeper for additional services and referrals

(c) to enhance quality of care by collaborating with other service providers and incorporating treatment plans

(d) all of the above

6. Define population-based medicine.

(a) the expectation that doctors will serve all members of the community in which their practice is based

(b) the concept of PCPs being responsible with every patient in their patient list

     (c) the idea that physicians should belong to the populations they serve

     (d) the goal of providing medical care to all members of the U.S. population

7. Which of the following is an example of the chronic care model at work?

     (a) the referral of patients with chronic conditions to specialists for treatment

     (b) patient education and the creation of standard practice guidelines for chronic conditions and patient education

     (c) the provision of medications to manage chronic conditions

     (d) a and c

8. PCPs are under a great deal of stress. Which of the following are significant stressors?

     (a) ensuring continuity of care

     (b) increased patient load and primary care responsibilities

     (c) increased clerical responsibilities

     (d) all of the above

9. A primary care team is intended to relieve pressure on the physician, improve continuity of care, and allow a division of labor. Which of the following best represents such a team?

     (a) a group practice including PCPs, nurse practitioners, and other health care professionals, as wells as clerical support staff

     (b) multiple primary care doctors working in a single practice and coordinating their services with a local hospital for secondary care

     (c) a primary care doctor, working in a solo practice, who partners with an on-call service during off-hours to provide continuity of care

     (d) none of the above

10. Explain the primary reason for the confusion regarding who provides primary care.

     (a) the confusion is the result of the imprecise terms delineating medical functions; the terms *general practitioner, family physician,* and *primary care physician* all refer to PCPs. The names of other specialties—*general pediatrics* and *general internal medicine,* for example—compound the confusion by implying that specialists in these fields also provide primary care

     (b) the confusion is the result of the introduction of a primary care specialty in the late 1960s with the advent of managed care health plans; until then, no distinctions were made between primary and specialty care, and primary care was universally delivered; the managed care requirement of a gatekeeper—a generalist responsible for referring patients to specialists—was created for cost-saving reasons

(c) the confusion is the result of having no clearly defined boundaries regarding who performs primary care functions; currently primary care is provided by physicians in the three primary care specialties (family practice, general internist, general pediatrician), specialists in non–primary care fields (such as gynecologists or obstetricians), as well as nonphysician clinicians (nurse practitioners and physicians assistants, for example)

(d) the confusion is the result of the increasing number of nonphysician primary care providers, such as nurse practitioners and physician assistants, who are competing with PCPs for patients

11. Which of the following best illustrates the fluid nature of primary care in the United States?

(a) specialists providing primary care and generalists providing secondary care

(b) hospitalists and generalists providing inpatient care

(c) PCPs referring patients to secondary care physicians

(d) nurse practitioners replacing PCPs

12. Identify a significant difference between rural and inner-city HPSAs.

(a) lack of health care in rural areas generally relates to proximity of health care; access to care is compromised by an absence of physicians within a convenient distance; proximity is not a problem in metropolitan HPSAs

(b) rural HPSAs have difficulty attracting health care providers due to their location because physicians prefer to locate their practices in urban areas; inner-city HPSAs benefit from physicians locating in urban areas

(c) inner-city residents are more likely to go without health care because of lack of insurance

(d) none of the above

13. Federal and state governments as well as the medical education system seek to address HPSAs. How do they use physician characteristics in their strategic plans?

(a) they provide scholarships to students who express a willingness to practice in an HPSA

(b) they work to recruit minority students and those who grew up in underserved areas

(c) they provide monetary incentives to encourage medical school gradu-ates to locate in underserved areas

(d) all of the above

Applying This Chapter

1. Identify which health care model (primary care or specialty care) each of the following scenarios represents:

   (a) a parent discovers that a nationally recognized children's hospital specializes in the disease that her child has; she calls the hospital and sets up an appointment with a staff physician

   (b) after discovering a suspicious mole, a man consults his family doctor, who then refers him to a dermatologist

   (c) a girl breaks her arm playing soccer; her parents rush her to the emergency room of their local hospital

2. You are a PCP with many years of experience. Medical students at a nearby university are asking your advise about whether or not to pursue a primary care specialty. For each of the following students, indicate what advice you would give and why.

   (a) student 1 is a "big picture" thinker; she can easily coordinate large amounts of information and is highly organized; she is also highly motivated by the need to create personal relationships with her patients and to be accessible to them

   (b) student 2 thrives on detail; he prefers studying single systems (such as the respiratory system or the circulatory system) rather than general care, and is driven to find out everything he can about a particular issue or ailment; he has said that he wants to be the top in his field one day

3. Of the factors impeding the flourishing of the primary care model in the United States, identify two that you consider the most important and explain your reasoning.

4. Which characteristic(s) of the primary care model does the chronic care model address: accessibility, comprehensiveness, continuity, coordination of care, and/or accountability to the entire population?

5. Describe the team approach and explain what problems it addresses in how the primary care model functions in the United States.

6. What single factor, if remedied, would have the biggest positive impact on eliminating HPSAs?

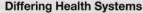

YOU TRY IT

Differing Health Systems

Your British guest feels under the weather and seeks medical care in the United States. You find yourself explaining to him how the U.S. health care system differs from the U.K. system. Indicate how you would clarify the difference in primary care between the two systems.

Primary Care Benefits

You find yourself on a panel as a proponent of the primary care model. Another speaker has just made the argument that the specialty care based system in the United States provides world-class health care to the U.S. population. Indicate how you would respond.

Variety of Primary Care Providers

No single medical specialty is responsible for primary care in the United States. Evaluate the impact that having a variety of primary care providers has had on the development of a comprehensive primary care system.

Health Care Access Plan

Your pediatric office is expanding and overwhelmed; you've noticed a large increase in the number of children being sent to you for diagnosis of special conditions, such as ADHD, depression, autism spectrum disorders, and so forth. As the sole physician with a single receptionist and two nurses, you're looking for ways to improve access to care for your patients and quality of life for yourself and your staff. Put together a plan.

Finding a New Doctor

You live in a small town that is losing its only family practice doctor. You're charged with finding someone to fill his shoes. Address the challenges you face in your search, indicating which you can change and which you can't, and suggest ways to address the ones you can.

73

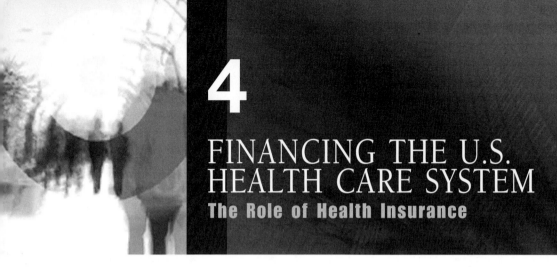

4

FINANCING THE U.S. HEALTH CARE SYSTEM
The Role of Health Insurance

Starting Point

Go to www.wiley.com/college/pointer to assess your knowledge of financing the U.S. health care system.
Determine where you need to concentrate your effort.

What You'll Learn in This Chapter

▲ Who finances health care and where the money goes
▲ The types of insurance plans most people in the U.S. have
▲ The difference between voluntary, social, and public welfare insurance
▲ Key components and types of voluntary health insurance
▲ The important differences between Medicare and Medicaid
▲ Types of health maintenance organizations

After Studying This Chapter, You'll Be Able To

▲ Demonstrate how economic factors impact the cost of health care
▲ Examine the major funding sources of and recipients for health care dollars
▲ Analyze the relationship between general economic factors and the rate of the uninsured
▲ Analyze the factors impacting who does and doesn't have insurance
▲ Distinguish the important features of voluntary insurance plans
▲ Differentiate between Medicare and Medicaid
▲ Examine how health maintenance organizations seek to control health care costs

Goals and Outcomes

▲ Master the terminology relating to the various types of insurance plans and their categories
▲ Identify the key components of each type of insurance
▲ Represent the flow of funds through the health care system
▲ Articulate the impact economic factors have had on health care funding and predict future trends
▲ Evaluate the relationship between economic factors and number of uninsured
▲ Compare health care plans in terms of financial risk management and cost control
▲ Evaluate the affect rising costs will have on the voluntary health insurance, government programs, and health maintenance organizations

INTRODUCTION

The United States spends more on health care than any other industrialized country in the world. According to the March 2006 Report To The Congress on Medicare Payment Policy by the Medicare Payment Advisory Commission (MedPAC), "by certain measures of health status, the United States does not compare favorably to other industrialized countries . . . having higher rates of infant mortality, higher standardized rates of all-cause mortality and life expectancy about the same"[1]. The financing of health services in the US is fragmented. Public and private health insurance are the key funders of the health care system through employers, citizen taxes and individual funds. As health care costs have increased, the burden of the cost is shifting with higher out of pocket costs for individuals. Individuals,, employers, and taxes through state and federal government all pay some part of these health care costs. Still, not all people in the U.S. have health insurance coverage. The MedPac 2006 report states that "During 2004, nearly 46 million people or 15.7 percent of the US population, were uninsured at any one period of time"[2]. This high rate of uninsured puts a strain on both the public and private insurers. The U.S. system includes several different types of insurance plans. Voluntary health insurance refers to private insurance plans that individuals and employers purchase. Government insurance programs fund health care for the needy and special populations, such as older Americans and the disabled. And a relatively new player in the insurance fields, the health maintenance organization (HMO), is changing not only the way health care is paid for, but also how it's provided.

4.1 Changing Economic Dynamics

From the end of World War II through the early 1990s, individual patients sought care from physicians and hospitals for distinct episodes of illness. Patients either paid directly for this care or (increasingly) through health insurance provided by their employers—and, after 1966, with the implementation of Medicare and Medicaid, by government funding. Those with coverage were relatively price-insensitive because they bore little or none of the costs for the services they used. Voluntary (private) and government health insurance plans paid providers full rates, either incurred costs or billed charges. As providers increased their activity (patient days, visits, and procedures), they produced greater revenues.

From 1965 through the early 1990s, health care costs and expenditures increased dramatically (as explained in 4.1.1), seriously eroding the global competitiveness of businesses and overwhelming federal, state, and local government budgets. Being eaten alive by increasing costs, businesses and government became increasingly price-sensitive. They wanted to predict and control their expenditures for health care and shift some of the financial risk to health insurers and providers. For a set price, they demanded a comprehensive or integrated package of services where providers were paid set rates per beneficiary, irrespective of the costs they incurred to offer the service.

By the late 1980s, the purchaser side of the market was dominated by large organizations (corporations and federal and state governments) who paid for health care coverage for groups of beneficiaries (employees, or Medicare or Medicaid recipients). At the same time, purchasers were beginning to question what they were getting for their money. Even though the United States had the highest per capita health care expenditures in the world, its citizens were considerably less healthy than those in most other industrialized countries. Pressure for making significant changes in the nation's health care system increased.

4.1.1 Increasing Expenditures

Health care is the nation's second largest industry, exceeded only by durable goods manufacturing. In 2004, total industry expenditures were $1.9 trillion, accounting for 16 percent of the gross domestic product (GDP)[3] Expenditures for personal health care services and products include

▲ **Institutional services:** For example, hospital and nursing home care.
▲ **Professional services:** From physicians, dentists, podiatrists, chiropractors, and many other outpatient service providers.
▲ **Nontraditional services:** For example, acupuncturists, massage therapists, naturopaths.
▲ **Products:** Durable medical equipment and so on.
▲ **Supplies:** Notably, pharmaceuticals.

Compare the 2004 expenditures with the health expenditures in 1960 to get an idea of just how much health care costs have increased in four decades:

Item	1960	2004
National health expenditures	$27 billion	$1,678.9 billion
Per capita spending	$126 per person	$6280 per person
Percentage of GDP	5%	16%

The increases in expenditures from 1960 to 2004 translate into sharp inclines in both per capita spending (as shown in Figure 4-1), as well as health care costs as a percentage of the gross domestic product (GDP).

The money to pay for health expenditures comes from two main sectors: private funds and government funds (read more about these sources that pay for health care in Section 4.2).

Figure 4-1

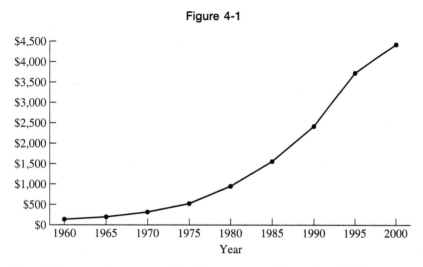

Growth in per capita personal health care expenditures from 1960 to 2000.

As expenses have increased over the years, the distribution of how much each of these sources pays has changed dramatically. In 1960, 75 percent of total expenditures came from private sources and 25 percent came from government; by 2003, 55.2 percent came from private funds and 44.8 percent from the federal government (see Figure 4-2).

4.1.2 Reasons for the Increase

The causes of the increase in U.S. health care expenditures are

▲ **Inflation in the economy as a whole:** As prices go up in general, costs of medical care also go up.

Figure 4-2

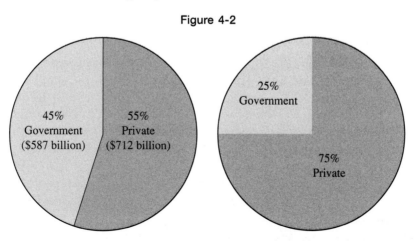

Source of health care expenditure funds: 1960 (*left*) and 2003 (*right*).

Figure 4-3

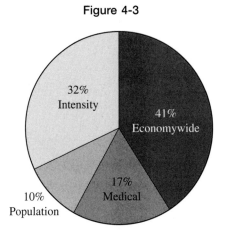

Causes of increases in personal health care expenditures, 1960–2003.

▲ **Inflation in the medical component of the consumer price index:** Even when adjusted for inflation, medical prices still show an increase
▲ **Overall growth in the population:** More people means more dollars spent on health care, assuming no other factors change.
▲ **Changes in the type and quality of health care services provided:** As health care services grow more sophisticated and comprehensive, the prices rise accordingly.

Figure 4-3 illustrates how much each of these factors contributed to the overall increase in health care expenditures.

FOR EXAMPLE

Keeping Down Costs

To keep costs down in this era of burgeoning health care expense, Regence BlueCross BlueShield of Utah gives its members a "how-to" pamphlet that offers suggestions and advice on using its policy in a way that saves the insurer money. In addition to explaining why its members should pay attention to cost (increased expenses mean increased premiums), the pamphlet also offers money-saving suggestions, including general lifestyle and safety tips (eat properly, wear a helmet when riding a bike, etc.), medical advice (don't agree to tests you don't need, take medications you don't need, or go to the emergency room for general care), and cost-cutting measures (buy generic drugs and use in-service doctors and hospitals). As insurance companies come under increasing financial strain, such communications are the now the norm.

4.1.3 Affecting How Health Care Is Financed

As the data in the preceding sections illustrate, the underlying "economic calculus" of health care is undergoing significant change. The most recent round of changes began in the mid-1980s and will fundamentally reshape the industry over the next several decades. These changes, summarized in Table 4-1, are purchaser driven and concern who the purchasers are, what they want and expect, and how they pay.

In the U.S. health care industry today, unlike in other industries, the purchaser is not generally the one who receives the service. In other words, the patient who receives the care is not the "purchaser"—that is, the one who pays for the service. This distinction is important in understanding the changes in health care financing and the natural tension between the consumers (the patients), the purchasers (the insurance companies or government), and the providers (the hospitals, physicians, and so on, who provide the services).

Employers purchase health insurance plans for their employees. Health premiums, many economists argue, are a substitute for cash compensation that would otherwise be paid to the worker. In response to rapid increases in premiums, many employers have raised the cost sharing requirements for their employees, asked them to contribute a larger share of premiums or, particularly for smaller firms, reduced the availability of coverage."[4]

Table 4-1: Drivers of Economic Change in the Health Care Industry

	Past	Present and Future
Purchasers are	Individuals	Employers
	Cost insensitive	Price sensitive
Health care demands	Service/treatment on an individual basis, as needed for a specific occurrence of a health issue	A comprehensive and integrated package of services to be available regardless of need
Financial risk is	Assumed by purchaser only	Shared by the purchaser and parties plus providers
Payment is made	As care is provided	As an output and outcome of the care process
	For incurred costs or billed charges	Based on negotiated rate, irrespective of the actual cost of the service

- List the reasons for the increasing health care costs.
- Describe how the increasing cost of health care changed the way health care is financed.
- Distinguish between the purchaser and the consumer of health care.

4.2 Flow of Funds through the System

Paying for health care involves private citizens, employers, charitable organizations, and county, state, and federal government. The following lists arranged these contributors from those who bear the greatest burden in paying for health care to those who bear the least:

▲ Private health insurance.
▲ Federal government.
▲ Individuals.
▲ State government.
▲ Other private sources.

Just as the preceding groups share the burden of the cost, the expenditures themselves are divided among private health care providers:

▲ Health care organizations, such as hospitals, nursing homes, home health agencies, and hospices.
▲ Health care professionals, such as physicians, dentists, chiropractors, podiatrists, and optometrists.
▲ Pharmaceuticals, supplies, and equipment.
▲ Nontraditional or alternative health services and products.

Sections 4.2.1 and 4.2.2 explain in more detail how the burden of health care cost is shared and the distributions of the money among the various health care services. As you read this information, however, keep in mind the difference between private health care services (involving the health and well-being of the individual) and public health care services (involving the health and well-being of populations). The following sections relate solely to private health care expenditures.

4.2.1 Where the Money Comes From

As stated in Section 4.2, money for health care expenditures comes from both the private sector and the public sector. To more fully understand exactly who bears the burden of health care costs, however, one needs to keep in mind who comprises these sectors. The private sector includes households *and* businesses, and the public sector includes federal, state, and local governments.

Individuals and employers typically pay for health insurance coverage. The insurance provider then makes payments through a variety of mechanisms (described

Table 4-2: Estimates of Purchaser Contributions for Health Care

Category	Amount (in Billions)	Percentage of Category
Household, via	$323	37
Individual out-of-pocket payments for the direct purchase of services		
Purchase of individual health insurance policies (primary and supplemental)		
Employee premiums for employment-based health insurance		
Deductible and coinsurance payments		
Balance billings		
Premiums paid for Medicare Part B coverage		
Employers, via	$250	29
Contributions to health insurance premiums		
Contributions to Medicare		
Workers' compensation payments		
Government, via	$203	23
Contributions to private health insurance premiums		
Medicaid		
Other	$90	11
Total expenditures for personal health care	**$866**	**100**
Direct provision of services by state, local, and federal government, via	$158	100
Department of Veterans Affairs		
U.S. military		
Indian Health Service		
State and local public hospitals		
Etc.		

in Section 4.2.3) to health care professionals and organizations, in addition to paying for drugs, medical supplies, equipment, and alternative medical treatments. The government, on the other hand, finances health care through government programs or by providing services directly (through public organizational providers). Table 4-2 outlines approximately how much each contributor—individuals, employers, and government—makes to the total cost for personal health care services.

4.2.2 Where the Money Goes

The $1.6 trillion that individuals, businesses, and government spend on health care services and supplies in 2003 is distributed in the following way (Figure 4-4 illustrates this distribution graphically):

▲ Hospital care: 33 percent.
▲ Professional services (such as physicians, dentists, podiatrists, and optometrists): 34 percent.
▲ Nursing home and home health care: 10 percent.
▲ Retails sales of medical products (primarily pharmaceuticals): 13 percent.
▲ Government public health activities: 4 percent.
▲ Other: 6 percent.

As you can see in Figure 4-4, 90 percent of health care expenditures goes to hospitals, professional services, and retail health products.

4.2.3 How It Gets There

Households, employers, and federal, state, and local governments share the burden of paying for private health care. The following list outlines the way in which

Figure 4-4

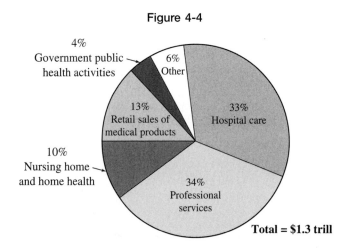

Distribution of expenditures for health care services and supplies.

FOR EXAMPLE

Shifting Costs to Employees

Employers, struggling under the burden of double-digit increases in health care costs, have managed to slow the increases significantly by shifting the cost of health care to their employees. According to a 2003 survey conducted by Mercer Human Resource Consulting, businesses are managing this cost savings by reducing the number of health plans offered to their employees and by requiring higher employee contributions, higher copayments, and higher deductibles.

---

these groups contribute funding (this flow of expenditures is graphically represented in Figure 4-5):

▲ **Households:** Individuals and families pay for health care by:
  • Purchasing health insurance.
  • Paying portions of premiums to supplement contributions that their employers and government make.
  • Making coinsurance and deductible payments.
  • Purchasing health care services directly.
▲ **Employers:** Employers purchase health insurance coverage for their employees.

Figure 4-5

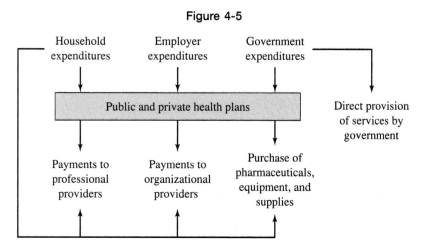

The flow of funds through the health care system.

▲ **Federal, state, and local governments:** These agencies finance health care through the following:

- Paying all or a portion of coverage for certain designated populations (for instance, older and poor people).
- Providing services directly; for example, through public, Veterans Administration, and military hospitals and clinics.

SELF-CHECK

- Identify how much money each of the following sectors contributes to the total amount spent on health care: (a) individuals, (b) government, and (c) private businesses.
- List the ways in which each of the following contribute to health care financing: (a) individuals, (b) government, and (c) private businesses.

4.3 Examining Who Has Health Insurance

Approximately 84 percent of the population is covered by some form of health insurance, although benefits vary widely. Table 4-3 shows the number of enrollees and what type of insurance they have.

As the data in Table 4-3 suggest, quite a sizeable number of people have no health insurance. Between 1985 and 2000, the number of uninsured people below age 65 increased by more than one-third, from approximately 14.5 percent (32 million people) in 1987 to 17 percent (41 million people) in 2000 (see Figure 4-6). In 2004, the number of uninsured increased again. The Census Bureau estimates that those without health insurance will grow to 53 to 60 million by 2007, representing 21 to 25 percent of the nonelderly population.

Table 4-3: Health Insurance Coverage

Type of Insurance	Number of Enrollees (in Millions)	Percentage of Population Covered
Voluntary health insurance (nonprofit and commercial plans)	174	59.8
Social insurance (Medicare)	41	14.3
Welfare insurance (Medicaid)	38	12.9

Table 4-3: Health Insurance Coverage (Continued)

Percentage of Population That Has Coverage Through:

Private health insurance (those under age 65)	72
Private health insurance provided by employer	59.8 (those under age 65)
Enrollment in a health maintenance organization	34 (those under age 65)
Medicare	14.3
Medicaid	12.9

The growth in the number of uninsured Americans over the past decade is due to these economic circumstances:

▲ **Rising health care costs:** An increase in health care costs relative to average family income, thus making insurance less affordable.

▲ **More families at or below the poverty level:** An increase in the absolute number of families living at or below the federally specified poverty level (the poverty level is established by the federal government on the basis of a number of factors: family size, annual income, and so on). These individuals account for 30 percent of the uninsured, and Medicaid covers only about 50 percent of them.

▲ **Fewer employers providing insurance plans to employees:** A decrease in the number of firms that provide health insurance for their employees. Fully 65 percent of uninsured people live in families headed by a full-time, full-year worker. The percentage of the nonelderly population with

Figure 4-6

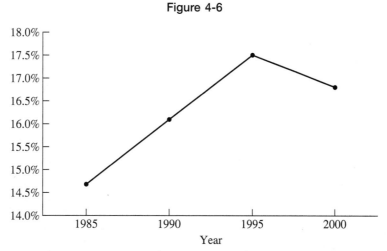

The percentage of people younger than 65 with no health insurance.

employment-linked health insurance decreased from 69 percent in 1987 to 64 percent in 1997.

Several factors—age, race, income, and so on—affect the rate of the uninsured, as shown in Table 4-4.

Table 4-4: Description of the Uninsured, by Category

Attributes	Percentage of Population (Less than Age 65) Uninsured
Age	
Under 18	12
18–24	29.6
25–34	24.9
35–44	17.7
45–64	13
Gender	
Male	16.7
Female	13.9
Race and Ethnicity	
White	10.7
Black	20.2
Hispanic	32.4
Asian	18.4
Poverty Level*	
Below 100%[†]	34
100–149%	37
150–199%	27
200% and above	9
Residence	
In urban areas	16
Outside urban areas	19

*Determined by U.S. Census Bureau criteria, including family income; family size; number of children in the family; and, for families with two or fewer adults, their age.

[†]The poverty level is set at 100%; thus, for example, 200% is an income of twice the poverty level.

FOR EXAMPLE

Insurance Coverage in the West

According to a report released in 2005 by the U.S. Bureau of Labor Statistics, employees in Alaska, Hawaii, California, Oregon, and Washington are more likely to be offered a health insurance plan through their employers than their peers in other regions of the United States. Seventy-three percent of employers in these states offer health plans, compared with 70 percent of the country as a whole. They are the least likely to extend these benefits to their retirees, however.

SELF-CHECK

- Indicate what percentage of the population has each type of insurance: (a) voluntary health insurance, (b) Medicare, and (c) Medicaid.
- How many people in the United States are uninsured?
- Of age, race/ethnicity, or income, which is the biggest predictor of who does and doesn't have health insurance?

4.4 Categorizing Health Insurance Plans

Strictly speaking, **insurance** is protection against the risk of financial loss associated with an event among members of a group and is provided (underwritten) only when the potential loss is large (catastrophic) and beyond the ability of a group member to pay in the short run. "Health insurance" is an umbrella term used to describe a variety of methods for paying for health care services.

Although some health insurance policies fit this description, most of today's plans don't. The reason is that today, health insurance isn't merely used a protection against catastrophic illness, but as the payment method for general health care as well. In the past, insurance was used to cover the cost of catastrophic illnesses or accidents, but for all other health care costs the individual paid. Today, insurance covers routine health care expenditures—which are small, discretionary, and often predictable—for an individual or family. As such, health insurance is not pure insurance, but rather a form of prepayment: Small periodic outlays are made on the basis of the likelihood of expenditures by members of a group.

To help make sense of the types of insurance available, health insurance is categorized by who provides the insurance and by what the contractual agreement is between the various parties.

All insurance plans, regardless of the contractual agreement of the plan itself, fall into one of three categories:

▲ **Voluntary health insurance:** This type of insurance is provided by non-profit and commercial (for profit) health plans, such as BlueCross BlueShield, Aetna, Cigna, and others. Individuals buy these plans for themselves, and employers purchase them for their employees or retirees.

▲ **Social insurance:** The government provides social insurance (for example, Medicare) as a benefit that is earned. In other words, workers pay into the Medicare fund and then are entitled to Medicare benefits when they meet certain criteria (age, for example).

▲ **Public welfare insurance:** The government provides public welfare insurance (namely, Medicaid) on the basis of need.

Each of these types of plans can, in turn, include any of the contractual agreements outlined in Section 4.4.1.

Once it is understood whether the insurance plan is a voluntary plan, a social insurance plan, or a public welfare plan, one can look at the contractual agreement outlined in the plan. This agreement determines which of the following categories the plan falls into:

▲ Indemnity plan.
▲ Service benefit.
▲ Managed care.

All insurance plans (whether social, voluntary, or welfare) define a contractual relationship among four parties:

▲ **Purchasers:** The primary payers (typically employers and federal, state, and local governments).

▲ **Beneficiaries:** The users of health care services.

▲ **Health plans:** The organizations that collect premiums, reimburse providers, and perform other administrative functions.

▲ **Providers:** The health care organizations and individual professionals who deliver health care services.

There are general characteristics that describe these indemnity, service benefit, and managed care plans. Keep in mind, however, that numerous variations exist.

4.4.1 Indemnity Plan

Indemnity plan is a contract between a beneficiary and a health plan in which the beneficiary pays a premium to the health plan (sometimes in addition to a

Figure 4-7

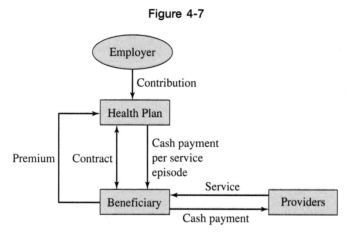

The indemnity plan structure.

contribution made by that person's employer). When the individual uses covered service, the health plan reimburses the beneficiary, who then pays the provider.

Following are the key features of this type of plan (shown in Figure 4-7):

▲ There is no contractual relationship between the health plan and providers.
▲ The payment by a health plan to the beneficiary is a set dollar amount for a specific service (for example, $400 for each day of hospital stay, or $40 per physician office visit) regardless of what the provider actually charges.
▲ The beneficiary pays the provider directly.

4.4.2 Service Benefit Plan

The most common arrangement is the service benefit plan (see Figure 4-8). In a **service benefit plan**, the purchaser (employer) contracts with a health plan and pays it a premium for each beneficiary (employee and family members); beneficiaries, in turn, usually make contributions that cover a portion of the premium.

The health plan contracts with provider hospitals or professionals to offer a specific array of services to beneficiaries for a negotiated payment (cost, charges, discounted charges, or set rate). Beneficiaries usually make deductible and coinsurance payments to providers when they receive service, but they are not liable for any other charges associated with covered benefits.

The key features of this type of plan are that

▲ Payments are made to providers by the health plan on behalf of beneficiaries for covered services.
▲ Beneficiaries receive services rather than cash payments (as in an indemnity plan).

Figure 4-8

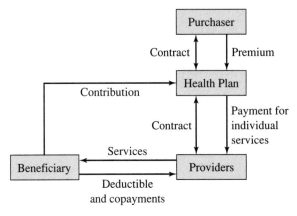

The structure of a service benefit plan.

Examples of service benefit plans include health maintenance organizations (HMOs), federal employee plans, and some BlueCross BlueShield plans.

4.4.3 Managed Care Plan

Managed care is a special type of service benefit plan that combines health insurance and provider functions (see Figure 4-9). The purchaser contracts with a health plan for a package of services on behalf of a beneficiary group for which it pays a set amount per enrollee per month.

The health plan has a contractual (and occasionally, ownership) relationship with a network of providers to whom it pays a fixed rate per member per month to provide covered services. Beneficiaries are often responsible for a copayment at the

Figure 4-9

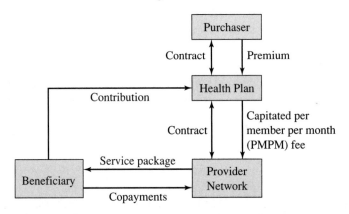

The structure of a managed care plan.

FOR EXAMPLE

Managing Managed Care

In order to hold down costs, managed care plans try to control both access to health care (requiring members to use in-care providers, for example) and cost of the care itself (by paying negotiating rates rather than actual costs). As physicians and patients begin to chafe under these conditions, arguing that health care decisions are no longer being made by health care professionals but by insurance companies, managed care reform has become a hot topic. At issue is how to best regulate health plans and at the same time ensure adequate protections for the consumers.

point of service, but not a deductible. Additionally, beneficiaries are subject to restrictions regarding choice of provider. Other than for the provision of emergency services, they must use providers within the health plan's network. When using out-of-network providers, they incur larger copayments or may have no coverage.

The distinctive features of a managed care plan are these:

▲ A comprehensive and integrated service package (rather than individual services) is provided to beneficiaries.

▲ The health plan's contract is with a network of organizations and professionals to provide all covered services for a fixed payment, regardless of whether participants use the service and irrespective of the actual costs of the service.

▲ As a consequence of the preceding arrangement, the health plan and/or provider network bears the financial risk associated with all covered care for a designated population over a period of time.

Examples of health delivery systems offering managed care plans are health maintenance organizations (HMOs) (see Section 4.7)

SELF-CHECK

• Describe the differences among voluntary, social, and public welfare insurance plans.
• Contrast an indemnity plan with a service benefit plan.
• Describe how managed care plans shift financial risk to the providers.

4.5 Private Insurance Coverage: Voluntary Health Insurance (VHI)

With voluntary health insurance (VHI), private (nonprofit and commercial) sources finance health care services. Businesses can offer this type of insurance as an employee benefit, or individuals can purchase it directly. It can serve as the sole source of coverage, or it can supplement benefits provided by social health insurance, such as Medicare (discussed in Section 4.6). Some of the largest and most well-known VHI plans are BlueCross BlueShield, Aetna, and Cigna, but there are many others.

Today, 72 percent of the population has some form of VHI. One can see in Figure 4-10 this percentage peaked at a little more than 80 percent in 1980 and then dropped by 1990 and has remained fairly stable since then.

VHI coverage is generally dependent upon, and linked to, employment. Of all the people who have this type of insurance plan, 88 percent receive their coverage through their place of employment. In fact, approximately 50 percent of private employers offer VHI to their employees.

4.5.1 Types of VHI plans

Several types of VHI plans exist, and, in general, they fall into the following categories:

▲ **Commercial:** These plans can be either nonprofit or for-profit; some are mutuals (that is, they're owned by their policy holders), others are stock corporations (owned and operated for the benefit of stockholders).

▲ **BlueCross BlueShield:** Commonly called simply *Blues,* these plans are closely tied to the hospital industry and medical profession. Blues were

Figure 4-10

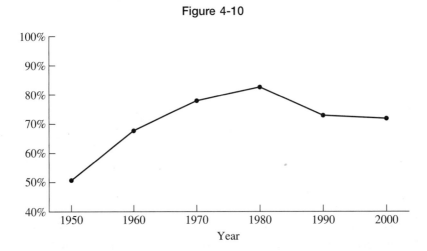

The percentage of people with voluntary health insurance.

> **FOR EXAMPLE**
>
> **Creating BlueCross BlueShield**
>
> Contemporary VHI plans date back to 1929, when Baylor Hospital in Dallas insured a group of public school teachers for inpatient hospital expenses; this was the first BlueCross plan. In 1939, the California Medical Society offered a VHI plan to cover in-hospital physician services; this was the first BlueShield plan. During the 1940s and 1950s, many of these plans merged their operations (typically in individual states) and were represented, at the national level, by the BlueCross BlueShield Association.

the first to offer service rather than indemnity benefits on the basis of communitywide ratings (which charge everyone the same premium regardless of their characteristics). Historically, they have been nonprofit entities; however, in recent years some have converted to for-profit status and many have commercial subsidiaries.

▲ **Health maintenance organizations (HMOs):** Part of the managed care movement (refer to Section 4.4), these plans combine the insurance function (underwriting) with delivery of health services through an owned or contracted network of providers. In its simplest form, an HMO links together (through contracts or ownership) into one entity a health plan, hospitals, and physicians. To find out about managed care and HMOs (as well as other managed care health systems) go to Chapter 11, which is entirely devoted to this topic.

▲ **Self-funded:** Self-funded plans are typically sponsored by employers, who bear the full financial risk of providing health care benefits to employees, dependents, and retirees. Employers with self-funded plans don't purchase insurance from, or pay premiums to, a health plan, although they may contract with an insurance company (commercial, Blue, or other entity) to provide administrative services.

Enrollment in VHI plans is split roughly in thirds among commercial, Blue, and HMO plans.

4.5.2 Coverage Variations in VHI Plans

The nature of VHI coverage varies by the following factors:

▲ **Benefit type:** Whether the benefits are either indemnity or service.
▲ **Contribution:** What proportion of the total premium is paid by beneficiaries (versus that contributed by others, such as an employer).

▲ **Coverage:** The type of benefits provided (hospital care, physician services, drugs, vision care, and so on) and how comprehensive or inclusive these benefits are (for example, number of routine physician office visits per year).

▲ **Deductible:** How much the beneficiary has to pay for health care service before plan payments "kick in."

▲ **Coinsurance rates:** The proportion of fees that are paid by beneficiaries for each service.

▲ **Exclusions and limitations:** The rules regarding when (and whether) coverage goes into effect; for example, waiting periods (having to wait a certain number of months of employment before the plan becomes active) and coverage of preexisting conditions.

SELF-CHECK

- List three characteristics of voluntary health insurance.
- Describe the four types of VHI plans: (a) commercial, (b) Blues, (c) HMOs, and (d) self-funded.

4.6 Government Insurance Programs: Medicare and Medicaid

People often confuse Medicare and Medicaid (another government program), but these two programs are very different in which populations they serve, how they are funded, and how they are administered. Table 4-5 outlines these differences.

4.6.1 Social Health Insurance: Medicare

Medicare is a federally sponsored program that provides health insurance to eligible Americans. Medicare was enacted in 1965 as an amendment (Title 18) to the Social Security Act.

Following are important facts about Medicare:

▲ Medicare is available to all Americans who meet the following criteria:
  - Those who are 65 or older.
  - Those who are disabled and receiving Social Security benefits.
  - Those with end-stage renal (kidney) disease.

▲ Individuals make contributions to the program through payroll deductions and are entitled to receive benefits. In this way, Medicare is not a welfare program.

Table 4-5: Comparing Medicare and Medicaid

Attribute	Medicare	Medicaid
Population served	People who are 65 or over, disabled and receiving Social Security benefits, or suffering from end-stage kidney failure	Those in need, as determined by individual states
Funding comes from	Federal government through contributions made via employee payroll deductions	57 percent from the federal government; the rest from state governments
How program is administered	Managed by the federal government	Sponsored by the federal government, but administered by state governments

▲ The program is managed by the Centers for Medicare and Medicaid Services (CMS).

Medicare is the health care industry's largest payer. In 2000, it covered 40 million people (14 percent of the population) and expended $227 billion (about $5500 per enrollee); $88 billion in Medicare funding went to hospitals, making up about 30 percent of their total patient revenues; and $37 billion went to physicians, accounting for about 20 percent of their total revenues.

Medicare is actually two separate, although coordinated, programs—Part A and Part B. **Medicare Part A** is a compulsory health plan that covers hospital-based services. Following are important facts to know about **Part A:**

▲ **Financing:** Part A hospital insurance is funded by a payroll tax paid into the Social Security (Medicare) Trust Fund. Employees contribute 1.45 percent of wages, matched equally by employers; self-employed individuals pay 2.9 percent of earnings.

▲ **Benefits:** The program provides 90 days of inpatient hospital care per episode of illness, a lifetime reserve of 60 days of inpatient hospital care that can be drawn upon when the maximum for an episode of illness is exceeded, skilled nursing facility care, home health visits following an inpatient admission, and hospice care.

▲ **Payments:** For each episode of illness, beneficiaries pay a deductible equal to the charge for one day of hospital care. They then make a copayment for each of the 65th through 90th days of inpatient hospital care equal to 25 percent of the deductible.

▲ **Provider reimbursement:** From the inception of the program until 1983, hospitals were reimbursed for their costs of providing care as defined by a complex set of regulations and formulas. Hospitals received estimated monthly payments, which were adjusted at year end on the basis of a cost report submitted to the Health Care Financing Administration (now the CMS).

Beginning in 1983, Medicare switched to a prospective payment system, in which a payment rate is assigned to 500 diagnosis-related groups (DRGs), on the basis of the patient's age, sex, principal and secondary diagnosis, procedure performed (if any), and discharge status. Certain costs, such as medical education and depreciation, are excluded from the DRG rate and reimbursed separately. Additionally, some hospitals (such as psychiatric, children's, rehabilitation, and long-term care) are excluded from the prospective payment system and reimbursed under different arrangements.

Medicare Part B is a voluntary, supplemental health plan that covers professional (primarily physician) services. Following are important points to know about Part B.

▲ **Financing:** Part B is financed 24 percent from premiums paid by enrollees and 76 percent from federal treasury funds. The monthly premium in 2002 was $54 per month, deducted directly from an enrollee's Social Security check. The monthly premium in 2006 is $88.50.[5]

▲ **Benefits:** Part B coverage includes physician care; physician-ordered supplies, durable medical equipment, and services provided by some other categories of health professionals; and outpatient hospital care, ambulatory surgical services, laboratory services, outpatient mental health services, and some preventative services.

▲ **Provider reimbursement:** Prior to 1992 physicians were paid fee-for-service on the basis of their "reasonable and customary" charges. In 1992, Medicare began making payments according to a resource-based relative value scale. Using this system, an index number is assigned to every physician encounter or procedure according to the amount of work required to perform it, in addition to practice expenses and malpractice insurance costs. To determine payment, the index number is multiplied by a standard conversion factor (or "going rate"), which is established each year. As an illustration, for a particular surgical procedure the index number is 15, the conversion factor is $40, and the fee is 15 times $40, or $600.

4.6.2 Welfare Insurance: Medicaid

Medicaid finances the provision of health care services to economically disadvantaged people. In a strict sense, Medicaid isn't health insurance; it's a welfare subsidy. Benefits aren't earned but provided to people in need. Medicaid was enacted in 1965 as Title 19 of the Social Security Act.

FOR EXAMPLE

Heading into the Red

Medicare is quickly going broke. By 2019, Medicare is projected to exhaust its hospital-care trust fund.[6] The situation is dire because Medicare, as a Social Security program, is affected by all the problems affecting Social Security, in addition to being affected by the rising costs of health care. Exacerbating Medicare's financial woes is the prescription drug provision included in the Medicare Modernization Act. In the past, Congress has addressed funding problems with Medicare by reducing payments to providers, increasing the wage base that's taxed to fund the program, and increasing the premiums that beneficiaries pay. Although currently no such measures on are the table, Medicare recipients are already seeing the effect of rising health care costs and tighter budgets: In 2005 they pay 17 percent more in monthly premiums for Part B coverage, and according to economists, these folks can expect double-digit premium increases for years to come.

In 2000, Medicaid covered 41 million individuals. Table 4-6 shows the scope of Medicaid coverage.

Funding for Medicaid comes from both state and federal coffers. Fifty-seven percent of its funding is federal, and the remainder comes from the states. Following are important facts to know about Medicaid:

▲ **Medicaid is not a federally mandated program:** States can choose whether to have the program. All states but Arizona have decided to do so.

▲ **States that choose to have a Medicaid program must offer certain minimum benefits (mandated by federal law):** Such benefits include physician services, nonpreventive dental services, hospital inpatient care, hospital outpatient care, nursing home care, home health visits, and laboratory and X-ray services.

▲ **Medicaid is federally sponsored and supported (overseen by the CMS) but state administered:** What this means is that the state can determine the following:

   • The financial, need-based criteria that individuals must meet to be enrolled in their state's Medicaid program.

   • Whether to offer optional benefits in addition to those mandated by the federal government (explained in the preceding bullet), such as inpatient psychiatric care, optometrist care and eyeglasses, routine dental care, and prescription drugs.

   • Utilization limits for both mandated and optional benefits (if offered).

   • The methods and rates for paying providers.

Table 4-6: Percentage of People Who Receive Medicaid

Attribute	Percentage
Total covered under the age of 65	9
Age	
Under 6	24
6–17	17
18–44	6
45–64	5
Gender	
Male	8
Female	11
Race	
White	7
Black	19
Hispanic	14
Poverty Level*	
Below 100%†	37
100–149%	20
150–199%	11
200% or greater	2

*Determined by U.S. Census Bureau criteria, including family income; family size; number of children in the family; and, for families with two or fewer adults, their age.

†The poverty level is set at 100%; thus, for example, 200% is an income of twice the poverty level.

SELF-CHECK

- Describe who qualifies for (a) Medicare benefits and (b) Medicaid.
- Define the purpose of the two Medicare programs, Part A and Part B.
- List three substantive points of difference between Medicare and Medicaid.

FOR EXAMPLE

Educating People about HMOs

HMOs, because of their differences from traditional health care plans, are often confusing to consumers. On the face of it, they look.—and work— like traditional service benefit plans, but there are important differences. In response to consumer confusion and HMO horror news stories, the California's Office of the Patient Advocate published a 67-page booklet, *California's HMO Guide*, which educates Californians about HMOs and outline their rights and responsibilities as patients and consumers.

4.7 Health Maintenance Organizations (HMOs)

A health maintenance organization, or HMO, is a hybrid health care insurance and provider mechanism that offers a type of managed care plan (refer to Section 4.4.3). In its simplest form, as defined earlier, an HMO links together (through contracts or ownership) into one entity a health plan, hospitals, and physicians.

Chapter 11 is devoted to the topic of managed care. For complete information on these types of health plans, go there.

4.7.1 HMO Growth

In 2000, approximately 80 million Americans, or 30 percent of the population, received their health care through an HMO. Growth in the number of HMO enrollees and percentage of the population covered by them are shown in Figures 4-11 and 4-12, respectively.

Obviously, the dramatic increase in the number of people enrolled in HMO plans indicates that the number of HMO plans also increased. In 1976, there were 174 HMOs. By 2000, there were 568, a 226 percent increase over the period.

4.7.2 HMO Models

There are five standard HMO models, preferred provider organizations (PPOs), and point-of-service (POS) plans (see more on managed care in Chapter 11).

Based on Rossiter, the five standard models of HMOs are:[7]

1. **Independent practice/physician association (IPA) HMO model:** Contracts with physicians in solo practice, and/or with independent

Figure 4-11

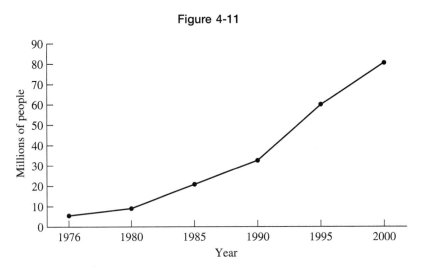

Number of Americans enrolled in HMOs.

practice/physician associations who, in turn, contract with their own member physicians. The majority of physicians in an IPA HMO model are in private practice and, in many cases, also have a significant number of patients who are not HMO members.

2. **Group HMO model:** Contracts with a single multispecialty medical group to provide care to HMO membership.
3. **Network HMO model:** Contracts with more than one medical group to provide services to its members.

Figure 4-12

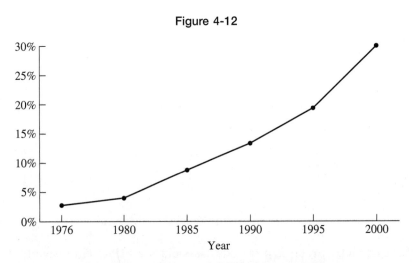

Percentage of the population enrolled in HMOs.

4. **Staff HMO model:** Employs physicians directly. Physicians are employees of the HMO and deal exclusively with HMO members.

5. **Mixed HMO model:** Is any combination of the model types described above.

PPOs are designed to supply services at a reasonable cost by providing enrollees incentives to use designated health care providers, while providing a lower level of coverage for services rendered by health care providers not part of the PPO network. Financial incentives for individuals to use preferred providers include lower copayments or coinsurance, and a maximum limit on out-of-pocket costs for in-network use. Unlike with HMOs, out-of-network usage is allowed by PPOs, though at a higher cost to the enrollee.[8]

POS plans are similar to PPOs in that they are characterized by a network of providers whose services are available to enrollees at a lower cost than the services of non-network providers. The difference is that whereas PPO enrollees are free to contact network specialists at their discretion, a POS participant must first receive authorization from a primary care physician (PCP) to receive full benefits. Also, the out-of-network benefits of a POS plan are typically less than those of a PPO.[9]

SELF-CHECK

- Define **health maintenance organization**, or **HMO**.
- List and describe the HMO models.

SUMMARY

In the United States much of the cost of private care—health care for individuals—is financed through either private insurance or public programs. As the health care system evolves and the expenses increase, the burden for these expenditures is shifting from the private sector (which before had been the primary source of health care funding) to the public sector. A variety of insurance options are available in the United States: Voluntary health insurance (purchased by individuals and employers) is the biggest category, funding the majority of private health care costs. A close second are the government programs, Medicare and Medicaid, which provide insurance to poor and elderly people, respectively. The third category, health maintenance organizations (HMOs), seek to manage costs by controlling access to care and are having a profound impact on the other two.

KEY TERMS

Beneficiaries	Individuals receiving health care services.
BlueCross BlueShield	Commonly called *Blues,* health insurance plans that are closely tied to the hospital industry and medical profession.
Combined HMO model	HMO model that includes both independent physicians (the IPA model), as well as physicians or groups employed by the HMO or under exclusive contract to it (group model).
Commercial plan	Commercial health insurance plans can be either nonprofit or for-profit; some are owned by their policy holders; others are stock corporations.
Group HMO model	HMO model in which professional services are provided by physicians who are employed by the HMO and/or by groups that are under exclusive contract to the HMO.
Health maintenance organizations (HMOs)	Managed care plans that combine the insurance function (underwriting) with delivery of health services through an owned or contracted network of providers.
Health plans	The organizations that collect premiums, reimburse providers, and perform other administrative functions.
Indemnity plan	An insurance plan in which the beneficiary pays a premium to the health plan, which in turn reimburses the beneficiary when the individual uses covered service. The beneficiary then pays the provider.
Insurance	Strictly speaking, protection against the risk of financial loss associated with an event among members of a group and is provided (underwritten) only when the potential loss is large (catastrophic) and beyond the ability of a group member to pay in the short run. In reality, health insurance plans in the United States are more akin to prepayment plans.
Independent practice association HMO (IPA HMO) model	HMO model in which services are provided by medical groups and physicians who are contract independent

Managed care	A special type of service benefit plan that combines health insurance and provider functions.
Medicaid	A federal/state program that provides health care services to poor people. Although federally sponsored, Medicare is administered by the state.
Medicare	A federally sponsored program that provides health insurance to eligible Americans who are elderly or disabled.
Medicare Part A	A compulsory health plan that covers hospital-based services.
Medicare Part B	A voluntary, supplemental health plan that covers professional (primarily physician) services.
Providers	The health care organizations and individual professionals who deliver health care services.
Purchasers	The primary payers (typically employers and federal, state, and local governments).
Self-funded plans	Insurance plans in which employers provide health care benefits without purchasing insurance from or paying premiums to a health plan.
Service benefit plan	An insurance plan in which a purchaser (employer) contracts with a health plan and pays it a premium for each beneficiary (employee and family members); beneficiaries, in turn, usually make contributions that cover a portion of the premium.

ASSESS YOUR UNDERSTANDING

Go to www.wiley.com/college/pointer to evaluate your knowledge of the basics of financing the U.S. health care system.

Measure your learning by comparing pre-test and post-test results.

Summary Questions

1. Health care is the largest industry in the United States, accounting for more than 15 percent of the gross domestic product. True or False?
2. The primary purchasers of health care today are
   (a) patients
   (b) insurance companies
   (c) government agencies and private employers
   (d) b and c
3. From 1960 to 2003, health care expenditures
   (a) stayed roughly the same
   (b) rose slightly
   (c) rose drastically
   (d) fell
4. Which of the following is *not* a cause of the increases in health care expenditures?
   (a) inflation
   (b) population growth
   (c) changes in health services
   (d) changes in the tax base
5. Arrange the following in order from those who bear the greatest burden for total health care expenditures to those who pay the least.
   (a) private insurance, federal government, state government, individuals
   (b) federal government, state government, individuals, private insurance
   (c) federal government, state government, private insurance, individuals
   (d) private insurance, federal government, individuals, state government
6. Arrange the following in order from those who receive the greatest portion of health care expenditures to those who receive the smallest.
   (a) physicians and other health professionals, nursing homes, hospitals
   (b) physicians and other health professionals, hospitals, nursing homes
   (c) nursing homes, physicians and other health professionals, hospitals
   (d) hospitals, nursing homes, physicians and other health professionals

7. Today, roughly 83 percent of the U.S. population has health insurance. According to the U.S. Census Bureau, how many people will have insurance by 2007?

   (a) 90–95 percent, given trends showing the cost savings of managed care programs

   (b) 75–79 percent, given trends showing that the uninsured rates continue to rise

   (c) 80–85 percent, given the tendency for the market to balance out and offset large increases or decreases

   (d) 87–90 percent, given projected increases in the number of government insurance programs

8. What economic circumstances have resulted in the increasing numbers of uninsured?

   (a) more families at or below the poverty level

   (b) fewer employers offering health insurance

   (c) higher out-of-pocket expenses

   (d) a and b

   (e) all of the above

9. Health insurance differs from other types of insurance (such as homeowner's insurance or auto insurance) in that it is essentially a payment plan for general health care rather than protection against catastrophic illness or injury. True or false?

10. Identify which type of insurance—voluntary, social, or welfare—each of the following is:

    (a) Aetna Health

    (b) Medicare

    (c) Medicaid

11. Insurance contracts involve four parties. Define each party.

    (a) beneficiary

    (b) purchaser

    (c) health plan

    (d) provider

12. Which of the following best characterizes voluntary health insurance plans?

    (a) VHI plans are typically offered as an employee benefit or purchased directly by individuals, and they can serve as a person's sole coverage or they can supplement other types of insurance coverage

    (b) VHI plans are offered by private businesses; as such they are solely for profit, rather than nonprofit

    (c) most people with VHI receive this coverage through their employers

      (d) a and c

      (e) all of the above

13. A type of voluntary health insurance plan, Blues

      (a) were the first service benefits plans offered in the United States.

      (b) were the first to base premiums on community ratings rather than individual characteristics.

      (c) are linked to the medical industry and are therefore nonprofit entities.

      (d) a and b.

      (e) all of the above.

14. Medicaid is

      (a) a federal health insurance program.

      (b) managed by state governments.

      (c) funded by employee contributions.

      (d) a and c.

      (e) all of the above.

15. Medicare is

      (a) funded through federal and state monies.

      (b) managed by the federal government.

      (c) available in all states.

      (d) a federal welfare program.

16. Medicare Parts A and B each provide funding for specific services. Identify these services.

      (a) Part A: Hospital care and physician services; Part B: Prescription drugs

      (b) Part A: Prescription drugs; Part B: Hospital care and physician services

      (c) Part A: Physician services; Part B: Hospital care

      (d) Part A: Hospital care; Part B: Physician services

17. A key characteristic of a health maintenance organization is

      (a) its growing popularity among health care providers.

      (b) its combining health plans and service providers into one entity.

      (c) its growing popularity among patients.

      (d) all of the above.

18. Of the different types of HMOs, which is the most popular?

      (a) IPA

      (b) group

      (c) combined

      (d) none of the above

Review Questions

1. Describe how health care in the middle of the twentieth century differs from health care today?

2. Until recent changes in health care financing, those who paid for health care bore the burden of financial risk. In what way have purchasers tried to shift risk to health providers?

3. Indicate which type of insurance (service benefit plan, indemnity plan, or managed care plan) you would want as each of the following. Explain your answers.
   (a) an individual patient
   (b) a health care provider
   (c) a purchaser

4. What is the difference between how private and public sectors finance health care?

5. Federal and state governments finance personal health care both directly and indirectly. Indicate for each of the following which represents direct financing and which represents indirect financing.
   (a) Medicaid
   (b) veterans' hospitals
   (c) state mental hospitals
   (d) subsidies for health insurance premiums

6. Identify why low income is the biggest predictor of who does and doesn't have insurance.

7. Sixty-five percent of uninsured people live in families headed by a full-time, full-year worker. Given what you know about the financing of health care, how is it possible that a fully employed person doesn't have health insurance?

8. Identify an important difference between an indemnity plan and a service benefit plan.

9. Define *managed care plan*.

10. What is a significant difference between HMOs and other voluntary insurance plans?

11. Given what you know about the characteristics of the different VHI plans, what type of plan offers employers the *least* amount of protection from financial risk?

12. To be eligible for Medicaid, what guidelines must a person fulfill?

13. Although Medicaid is a state program, what role does the federal government play?

14. What advantage do HMOs seek in combining health plans, hospitals, and physicians into one entity?

15. Why would a health care provider prefer to belong to an IPA rather than a group HMO?

Applying This Chapter

1. Identify the goals or aims of each of the following and explain how they create tension in the delivery of health care:
   (a) insurer
   (b) purchaser
   (c) provider

2. Using Table 4-2, indicate which of the following—self-purchased insurance, employer-supplied insurance, Medicare, Medicaid, or direct government programs—would likely finance health care for the following people.
   (a) a retired public school teacher
   (b) a private on active duty in the military
   (c) a low-income single parent
   (d) an employee on disability leave for a work accident

3. At work, your employer offers two insurance plans. A married coworker with two children asks your advice about which plan she should choose. She reveals that her daughter is autistic and requires special medication and counseling. Although you can't tell her which plan to choose, what advice will you give her about choosing?

4. Explain how economics impacts the number of people who lack health insurance in the United States.

5. Evaluate the various health care plans (indemnity, service benefit, and managed care) in terms of how well their structures enable them to control health care costs.

6. Evaluate the impact of the following events or circumstances on health care costs:
   (a) advances and discoveries in medical technology and research
   (b) aging U.S. population
   (c) general inflation

7. In each of the following situations, indicate how health care would be paid for (refer to Figure 4-6):
   (a) you're an individual paying out-of-pocket for care
   (b) your employer provides an insurance plan for which you pay a premium (to be part of the plan) and copayments (when you utilize health care services covered by the plan)
   (c) you're a veteran being treated at a VA hospital

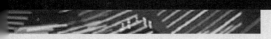

Changing Economic Dynamics

In 1960, 75 percent of total expenditures came from private sources and 25 percent came from government; by 2003, 55.2 percent came from private funds and 44.8 percent from the federal government. Explain this shift in burden from private to public health care funding.

Flow of Funds through the System

Explain how increasing poverty levels and rising health care costs impact the number of people who have insurance. Using Table 4-4, identify which groups are least likely to have health insurance.

Examining Who Has Health Insurance

Explain why income level is the most significant predictor of an individual's insurance status.

Categorizing Health Insurance Plans

Today, many Americans rely on employer-financed health insurance. Evaluate whether this system is sustainable in the future without any major changes in the way health care is financed.

Private Insurance Coverage: Voluntary Health Insurance (VHI)

Extrapolate why, of the VHI plans, the self-funded option is the least common of the employer-sponsored health plans.

Government Insurance Programs: Medicare and Medicaid

Using what you know about the purpose and function of Medicare and Medicaid, predict the impact that rising health care costs will have on the future of these programs.

Health Maintenance Organizations (HMOs)

Using what you know about the cost of health care and the purpose of managed care organizations, give a reason for why the group model is the least popular.

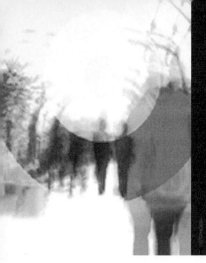

5

THE HEALTH CARE WORKFORCE
Doctors, Nurses, and Other Professionals

Starting Point

Go to www.wiley.com/college/pointer to assess your knowledge of the health care workforce.
Determine where you need to concentrate your effort.

What You'll Learn in This Chapter

▲ The scope of the health care workforce
▲ The role of specialist and generalist physicians
▲ How physicians are trained and licensed
▲ The scope of responsibilities and training for the different nursing professions
▲ The role and training of dentists, pharmacists, chiropractors, podiatrists, and optometrists
▲ The training and responsibilities of physical therapists and physician assistants

After Studying This Chapter, You'll Be Able To

▲ Provide examples of the health care workforce job classifications
▲ Differentiate between generalist and specialist physicians
▲ Identify and differentiate between RNs, LPNs, and other nursing professionals
▲ Assemble a health care team, identifying the roles of each participant
▲ Select an appropriate provider based on health care need
▲ Explain the relationship between the various health care providers

Goals and Outcomes

▲ Master the terminology relating to the various health care fields and their training requirements
▲ Recommend the best medical professional for various health care issues
▲ Analyze the impact an abundance of specialists and a shortage of generalists has on the health care system
▲ Organize the various professionals hierarchically, based on their job functions and the independence with which they work
▲ Make staffing suggestions, based on health organization need and health provider area of expertise
▲ Theorize what future impact the generalist shortage may have on the role of registered nurses and other health care professionals

INTRODUCTION

People in all areas of the health care workforce are vital to the U.S. health care system. This workforce numbers millions of workers, and includes professional, administrative, and support staff. Physicians, because of their training and expertise, are the main providers of health care in the United States. Nurses, however, make up the largest segment of the health care workforce and are a vital component in the delivery of care. The workforce includes other health professionals, such as podiatrists, chiropractors, physician assistants, and others who diagnose ailments, provide treatment, and provide preventive care.

5.1 Sizing Up the Workforce

The health care industry is one of the nation's largest employers. Nearly twelve million people hold jobs in health care (91 percent in the private sector and 9 percent in government); this comprises a little over 8 percent of the civilian workforce. The number of people in the medical field has grown dramatically since 1920, when only 1.5 percent of the U.S. population held a job in a health-related field (see Figure 5-1).

The health care industry hasn't finished growing, however. Consider these projections:

▲ By 2010, employment in health service is expected to increase 25 percent, outpacing the economy, which is expected to grow 16 percent as a whole.

Figure 5-1

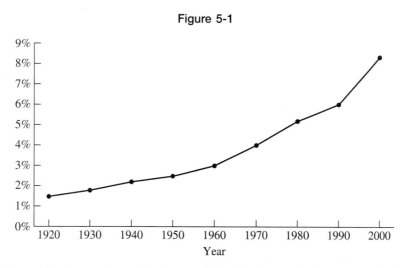

Employment in health care has increased significantly, particularly since 1960.

Table 5-1: Where the Health Care Workers Are

Type of Organization	Number of Employees	Percentage of Total Industry Employment
Hospitals	5,189,000	43
Nursing and personal care facilities	1,745,000	15
Physician offices and clinics	1,774,000	15
Dentist offices and clinics	668,000	6
Other	2,541,000	21

▲ Between 2000 and 2010, health care will account for 13 percent of all new jobs created.

▲ Nine of the top twenty occupations projected to be the economy's fastest growing over this period will be in health care.

To get an idea of how many people work in the health care industry and what their distribution is among the health care organizations, see Table 5-1.

The people who work in health care fall into three general categories, each of which has a particular role and is vital to the overall success of the health organization:

▲ **Professional and related occupations** (such as physicians, nurses, pharmacists, and other direct caregivers). The people in this group comprise 45 percent of the total health care workforce, and they're the providers who work directly with the patients. Table 5-2 shows the distribution of these professionals across the different fields.

The professionals in this category are responsible for performing critical and highly complex tasks; undergo a lengthy education process; master a large body of knowledge on which their practice is based; have a direct relationship with clients and serve as their agents; exercise a high level of autonomy and discretion regarding the nature of their practice and the context in which it occurs; control (with minimal outside influence) entry into, and preparation for, the profession; and are licensed or credentialed.

▲ **Service workers** (patient assistants, attendants, and aides; food preparation, maintenance, and housekeeping). These workers make up 30 percent of the workforce and offer support services to the health care providers and maintain the facilities in which the providers work.

Table 5-2: Distribution of Health Care Professionals

Professional	Number (Active)	Percentage of Total
Chiropractors	49,600	1
Dentists	168,000	4
Dietitians and nutritionists	97,000	3
Occupational therapists	55,000	1
Optometrists	29,500	0.7
Pharmacists	208,000	6
Physical therapists	144,000	4
Physicians	813,800	21
Podiatrists	11,000	0.3
Registered nurses	2,271,000	58
Speech therapists	97,000	3
Total	3,902,000	100

▲ **Administrative personnel** (including administrative support staff and managers): This group comprises approximately 25 percent of the health care workforce. These individuals are responsible for overseeing and managing the operation of the facility.

FOR EXAMPLE

Doctor Shortages in Rural America

Although health care is one of the largest industries in America with an overall surplus of physicians, rural America is facing a shortage. These shortages are bad for the residents of rural areas, as well as their health care providers. With few, if any, doctors and lacking adequately equipped medical facilities, rural residents find themselves waiting an inordinately long time for service, traveling long distances to obtain health care, or doing without. The physicians in these areas work longer hours, for less money, and in relative isolation than their urban counterparts. For many doctors, practicing in rural America is a money-losing proposition. Despite federal and local incentives designed to attract doctors to underserved areas, industry experts indicate that 1500 positions for doctors are currently vacant.

- Approximately how many people hold jobs in health care?
- What percentage of the health care workforce is employed in the private sector? Public sector?
- Describe the role for each of the following: (a) professional and related occupations, (b) service worker, and (c) administrative personnel.

5.2 Understanding the Role of the Physician

Most people are familiar with the job that physicians do: They diagnose and treat—through both medical and surgical means—illnesses and conditions that impair human functioning. They also supervise the interactions that their patients have with other health care professionals. What many people don't realize is that there are two types of physicians: allopathic and osteopathic.

Although their education and competencies are roughly equivalent, and both employ the full range of accepted diagnostic and treatment regimens (including prescribing drugs and doing surgery), there are some important differences:

▲ **Allopathic physicians,** or **Doctors of Medicine (MDs):** The medical designation that most people are familiar with, these doctors focus on treating disease—that is, any condition that impairs a person's functioning and well-being.

▲ **Osteopathic physicians,** or **Doctors of Osteopathy (DOs):** These doctors typically place greater emphasis on the neuromusculoskeletal system, preventive medicine, and holistic care; that is, they focus on the whole person rather than solely on the infirmity or condition that brought the patient to them in the first place. About 5 percent of active physicians are DOs.

The average physician works about 55 hours per week and has an annual net income (after expenses) of roughly $200,000.

5.2.1 Counting All Doctors

The number of physicians, whether allopathic or osteopathic, has increased significantly since 1950, when there were 135 practicing doctors for every 100,000 people. In 2000, that number was up to 258 per 100,000 (see Figure 5-2). Today, the United States has approximately 814,000 licensed physicians (only about 84 percent of whom currently practice medicine).

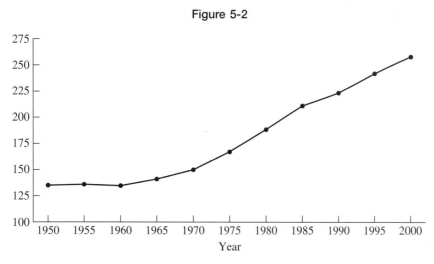

Figure 5-2

The increase in the number of physicians since 1950.

In addition, not all licensed physicians are active; and of those who are active, not all are personal care providers (that is, they work in some other capacity than patient care). Table 5-3 shows the status of doctors in the United States.

Table 5-3: Status of Physicians in the United States

Status	Number	Percentage of Total Physicians
Nonfederal	673,000	83
Involved in patient care	631,400	78
Office-based practice	490,400	60
Hospital-based practice	141,000	17·
Other professional activity	41,600	5
Federal	19,400	2
Involved in patient care	16,000	2
Other	3,400	0.4
Inactive	75,200	9
Not classified	45,100	6
Unknown	2,000	0.1
Total	813,800	100

Table 5-4: Distribution of Physician Specialists

Specialty	Percentage of Total Physicians
Anesthesiology	7
Dermatology	2
Emergency medicine	3
Family practice	14
Gastroenterology	3
Internal medicine	18
Neurology	2
Obstetrics and gynecology	7
Ophthalmology	3
Orthopedic surgery	3
Otolaryngology	2
Pathology	2
Pediatrics	9
Plastic surgery	1
Psychiatry	5
Pulmonology	1
Radiology	4
Surgery (general)	5
Urology	2
Other	7

5.2.2 Specialists

Approximately 95 percent of physicians are involved in some type of specialty practice, such as obstetrics and gynecology, neurology, internal medicine, and family practice. Table 5-4 shows the distribution across various specialties of doctors in office-based practices. (Note: The data in this table reflects physicians who don't work for the federal government.)

To specialize in a particular field, physicians must complete a residency program and pass a medical specialty exam (see Section 5.3.2). A **residency** is a period of advanced medical training and education that normally follows graduation from medical school and completion of an internship. Residency programs include supervised practice of a specialty in a hospital and in its outpatient department, as well as instruction from specialists on the hospital staff. A **specialist** is a physician who completes a residency program and passes a medical specialty exam, which qualifies him or her to specialize in a particular medical field.

This focused study gives them advanced knowledge and experience that translates into both status and earning potential. As a rule, specialists enjoy higher status and earn higher incomes than their nonspecialist peers.

By the nature of their practices, specialists concentrate on health issues relating specifically to their area of specialty. Oncologists focus on cancer; gynecologists focus on women's health issues; otolaryngologists focus on ears, noses, and throats.

Still, because many Americans rely solely on specialists for their medical care, some specialists—such as gynecologists—find themselves practicing some form of general medicine in addition to their specialty. Similarly, the functions of some specialties such as internal medicine (the field specializing in the diagnosis and treatment of illness in adults) and pediatrics (the field specializing in the treatment of children) are closely linked to general practice, albeit for special populations.

5.2.3 General Practitioners

General practitioners are doctors who focus their practice on primary care of individuals and families. Often considered "family doctors," they are personal physicians, oriented to the whole patient and not a particular biological system or illness. They

▲ Function as the primary point of contact for individuals and their families and serve as an entry point into the health care industry for all the patient's medical needs.

▲ Provide comprehensive health care, offering treatment themselves and, when needed, referring patients to specialists or other health care providers, such as physical therapists, dietitians, and coordinating the care provided.

▲ Often serve their patients for years—sometimes across generations.

Despite their place at the center of traditional health care, the number of general practitioners is dropping. In 1931, 112,000 physicians classified themselves as general practitioners. Today approximately 68,000 do.

As the population ages, as more people access health care, and as navigating through the health care system becomes more complex, this shortage is fast becoming a crisis. The term **generalist** is traditionally used to mean a general practitioner, as described in the preceding paragraphs. In the age of managed care, however, the term took on new meaning. In the context of managed care, a generalist is a physician—usually a primary care or family physician—who coordinates, or manages, the health services available to plan members.

> ## FOR EXAMPLE
>
> ### Calling All Generalists
>
> Although the United States has all the specialists it needs, it's currently experiencing a shortage of general practitioners, whose effects will only get worse as the U.S. population ages and navigating through the health care industry becomes from complex. To offset this shortage, experts recommend that half of all medical school graduates enter generalist fields (currently, less than half do). To that end, several medical schools, such as the University of Massachusetts Medical School and New York Medical School, have taken action to increase the number of students enrolling with the intention of practicing general medicine. Some of these changes involve changes in admission and experiences relating to generalist medicine and primary care.

5.2.4 Hospitalists

Saving money on health costs without compromising patient care has become the prime directive of today's hospitals, many of which are struggling financially under the burden of rising health costs and negotiated payment rates. Key to a hospital's bottom line is length of stay: The longer a patient remains in the hospital, the higher the cost of care, and the less money the hospital makes (because of the negotiated payment rates common to voluntary and managed care health plans, as well as government health programs; refer to Chapter 4). Enter the **hospitalist.** A hospitalist is a hospital-based general physician who takes over the care of hospitalized patients in the place of their primary care physician.

Although the hospitalist's primary goal is to maximize patient care, the ancillary goal is to reduce length of stay and keep down the hospital's costs. Although a relatively new phenomenon—at least as an officially recognized position—this movement is a fast-growing one.

SELF-CHECK

- Describe the difference between MDs and DOs.
- Compare a generalist to a specialist.
- What is the role of a hospitalist?

5.3 Training Doctors

The education and training of U.S. doctors is rigorous (and expensive). Physicians typically complete eleven to sixteen years of post–high school education, including four years as undergraduates, four years of medical school, and three to eight years of specialty (residency) and subspecialty (fellowship) training.

5.3.1 Medical School

The four years of medical school (referred to as undergraduate medical education) is divided into a pair of two-year blocks:

▲ **Preclinical:** During the first two years in medical school students study basic sciences that are fundamental to medical practice (anatomy, physiology, biochemistry, pathology, microbiology, pharmacology) and learn how to take patient histories and conduct basic physical examinations.

▲ **Clinical:** The last two years of training take place in patient care settings (hospitals and ambulatory care facilities) under the supervision of physician faculty members. Students learn to diagnose and treat patients and perform medical procedures by rotating through various clinical services: internal medicine, general surgery, obstetrics and gynecology, pediatrics, psychiatry, and family practice.

Upon graduation, students are awarded an MD or DO degree. After completing an examination and one year of postgraduate training, they are licensed by the states.

The United States has 144 medical schools, of which 125 are allopathic (that is, they grant MD degrees) and 19 that are osteopathic (they grant DO degrees). Total enrollment for these schools is about 76,000 students, but acceptance into medical school isn't ensured. The average application-to-admission ratio is 2.6:1. In other words, fewer than half of the prospective students who apply to a medical school are admitted for study. Table 5-5 shows who those students are, in terms of race and gender.

5.3.2 Residency and Fellowship

To specialize in a particular medical field, physicians have to undertake specialty training (referred to as **graduate medical education**). These residencies include some academic instruction, but most of the training involves caring for patients under the supervision of experienced physician specialists. The United States has 8000 residency programs offered by hundreds of hospitals. Nearly 100,000 students participate in these programs. Approximately 24 percent of all residents are graduates of non-U.S. medical schools.

After the residency period, a physician is **board-eligible,** meaning he or she completed the course of specialty study but has not taken or passed the medical board specialty exam. These exams often include both an oral and written component. Upon passing the exam, the physician is then **board-certified.**

Some physicians seek additional training in fellowships leading to subspecialty certification.

Table 5-5: Medical Student Characteristics

Attribute	Percentage of Total Enrollment
Race/ethnicity	
White	64
Asian	20
Black	8
Hispanic	7
American Indian	1
Gender	
Male	56
Female	44

FOR EXAMPLE

Most Common Medical Specialties

According to the National Resident Matching Program (NRMP), the following are the most popular specialty areas:

▲ **Emergency medicine:** Front-line emergency care for patients in response to acute illness and injury.

▲ **Family practice:** Total, long-term health care of an individual or family.

▲ **Internal medicine:** Long-term, comprehensive health care of adolescents, adults, and elderly people.

▲ **Obstetrics-gynecology:** Medical and surgical care of the female reproductive system and associated disorders.

▲ **Orthopedic surgery:** Medical and surgical care focusing on the form and function of the limbs, spine, and associated structures.

▲ **Pediatrics:** Preventive care for healthy children and medical care for those who are seriously or chronically ill.

▲ **Psychiatry:** Medical care relating to the prevention, diagnosis, and treatment of mental, addictive, and emotional disorders.

▲ **General surgery:** Medical care relating to the diagnosis and provision of care before, during, and after surgery, as well as managing the overall care of the surgical patient.

SELF-CHECK

- Describe the two phases of medical school.
- What must a person do to become licensed as a physician?
- What additional education is necessary to become a specialist?

5.4 Nurses

The function of nursing—caring for the ill and infirm—has been around since ancient times; the profession of nursing as we know it today is a relatively modern creation. Once a job that lacked any real formal training and considered fit only for prostitutes, nursing today requires rigorous training involving the sciences related to how the human body works, the cause and treatment of disease, and other things impacting patient care. Nursing is the largest health care profession, and nurses account for approximately 20 percent of the total health care industry's workforce.

5.4.1 Registered Nurses (RNs)

A **registered nurse (RN)** is a graduate trained nurse who has been licensed by a state authority (as a board of nursing examiners) after successfully passing examinations for registration.

RNs perform a broad array of tasks as patient advocates. They

▲ Observe, assess, and record symptoms to show the progression of the illness or the effectiveness of treatment.

▲ Develop and implement nursing care plans.

▲ Assist physicians in examining and treating patients.

▲ Administer medications and perform certain medical procedures.

▲ Supervise other personnel.

▲ Educate patients and their families about follow-up care.

Which of these tasks individual RNs perform depends on the licensing laws in the states where they work, as well as the environment in which they practice.

In addition to general practice, many RNs (about 7 percent) engage in some form of advanced practice:

▲ **Nurse practitioner:** Registered nurses who are licensed to perform physical exams and other medical services, including writing prescriptions, usually under a physician's supervision. Some nurse practitioners open their own practices and treat patients without physician supervision.

▲ **Clinical nurse specialist:** Registered nurses who diagnose and treat health problems.

▲ **Nurse midwife:** Registered nurses who oversee pregnancies and births and, in some cases, deal with other gynecological issues. Certified nurse midwives have completed additional training from an accredited institution and are licensed to practice in all 50 states.

▲ **Nurse anesthetist:** Registered nurses who, after extensive training and national certification, provide services similar to those provided by anesthesiologists.

The United States has approximately 2.7 million registered nurses, a number that has increased since 1980. Then, there were 541 nurses per 100,000 people; in 2000 there were 816 nurses per 100,000. So, who are the RNs that take care of the U.S. population? Table 5-6 shows you.

Table 5-6: Profile of RNs in the United States

Descriptor	Percentage of RNs
Work	
Work full-time	59
Work part-time	23
Professionally inactive	18
Age	
Under 40	32 (average age is 45)
Gender	
Male	6
Female	94
Family	
Married	72
With children at home	53
Race	
White	86
Black	5
Hispanic	4
Average annual income	$45,000

5.4.2 Training Requirements

To prepare for these duties and to qualify for certification to practice nursing, a person must undergo rigorous training and be educated in at least one of three ways:

▲ **Associate Degree in Nursing (ADN) programs:** These two-year programs are offered by community colleges.

▲ **Diploma programs:** These three-year programs are offered by hospital-based schools of nursing. Although a degree is not awarded, undergraduate credit is often earned. Because of the high cost of these programs, they are becoming less common.

▲ **Bachelor of Science in Nursing (BSN) programs:** These four-year programs are offered by colleges and universities.

RN education consists of classroom instruction (in the biomedical and social-behavioral sciences) and supervised clinical experience in hospitals, doctors' offices, and community settings. Although the breadth and depth of study and experience vary by type of program, all graduates, regardless of the program they completed, are eligible to take the same national exam and receive identical licenses to practice granted by the states.

Registered nurses who want to go on to perform specialized nursing tasks (nurse midwife, for example, or nurse anesthetist) must complete additional course work leading to a master's or doctorate degree, and in most cases, pass a certification exam for their area of specialization.

5.4.3 Where the Nurses Are

After being licensed, RNs can practice in a number of different settings: hospitals, public or private health care organizations, nursing homes, and so on. Table 5-7 outlines where the nurses are.

Table 5-7: Where Registered Nurses Work

Practice	Percentage of Employed RNs
Hospitals	59
Public and community health organizations	18
Ambulatory care	10
Nursing homes and extended care facilities	7
Nursing education	2
Other	4

5.4.4 Other Nursing Personnel: LPNs and LVNs

In the field of nursing, **licensed practical nurses (LPNs)**—called licensed vocational nurses (LVNs) in California and Texas—make up the biggest group. LPNs provide basic, nonprofessional nursing care. They

▲ Observe patients.
▲ Take vital signs.
▲ Keep records.
▲ Change dressings.
▲ Assist patients with personal hygiene, getting around, and eating and bathing.
▲ Administer certain medications, in some states.

To become an LPN, candidates complete 12- to 14-month training programs offered by community colleges and technical or trade schools. There are 1100 such programs in the United States. In addition, all states require that LPNs possess a high school diploma (or equivalent) and pass a licensing exam.

Table 5-8 shows where the approximately 700,000 LPNs work. On average, LPNs make $29,000 annually.

FOR EXAMPLE

A Nurse's Typical Day

What is a typical day for a nurse? Obviously, the answer depends on where the nurse works. The typical day of a nurse who works in a family practice office is very different from an emergency room nurse's typical day. Even in hospitals, the various departments offer different challenges for their nurses. Still, a typical day on a typical inpatient floor in a hospital looks like this: First, the nurses work round-the-clock in shifts. When they arrive, they clock in and receive reports from the nurses going off duty. They then spend their time preparing meals, feeding patients, giving medications, recording vital statistics, admitting patients, discharging patients, educating patients, consoling families, comforting the dying, dressing wounds, answering patient calls, consulting with physicians, filling out medical reports, dealing with insurance companies, documenting doctors' orders, carrying out doctors' orders, overseeing LPN and nurse assistants, reacting to emergencies, and so on. They perform these duties with and without help, and for anywhere between a few and several patients.

Table 5-8: Where Licensed Practical Nurses Work

Practice	Percentage of Employed LPNs
Hospitals	28
Nursing homes	29
Doctors' offices and other ambulatory care settings	14
Residential care facilities and home health care agencies	29

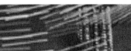

SELF-CHECK

- Identify the differences between an RN and an LPN in terms of education.
- List the functions that an RN can perform that an LPN can't.

5.5 Other Independent Health Professionals

The health care workforce includes several other professionals who provide care independently of physicians. The following sections discuss five of the more common ones—dentists, chiropractors, optometrists, podiatrists, and pharmacists—and describe the education required for each, as well as the services they offer. Table 5-9 gives a brief overview of how many people in each profession are actively practicing in the United States and what their average incomes are.

Table 5-9: Other Health Professionals

Professional	Number Practicing	Average Annual Income
Dentist	168,000	$129,000
Chiropractor	50,000	$67,000
Optometrist	30,000	$120,000
Podiatrist	12,000	$107,000
Pharmacist	208,000	$71,000

5.5.1 Dentists

Dentists prevent, diagnose, and treat diseases of the mouth, teeth, gums, and associated structures. To become a dentist, candidates, after receiving a bachelor's degree, must complete four more years of degree work at an accredited dental school. The first two (preclinical) years are spent on the basic sciences, such as dental anatomy, physiology, microbiology, and pathology. During the second two (clinical) years, students treat patients in teaching clinics under the supervision of faculty. Upon graduation, students receive their degrees: Doctor of Dental Surgery (DDS) or Doctor of Dental Medicine (DMD). Graduates must then pass a written and practical National Board Dental Examination before any state will grant them a license to practice.

Like physicians, dentists can take an additional two to four years of postgraduate education and specialize in any of nine areas:

▲ Orthodontics (straightening teeth and correcting misalignment).

▲ Oral and maxiofacial surgery (operating on the mouth and jaw).

▲ Pediatric dentistry (practice focused on children).

▲ Periodontics (treating gums and bones supporting the teeth).

▲ Prosthodontics (replacement of missing teeth).

▲ Endodontics (performing root canals).

▲ Public health dentistry (dental health promotion and disease prevention).

▲ Oral pathology (studying dental disease).

▲ Oral and maxiofacial radiology (diagnosing diseases of the mouth, head, and neck using imaging technology).

Of the 168,000 practicing dentists in the United States, 92 percent are in private practice (80 percent solo practice; 12 percent group practice). Some dentists (particularly specialists) are granted membership on a hospital medical staff, and many work in institutional settings, such as nursing homes and ambulatory care facilities (facilities that provide outpatient services).

5.5.2 Chiropractors

Chiropractors diagnose and treat problems of the nervous, muscle, and skeletal systems, especially the spine. Chiropractic is based on the theory that obstruction in these systems, in addition to impairing functioning, lowers resistance to certain diseases. Practitioners provide drugless and nonsurgical treatments by adjusting and manipulating the musculoskeletal system.

Chiropractors have a minimum of two years of undergraduate education (and increasingly, four), in addition to completing four years of chiropractic training at one of the sixteen chiropractic colleges in the United States. The first two years of education focus on basic sciences; the second two years involve course work in manipulative and adjustment techniques and training in clinical disciplines such as physical diagnosis, neurology, orthopedics, physiotherapy, and sports medicine. Graduation leads to award of the Doctor of Chiropractic (DC) degree. All practitioners must pass a state-administered exam before being granted a license to practice.

In the United States there are approximately 50,000 professionally active chiropractors. Virtually all work in ambulatory settings, which can be either solo practices or partnerships. Chiropractors are rarely granted staff privileges in hospitals.

5.5.3 Optometrists

Optometrists diagnose and treat vision problems and some diseases of the eye. They perform vision tests and prescribe eyeglasses, contact lenses, and other treatments; they can also prescribe certain drugs.

Be careful not to confuse optometrists with either ophthalmologists (physicians who provide a spectrum of medical and surgical eye care) or opticians (technicians who fit glasses according to the prescriptions of optometrists or ophthalmologists).

Optometrists typically have three or four years of undergraduate education in addition to four years of training in a school of optometry. Like other health professional schools, optometry education consists of two components: study of the basic sciences and supervised clinical training. There are seventeen schools of optometry in the United States, with a total first-year enrollment of approximately 1400 students. Upon graduation, students must pass an exam before being granted a license to practice by the states.

All optometry care is provided on an outpatient basis and the approximately 30,000 professionally active optometrists practice in various places and arrangements:

▲ Independent solo practice.
▲ Small group practice.
▲ Employment in retail vision care centers, medical groups, clinics, and hospitals.

5.5.4 Podiatrists

Podiatrists diagnose and treat diseases and injuries of the foot and lower leg, in addition to providing preventive care. They take X-rays, prescribe certain drugs, set fractures, apply casts, fit prosthetic devices, and perform surgery.

Entrants to the seven schools of podiatry (with a total enrollment of about 2000 students) typically possess an undergraduate degree. The training program, consisting of instruction in the basic sciences and supervised clinical training, lasts four years. Upon graduation, students are awarded a Doctor of Podiatric

Medicine (DPM) degree. Before granting a license, all states require that the podiatrists successfully complete a written and oral examination.

Most graduates complete a one-year general residency prior to entering practice. Postgraduate training (lasting up to three years) is available in such areas as anesthesiology, pathology, radiology, emergency medicine, surgery, and sports medicine.

Most of the 12,000 practicing podiatrists are in solo practice. Some hospitals grant podiatrists staff privileges.

5.5.5 Pharmacists

Pharmacists provide consultation to, and dispense drugs ordered by, physicians and other practitioners. They understand drug biochemical properties, effective dosages, methods of administration, interactions, and side effects. Pharmacists also counsel patients about the medications they've been prescribed and their appropriate use.

There are 82 colleges of pharmacy in the United States with a total enrollment of 29,000 students; the number of graduates per year averages 7300. Historically, there have been two types of pharmacy training programs:

▲ **Undergraduate:** This type of program, which has been phased out, led to a BS degree in pharmacy.

FOR EXAMPLE

The Conscience Clause and Legal Rights

Can a pharmacist refuse to fill a valid prescription based on moral or ethical beliefs? It's an interesting question and one that has gotten recent attention because of news stories about women whose pharmacists refused to dispense contraceptives based on their personal or religious convictions. In two of the most widely spread stories, one woman was a married mother of two with a prescription for birth control; the other was a rape victim with a prescription for the morning-after pill. But contraception isn't the only hot-topic issue. In Oregon, where assisted suicide is legal, pharmacists can object to filling a prescription that would lead to suicide, based on conscience, and pharmacists in other states could do the same in dispensing drugs used in lethal injections. The American Pharmacists Association policy states, "The pharmacist has the right to conscience, and the patient has the right to legally prescribed medication." As state legislatures weigh in—some introducing or passing laws that protect the pharmacist from legal action; others passing laws that protect the rights of patients denied—the issue is only likely to get more interesting.

▲ **Professional doctorate:** These programs are four years in length; students enter with at least two years of undergraduate study, but most have a college degree. After obtaining their Doctor of Pharmacy (PharmD) degree, some students pursue postgraduate (either Master of Science [MS] or Doctor of Philosophy [PhD]) programs preparing them for teaching and research roles; one- or two-year postgraduate residencies are available in areas of specialty practice.

Of the 208,000 practicing pharmacists, 60 percent work in community pharmacies, retail chains, grocery stores, pharmaceutical wholesalers, or mass merchandisers; 20 percent are employed in hospitals.

SELF-CHECK

- Define what each of the following professionals do: (a) dentists, (b) optometrists, (c) chiropractors, (d) podiatrists, and (e) pharmacists.
- Name and describe four dental specialties.

5.6 Working in Concert with Physicians

In addition to the independent providers, several health care providers work under the direction of or with referrals from physicians.

5.6.1 Physical Therapists

Physical therapists focus on the musculoskeletal system and provide services that restore functioning, improve mobility, and prevent or limit disabilities. They treat patients through non-drug or non-surgical therapies, using instead strategies such as exercise, stimulation, massage, ultrasound, adaptive devices (crutches and braces), and prostheses (artificial limbs).

Patients can seek out physical therapists on their own, or a physician can refer them to a therapist. All physical therapy training was required to be at the graduate level. Currently, there are 198 accredited programs; 165 offer a master's degree and 33 offer a doctorate. The curriculum includes training in the following:

▲ The basic sciences.
▲ Physical diagnosis and examination.
▲ Therapeutic procedures.

Classroom instruction is accompanied by supervised clinical experience. All graduates are required to pass a licensing examination before they can practice.

Physical therapists who want to secure a teaching or research position must complete a doctoral program. Similarly, those who want to specialize in the following areas require a doctoral degree as well:

▲ Pediatric physical therapy, specializing in treating children.

▲ Geriatric physical therapy, specializing in treating elderly people.

▲ Orthopedic physical therapy, specializing in treating patients with impaired movement caused by problems with the bones, joints, ligaments, muscles, and nerves.

▲ Sports medicine, specializing in preventing sports injuries and rehabilitating patients who suffer from them.

▲ Neurology, specializing in treating neurological diseases and studying how they affect human movement.

▲ Cardiopulmonary physical therapy, specializing in treating and rehabilitating people with heart and lung problems.

There are approximately 144,000 professionally active physical therapists; 25 percent work part time. You find physical therapists employed in hospitals, nursing homes, home health agencies, clinics, and physician offices (particularly those of orthopedic specialists); some are engaged in independent solo practice. Their median annual income is $55,000.

5.6.2 Physician Assistants

Physician assistants (PAs) provide a broad range of diagnostic and therapeutic services. They take histories, conduct examinations, order and interpret tests, make diagnoses, and perform procedures (such as suturing, splinting, and casting); in all but three states they can prescribe certain medications.

A physician assistant's practice must be linked to, and supervised by, a physician; however, it need not be immediate or direct. For example, in hospitals and clinics, PAs see patients without a physician being present; in rural areas, they often function as primary care providers, consulting with supervising physicians by telephone and during periodic visits. Historically, the development of this profession was based on the training and practice of medics and pharmacist mates in the military.

There are 129 accredited PA training programs (with a total enrollment of about 6000 students), which award associate, baccalaureate, and master's degrees; training takes at least two years. Students receive classroom instruction in the basic sciences in addition to supervised clinical experience in hospitals and ambulatory care settings. All states require PA graduates to take a national certifying examination; after passing this exam, they can use the PA-C credential

FOR EXAMPLE

Serving Underserved Populations

The federal government has designated some areas to be "Primary Care Health Professions Shortage Areas"—that is, areas in which the population lacks access to necessary health care because of distance (doctors are too far away), overutilization (there are too few doctors to adequately serve the population), or access barriers (such as low income or lack of health insurance). The shortage of physicians—particularly general internists, pediatricians, and obstetricians, who more often than not set up practice in economically healthy areas in cities—only exacerbates the problems. An interesting study published in the *Annals of Family Medicine,* however, indicates that physician assistants, followed closely by family physicians, nurse practitioners, and nurse midwives, are more likely to work in underserved areas.

(certified physician assistant). Postgraduate education programs are available in internal medicine, primary care, emergency medicine, surgery, pediatrics, and occupational medicine.

Approximately 40,000 PAs practice in the United States, earning an average annual salary of $65,000.

SELF-CHECK

- Describe what type of health care each of the following provide: (a) physical therapist and (b) physician assistant.
- Describe the working relationship between physicians and (a) physical therapists and (b) physician assistants.

SUMMARY

Without the health care workforce, there would be no health care system in the United States. This workforce is the second largest workforce in the country, and relies on health care professionals as well as administrative and support staff. Physicians, whether they are generalists or specialists, are the hub of the health care workforce. Nurses comprise the largest group and are often the most available of the direct care providers. Other health professionals, such as podiatrists, chiropractors, and physician assistants, provide additional services either independently or in conjunction with physicians. All together, these professionals are on the front lines of the U.S. health care system.

KEY TERMS

Administrative personnel	Administrative support staff and managers responsible for overseeing and managing the operation of a health care facility.
Allopathic physicians	A medical designation for physicians who graduate from allopathic schools of medicine and focus on treating disease. Known as MDs.
Board-certified	A physician who has passed the medical board specialty exam.
Board-eligible	To complete the course of specialty study but has not taken or passed the medical board specialty exam.
Chiropractors	Medical professionals who diagnose and treat problems of the nervous, muscle, and skeletal systems, especially the spine, by adjusting and manipulating the musculoskeletal system.
Clinical education	The last two years of medical training that takes place in patient care settings (hospitals and ambulatory care facilities) under the supervision of physician faculty members. During this phase of their education, future doctors learn to diagnose and treat patients and perform medical procedures.
Clinical nurse specialist	Registered nurse who, after receiving additional training and certification, is able to diagnose and treat health problems.
Dentists	Medical professionals who prevent, diagnose, and treat diseases of the mouth, teeth, gums, and associated structures.
Generalist	Traditionally, a general practitioner. Today, a physician—usually a primary care or family physician—who coordinates, or manages, the health services available to plan members.
General practitioners	Doctors who focus their practice on primary care of individuals and families.
Graduate medical education	Specialty training that includes some academic instruction, but mostly caring for patients under the supervision of experienced physician specialists.

Hospitalist	A hospital-based general physician who takes over the care of hospitalized patients in the place of their primary care physician.
Licensed practical nurses (LPNs)	Provide basic, nonprofessional nursing care, such as observe patients, take vital signs, and keep records.
Nurse anesthetist	Registered nurse who, after extensive training and national certification, provides services similar to those provided by anesthesiologists.
Nurse midwife	Registered nurse who, after additional training and certification, oversees pregnancies and births and, in some cases, deals with other gynecological issues.
Nurse practitioner	Registered nurse who, after additional training and certification, is licensed to perform physical exams and other medical services, including writing prescriptions, usually under a physician's supervision.
Optometrists	Medical professionals who diagnose and treat vision problems and some diseases of the eye.
Osteopathic physicians	Physicians who graduate from an osteopathic medical school and place greater emphasis on the neuromusculoskeletal system, preventive medicine, and holistic care. Known as DOs.
Pharmacists	Medical professionals who provide consultation to, and dispense drugs ordered by, physicians and other practitioners, as well as counsel patients about the medications they've been prescribed and their appropriate use.
Physical therapists	Medical professionals who focus on the musculoskeletal system and provide services that restore functioning, improve mobility, and prevent or limit disabilities.
Physician assistants (PAs)	Non-physician medical professionals who provide a broad range of diagnostic and therapeutic services, and in all but a few states, prescribe medications. They work under the supervision of a physician.
Podiatrists	Medical professionals who diagnose and treat diseases and injuries of the foot and lower leg, in addition to providing preventive care.

Preclinical education	Also called academic education, the period during the first two years in medical school when students study basic sciences that are fundamental to medical practice (anatomy, physiology, biochemistry, pathology, microbiology, pharmacology) and learn how to take patient histories and conduct basic physical examinations.
Professional and related occupations	Health care providers (such as physicians, nurses, pharmacists, and other direct caregivers) who work directly with the patients.
Registered nurse (RN)	A graduate trained nurse who has been licensed by a state authority (as a board of nursing examiners) after successfully passing examinations for registration.
Residency	A period of advanced medical training and education that normally follows graduation from medical school and completion of an internship. Residency programs include supervised practice of a specialty in a hospital and in its outpatient department, as well as instruction from specialists on the hospital staff.
Service workers	Medical support staff (such as patient assistants, attendants, and aides; food preparation, maintenance, and housekeeping) who offer support services to the health care providers and maintain the facilities in which the providers work.
Specialist	A physician who completes a residency program (a period of advanced knowledge and supervised experience in a particular medical field) and passes a medical specialty exam, which qualifies him or her to specialize in a particular medical field.

ASSESS YOUR UNDERSTANDING

Go to www.wiley.com/college/pointer to evaluate your knowledge of the health care workforce.

Measure your learning by comparing pre-test and post-test results.

Summary Questions

1. Professional and related occupations personnel are all health care providers—doctors, nurses, pharmacists, and so forth, who come into direct contact with patients. True or False?

2. Of all the health care professionals, physicians comprise the largest group. True or False?

3. Compared to an osteopathic physician, an allopathic physician is one who
    (a) focuses on treating disease.
    (b) focuses on the whole person.
    (c) is more likely to suggest traditional treatment options.
    (d) b and c.

4. Which of the following statements is true of osteopathic physicians?
    (a) osteopaths are more highly educated than allopaths
    (b) there are more osteopathic physicians than there are allopathic physicians
    (c) osteopaths receive essentially the same training and education that allopathics receive
    (d) osteopaths are primarily interested in the causes of disease

5. Hospitalists assume the role of specialists in hospital settings. True or False?

6. Physicians receive either preclinical or clinical education. Define *preclinical education.*
    (a) classroom education during first two years of medical school, focusing on basic health sciences
    (b) n-site education during last two years of medical school focusing on patient care
    (c) all training prior to residency training
    (d) a and c

7. Define *clinical education.*
    (a) classroom education during first two years of medical school, focusing on basic health sciences

      (b) on-site education during last two years of medical school focusing on patient care

      (c) all training following residency

      (d) b and c

8. In addition to graduating from medical school, physician licensing requires that doctors

      (a) complete a residency.

      (b) pass an examination.

      (c) perform a year of postgraduate training.

      (d) b and c.

      (e) all of the above.

9. Registered nurses in advanced practice differ from other registered nurses in what way?

      (a) they receive additional training in specialty areas

      (b) they can perform tasks that a physician would otherwise have to perform

      (c) they can set up their own practices

      (d) all of the above

10. To become an RN a candidate must

      (a) complete a nursing program at an accredited school.

      (b) complete a period of supervised, on-the-job training in a health care setting.

      (c) pass a national exam and receive a license.

      (d) all of the above.

11. Referring to Table 5-9, which health professional receives the greatest annual income on average? The lowest income?

12. Referring to Table 5-9, which health profession has the most members? The fewest members?

13. Identify the health professional you would go to—pharmacist, dentist, podiatrist, chiropractor, optometrist—for each of the following:

      (a) trouble seeing at night

      (b) sore gums

      (c) information on drug interactions

      (d) ankle pain

      (e) sore neck

14. Physical therapists are trained to

      (a) diagnose and treat musculoskeletal problems.

      (b) prescribe medication to improve functioning.

   (c) restore functioning of limbs and muscles, as well as prevent or limit disabilities.

   (d) a and c.

   (e) all of the above.

15. Which of the following is true about physician assistants?

   (a) they can provide diagnostic and therapeutic services, as a doctor would

   (b) in most states, they can prescribe medication

   (c) they work directly under the supervision of a physician

   (d) a and b

   (e) all of the above

Review Questions

1. Identify which category (professional and related occupations, service worker, and administrative personnel) each of the following belongs to:

   (a) hospital president

   (b) director of surgery

   (c) custodian

   (d) account manager

   (e) human resources manager

   (f) registered nurse

   (g) physical therapist

2. Identify whether you would be more inclined to go to a generalist or specialist for the following problems:

   (a) aching joints

   (b) back pain

   (c) the flu

   (d) immunizations

   (e) cancer

   (f) broken leg

3. Describe the difference between osteopathic physicians and allopathic physicians.

4. Outline the educational path that a pediatric cardiologist would have to take to certification.

5. How does a general practitioner's training differ from a specialist's training?

   (a) general practitioners receive additional preclinical training and less clinical training

   (b) general practitioners perform their residencies in hospital settings.

    (c) general practitioners perform residencies in a variety of specialty areas rather than a single specialty area

    (d) general practitioners' training includes four years of medical school and a year of postgraduate training.

6. Identify whether the following are most likely to be performed by a registered nurse, a registered nurse in advanced practice, or a licensed practical nurse.

    (a) take a patient's vital signs (all)

    (b) administer medications (RN and some LPNs)

    (c) supervise other personnel (RN)

    (d) provide info to families on follow-up care (RN)

    (e) diagnose and treat health problems (RN in advanced practice)

    (f) write prescriptions (RN in advanced practice)

    (g) perform physical exams (RN in advanced practice)

    (h) assist patients with personal hygiene, getting around, and eating and bathing (LPN)

7. Describe three ways a nurse practitioner can ease a physician's workload.

8. In what way are the dentists, optometrists, chiropractors, and podiatrists similar to MDs and DOs?

    (a) they must complete years of postgraduate study involving both academic and clinical experiences; some can specialize

    (b) they diagnose, treat, and provide follow-up care to their patients

    (c) they can work in solo or group practice; some are given hospital privileges

    (d) a and b

    (e) all of the above

9. Most, but not all, candidates to schools of optometry, chiropractics, podiatry, dentistry, and pharmacy receive a four-year degree prior to enrolling. Which of these fields *requires* a four-year degree?

    (a) optometry

    (b) chiropractics

    (c) podiatry

    (d) dentistry

    (e) pharmacy

10. Identify which physical therapy specialist (pediatric, geriatric, orthopedic, etc.; refer to Section 5.6.1) you would go to with the following conditions:

    (a) a tennis player recovering from a torn tendon (sports medicine)

    (b) a patient recovering from a heart attack (cardiopulmonary)

(c) an elderly patient following a knee replacement surgery (geriatric)

(d) a young woman recovering from brain injury (neurology)

11. Describe the type of supervision a physician assistant must receive from a physician.

(a) the supervision must be direct and routinely scheduled

(b) the physician must approve all prescriptions the PA writes

(c) the supervision period ends after a certain amount of time, specified by state licensing laws

(d) a and b

(e) none of the above

Applying This Chapter

1. Describe the people you would need if you want to staff a small (two- to three-doctor) office that provides family health care. Be sure to indicate what category (professional, service, or administrative) that each person fits into.

2. Given what you know about the specialists in comparison to generalists, explain why the United States has so few generalists.

3. Explain why it makes sense that there would be more LPNs than RNs in a nursing home or extended care facility.

4. Of the health care professionals who are independent of physicians, chiropractors, on average, make the least (refer to Table 5-9). Explain why you think this is so.

5. Arrange the health care professionals in hierarchical order, based on the degree to which they work independently. Include generalists, specialists, the three types of nurses, physical therapists, and physician assistants.

YOU TRY IT

Sizing Up the Workforce

By 2010, growth in the health care workforce is expected to outpace growth in the general workforce. Using Table 5-1, identify which health organizations are most likely to see the greatest growth. Explain your reasoning.

Understanding the Role of the Physician

You are in your last year of medical school and are debating whether to start a practice or begin a residency. List the factors that you'll consider as you make your decision.

Training Doctors

You (or someone you know) are expecting a child. Identify the health care providers who could care for you during this time and list the factors you would take into account as you decide which provider to choose.

Nurses

Some health professionals are allowed to work independently of physicians; others' work must be supervised by a physician. What do you think the rationale is behind these guidelines mandating (or not) physician oversight of other professionals? Are there any similarities (in training or job responsibilities) between those who must work under physician supervision and those who can work independently?

Other Independent Health Professionals

Assuming that the shortage of general practitioners continues, how would you utilize the other health care professions to alleviate some of the shortage?

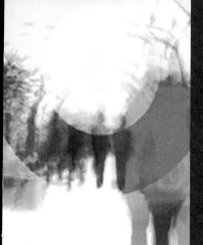

6

RESEARCH AND TECHNOLOGY
Advances in Medical Science

Starting Point

Go to www.wiley.com/college/pointer to assess your knowledge of the medical and technological breakthroughs in the U.S. health care system. *Determine where you need to concentrate your effort.*

What You'll Learn in This Chapter

▲ Noteworthy medical advancements
▲ The function and characteristics of different types of research facilities
▲ Sources of funding for medical research
▲ The challenges medical and technological advancements introduce into the U.S. health care system

After Studying This Chapter, You'll Be Able To

▲ Analyze how medical breakthroughs are changing medical care
▲ Understand and apply the principles of scientific research
▲ Assess the impact of changes on the delivery and coordination of care
▲ Discuss how the source of medical research funding impacts the research performed
▲ Identify public and private research facilities
▲ Discuss challenges facing medical research

Goals and Outcomes

▲ Master the terminology relating to the medical research
▲ Assess impact of medical and technological advances on cost of health care
▲ Extrapolate the impact that a shift from publicly funded to privately funded may have on research results
▲ Understand the discrepancy between how Americans view health care and medical research and predict how this discrepancy may impact future care

INTRODUCTION

The care of both outpatients and inpatients at the beginning of the twenty-first century is almost unrecognizable compared with the treatments offered just 25 years ago; to understand how profound these changes have been, you need to know about medical research. Medical research questions and probes all areas related directly or indirectly to health and wellness: the human body; treatment and diagnostic strategies; the effect and use of technologically advanced tools and communication and data systems; and more. Research facilities, each with a different focus, exist all across the United States. These facilities and the studies they conduct require significant funding, which comes from both private and public sources. As medical knowledge continues to advance, it will also continue to change the care people in America receive and how they receive it.

6.1 Understanding Medical Research

Since human prehistory, humankind has taken care of the ill, the infirm, and the injured. Of course, the earliest tools of the medical trade included spells, incantations, potions, and talismans. For centuries thereafter, medical "science" blurred the line between science and superstition. Consider, for example, that in the early Middle Ages, when the plague overwhelmed Europe, people were divided about the cause of the epidemic: some contaminating agent (for example, infected air) or divine displeasure. The more "scientific" minded (those in the contaminating agent group) believed that protection lay in avoiding or expelling the agent; hence, they recommended carrying things—namely posies or human excrement, with their own powerful smells—to block the infected air. The less scientific group recommended self-flagellation, in the hopes that their self-punishment would appease an angry God.

Medical science, fortunately, has taken many steps forward since then. One of the most fundamental breakthroughs has been the development and application of the **scientific method** as a way to study and understand human wellness. The scientific method relies on the following, marking a dramatic shift from the superstition-bound ideas of centuries past:

▲ **Observation:** Observe some aspect and describe what you see. For example, a medical researcher looking into what causes the flu may observe that when an ill person with the flu is with a well person without the flu, the well person gets the flu within a few days after being exposed. The observer watches this phenomenon happen and becomes curious.

▲ **Inquiry:** Ask questions about your observation. For example, the same researcher then might ask questions about the nature of spreading the flu. Did the two people touch? Did the sick person sneeze on the well person? Did he or she cough?

▲ **Hypothesis:** Formulate a hypothesis (a proposition capable of being tested) that offers a causal relationship about what you're observing. For example, the medical researcher may then, based on the questions asked earlier, say "Coughing causes the flu to be spread."

▲ **Experimentation:** Test your hypothesis, thus either confirming or falsifying it. In our example, the researcher might test this hypothesis by having two groups intermingle (but not touch) in a closed room. One group would have the flu and the other would not.

▲ **Theory:** Create a *theory*. A **theory** is a judgment, concept, or formula that is considered true or accurate based on experimental evidence and generalizations of fact, but not yet accepted as a law. For example, the researcher might, based on his or her observations in the experiment, develop a theory on the spread of influenza in closed spaces.

Without such a systematic process, meaningful medical advancement would be impossible. With this process, medical researchers have fundamentally altered the way health care is provided. An important thing to keep in mind is that the result of all this research is that not only is the process of care better, but so are the outcomes. Technological advances have extended the lives of countless patients and have improved the quality of life for countless more. The following sections outline some of the areas that have seen particular growth.

6.1.1 Advances in Knowledge

When Leonardo da Vinci drew pictures of the human body, he did so more accurately than any artist or scientist before him because he differed from his peers and predecessors by actually studying the human form—and dissecting human corpses. Until then, early physicians extrapolated how the human body worked and looked by studying animals; to illustrate how problematic this approach was, consider that some early medical sketches show humans with two stomachs (similar to a cow's). Obviously, understanding the human body is the first key in providing effective health care. Modern research in this area focuses on these areas:

▲ **How the human body works:** Computer imagery and microvision equipment have made it possible to actually see inside the body in real time. High-resolution imaging equipment along with computer programs and radioactive dyes enable us to see and map every millimeter of a human body. Advanced computed axial tomography (CAT), positron emission tomography (PET), and magnetic resonance imaging (MRI) tests can help us see the body systems in motion. Microscopic cameras, swallowed in pill form, can travel through the body, sending back dynamic views of the inner workings of organs.

▲ **How environmental, biological, and psychological conditions affect the human body:** Advances in computer diagnostic technology have helped medical professionals determine how a variety of conditions affect the human body. Triangulation of results from computer imaging, sound resonance, and so on, of sources combine both quantitative and qualitative data to give an overall, big-picture view of how all of these conditions interact within the body and on our psyche.

▲ **How the body responds to injury and illness and how the body responds to treatment or therapeutic interventions:** A variety of sophisticated biofeedback technologies combined with computer modeling can closely simulate how a body will respond to various injuries, illnesses, and treatments.

Beyond understanding the body, understanding disease is also vital in improving health care. Consider the plague of the Middle Ages. Those who took a more scientific approach attributed the disease to some contaminating agent. They were on the right track, but they had no better luck in avoiding the disease than those who saw it as punishment for sins. The reason is that they misidentified what actually caused it (infected fleas rather than infected air) and how it was spread. (It wasn't until the late nineteenth century that Louis Pasteur confirmed that bacteria caused diseases.) Hence, another key in improving health care is understanding how **disease agents** function:

▲ **Their genesis:** How they form and where they come from. At the turn of the twentieth century, for example, no one knew what caused yellow fever; by discovering that mosquitoes were the culprit, health officials could institute health policies (spraying ponds and other bodies of still water, for example) to significantly reduce or eradicate the disease. In a more contemporary example, health officials are worried about a pandemic caused by avian flu. Because health professionals know how a flu that affects primarily birds can mutate into a strain that can affect and be transmitted by humans, their first line of defense could be recommendations of health policies (general inoculation, for example) that would reduce the likelihood that the virus could mutate to a human–human strain.

▲ **Their transmission:** How (and whether) they can spread from person to person. In the late 1970s and early1980s, HIV, the virus that causes AIDS, was discovered. At first, it was thought that HIV could only be spread through sexual contact. As the years progressed, aggressive efforts were made toward teaching people how to protect themselves during sexual activity. Parallel to these efforts, more discoveries were made on the specifics of HIV's transmission. It was found that any bodily fluid of a HIV-positive person, such as blood, could transmit HIV to another. This caused further efforts to protect health and safety workers and officials. It also caused more public efforts to educate people on the transmission of HIV. Policies and procedures were established in the United States at organizational, local, state, and federal levels, and informational campaigns were conducted. The previously growing number of new infections each year finally leveled off in this country as more and more of the public understood how the disease was transmitted.

▲ **Their life cycle:** How a disease agent grows and develops in the human body. Understanding the incubation, infectious stage, and the life cycle of diseases can help keep diseases from contaminating others and spreading through populations. For example, knowing how long a child with chickenpox is contagious is vital in knowing how long to keep that child out of school or away from other siblings. Additionally, knowing the incubation period and lifespan of chickenpox helps one know when others exposed to the virus will begin to show signs. In the cases of large-scale epidemics, knowing this information can go a long way in curbing the spread of the disease to large populations.

6.1.2 Advances in Diagnostic Techniques

Diagnosis techniques for everything from common conditions (sore throat and tonsillitis) to chronic conditions (diabetes and heart disease) to catastrophic illnesses (lung cancer or Lou Gehrig's disease) have advanced a great deal in the late twentieth century. These techniques are generally less invasive and more reliable. Consider these common diagnostic tools:

▲ **MRI scans:** Magnetic resonance imaging (MRI) systems enable physicians to see images of internal bodily systems and organs. They can be used to look for tumors, abnormalities in organs and tissues, as well as a host of other applications.

▲ **CT scans:** Computed (axial) tomography (CT; also called CAT scans) takes X-ray images of various angles around the body and then uses computer data analysis to show cross sections of various organs and tissues within the body.

▲ **Interventional radiology:** This is a specialty type of radiology that uses CT, ultrasound, and fluoroscopy (X-ray of deep bodily structures using a fluoroscope) to conduct (through punctures in the skin) biopsies, drainage, catheters, or stents.

As notable as these preceding advances are, diagnosis has moved beyond the identification of an existing disease. Today, physicians can identify predispositions for a host of diseases, conditions, and infirmities through genetic testing. Genetic testing is the testing of DNA from blood or other bodily fluids for abnormalities that may signal disease or conditions. This can take the form of a missing or added chromosome, or it may be a change in the chemical base of the DNA itself.

> ## FOR EXAMPLE
>
> ### Human Genome Project
>
> In 2003, the Human Genome Project was completed. Coordinated by the U.S. Department of Energy and the National Institutes of Health with contributions from countries all over the world, the project goals included identifying all the genes in the human DNA and storing the resulting information in databases for further research. Specifically, scientists are looking to discover, among other things, the number of genes, their exact locations, and their functions; predict how susceptible people are to disease, based on the variations in the gene sequence; and identify genes involved in complex traits (diabetes) and multigene diseases (cancer). From this information, researchers hope to someday gain an unprecedented understanding of human biology—resulting in unprecedented advances in health and medical science.

6.1.3 Advances in Treatment Options and Therapeutic Interventions

Medical research has advanced the course of treatment and therapeutic interventions. Not only are everyday treatments for common conditions (such as bed rest for low-back pain) used more precisely and effectively, but there have also been dramatic changes in how patients with chronic or acute medical conditions are cared for. Consider the following advances:

▲ **Minimally invasive procedures:** These procedures, such as **arthroscopic surgery,** where a small scope is inserted into a tiny incision to examine and repair an area (usually a joint), are less traumatic to the body and require less recuperation time.

▲ **Development of devices and techniques that allow interventions to be performed without major surgery:** An example is the **fluoroscope,** a real-time imaging system used to see and record what is happening inside a patient. Fluoroscopes utilize X-rays, fluorescent screens, and CCD cameras to take the images. Another example is the **arthroscope,** a specific type of endoscope that is inserted into a joint through a tiny incision to examine, record, and treat.

▲ **Gene therapy:** Using site-specific gene "implants" to change the course of, or eliminate, diseases. In other words, gene therapy is the insertion of genes into a person's cells and tissues to treat disease, particularly hereditary diseases. An example is gene therapy for myocardial angiogenesis, in which gene therapy is used to make or build new blood vessels from preexisting ones.

▲ *Xeno*-**transplantation:** Using animal cells, tissues, and organs as a source for human transplants. And example of this is transplanting a baboon heart into a man.

▲ **Organ/tissue transplantation:** The transplantation of one organ or tissue from one body to another. For example, a patient with a failing kidney may be able to receive a kidney from another person (alive or recentl deceased).

6.1.4 Advances in Pharmaceuticals

Before modern pharmaceuticals, physicians and patients relied on herbal remedies, poultices, and very basic (and often addictive) pain relievers such as morphine and laudanum (an opium preparation, often involving alcohol). In fact, it wasn't until the 1940s when penicillin, discovered by Alexander Fleming in 1928, was used to fight bacterial infections in people. This event marked a fundamental shift in the way medications were viewed. Instead of seeing pharmaceuticals as being primarily palliative (that is, easing symptoms and discomfort, but offering no cure), people began to imagine the curative potential of medications. Since then—and as evidenced by the huge business of marketing medications directly to consumers— drugs have become a major component of the U.S. health care pie.

The advances in pharmaceuticals today have resulted in drugs that are more effective and have fewer side effects, as well as drugs that can totally replace current forms of treatment; for example, "Drano-like" drugs that remove plaque from coronary arteries, making bypass surgery or surgery to implant stents unnecessary. In addition, new drugs, such as the following, have been introduced:

▲ **Superstatins**, which promise to lower cholesterol by up to 60 percent, should significantly contribute to lower and lower heart disease related medical costs.

▲ **Selective serotonin reuptake inhibitors (SSRIs),** which increase the level of serotonin in the body, help reduce anxiety disorders and depression within patients. This should lead to lower associated health care costs over time.

▲ **Quinolone antibiotics**, a class of antibiotics that are effective against a larger *microbial spectrum* (range of bacterial microbes that are similarly related in structure). This gives physicians the ability to prescribe these drugs that treat a wider array of infections and treat more people in more varied ways, which ultimately lowers health care costs.

6.1.5 Advances in Information and Communication Technologies

A revolution in information and communication technologies has already transformed much of the nation's business community. Health care has not been in the forefront of these changes, but it will not be far behind. New technologies are already bringing electronic clinical data systems to physicians by means of handheld computers, and electronic communication between patients, physicians, and consultants is transforming the process of care in ways unimagined only 10 years ago.

The Institute for the Future predicts that these information and communication technologies will affect health care in three principal areas:

▲ **Process-management systems:** These systems merge the many processes of a health care facility into one system. For example, a patient going into the hospital has to be admitted, take tests, be seen by a doctor, be treated, be discharged, and then be billed for services. Up until very recently in most health care organizations, all of these processes were their own separate system. Each worked independently of one another and did not communicate. With the advent of process-management systems in health care, these processes can now work together in one seamless system. This means more efficiency for the health care system and less cost, as well as a more pleasant and seamless system for the patient from admission to the final bill.

▲ **Clinical information interfaces and data analysis:** Much like process-management systems, clinical information systems and data analysis work in the same way by combining all the clinical data for a patient or group of patients in one central system. In this way, a patient's X-rays, MRI images, blood test results, surgery information, and so on are all in one Master Patient Index and can be accessed and analyzed via computer by the appropriate health care worker.

▲ **Telemedicine and remote monitoring:** Telemedicine is an emerging technology that would enable people in areas with few medical resources (physicians, clinics, hospitals, and so on) to access health care long distance. Telemedicine has enormous potential for alleviating the effects of the geographic maldistribution of health professionals. The current state of telemedicine is relatively unstructured, with a wide variety of public and private sector experiments proceeding simultaneously. Some applications, such as reading electrocardiograms at a distance, have become commonplace. Others, such as dermatology consultations, are being performed in many different places but without standard procedures for transmission, interaction, evaluation, or charging. Still other applications, such as doing an appendectomy at a distance, remain in the realm of science fiction, if just barely.

Although telemedicine has a legitimate, important, and growing role in rural medicine, the path to the future is uncertain. Several significant obstacles exist that make the current efforts uncoordinated, expensive, and sometimes inaccessible. For example, one obstacle is the availability (or lack thereof) of standard, like technologies at both telemedicine sites. A rural hospital that cannot afford high-paid specialists may be unable to participate because of the unavailability of high-speed Internet access in its remote area. Another obstacle is cost. Although telemedicine helps reduce costs and adds to services in the long term, the short-term initial cost investment in technology is still relatively high. Additionally, telemedicine and its offshoots are threatening to many in the health care establishment who see it as eroding their profession and time availability even more.

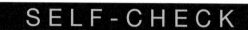

SELF-CHECK

- Describe the scientific method.
- Explain how perceptions of medication changed between the early twentieth century and the mid-twentieth century.
- List the areas in which medical knowledge has advanced.

6.2 Research Facilities

Da Vinci performed his human dissections by candlelight in a scene that he described as "living through the night hours in the company of quartered and flayed corpses fearful to behold." Fortunately, modern researchers have more suitable and accommodating facilities.

6.2.1 Public Research Facilities: National Institutes of Health

The **National Institutes of Health (NIH)** is part of the U.S. Department of Health and Human Services. It conducts and supports medical research and is composed of 27 institutes and centers, including the following:

- ▲ **National Cancer Institute:** Focuses on cancer prevention, diagnosis, and treatment.
- ▲ **National Eye Institute:** Focuses on prevention and treatment of eye disease and other disorders.
- ▲ **National Heart, Lung, and Blood Institute:** Focuses on prevention and treatment of diseases and disorders of the heart, lungs, and blood. Also researches sleep disorders.
- ▲ **National Human Genome Research Institute:** Supports the NIH contribution to the international Human Genome Project.
- ▲ **National Institute on Aging:** Studies the biomedical, social, and behavioral aspects of aging.
- ▲ **National Institute on Alcohol Abuse and Alcoholism:** Focuses on prevention and treatment of alcohol abuse and alcoholism.

▲ **National Institute of Allergy and Infectious Diseases:** Focuses on understanding and treating infectious, immunologic, and allergic diseases.

▲ **National Institute of Arthritis and Musculoskeletal and Skin Diseases:** Studies causes, treatment, and prevention of arthritis and musculoskeletal and skin diseases.

▲ **National Institute of Biomedical Imaging and Bioengineering:** Focuses on the design, development, and assessment of technological capabilities in biomedical imaging and bioengineering. (*Biomedical imaging* is the medical field concerned with the development and use of imaging devices that create and analyze images of internal organs and tissues. *Bioengineering* integrates engineering sciences to advance biology and health care; examples include the development and use of artificial organs, tissue engineering and transplant medicine, etc.)

▲ **National Institute of Child Health and Human Development:** Focuses on fertility, pregnancy, and child growth and development.

▲ **National Institute on Deafness and Other Communication Disorders:** Researches the prevention and treatment of diseases and disorders of hearing, balance, smell, taste, voice, speech, and language.

▲ **National Institute of Deafness and Craniofacial Research:** Focuses on the prevention and treatment of infectious and inherited craniofacial-oral-dental diseases.

▲ **National Institute of Diabetes and Digestive and Kidney Diseases:** Studies the prevention and treatment of diabetes, endocrinology, and metabolic diseases; digestive diseases and nutrition; and kidney, urologic, and hematologic diseases.

▲ **National Institute on Drug Abuse:** Focuses on prevention and treatment of drug abuse and addiction.

▲ **National Institute of Environmental Health Sciences:** Researches how environmental exposures, genetic susceptibility, and age interact to affect a person's health.

▲ **National Institute of General Medical Sciences:** Focuses on basic biomedical research not targeted to specific diseases, such as genes, proteins, and cells; fundamental processes like communication within and between cells; how bodies use energy; and how the human body responds to medicines.

▲ **National Institute of Neurological Disorders and Stroke:** Studies the normal and diseased nervous system to improve prevention, treatment, and diagnosis of neurological disorders.

▲ **National Institute of Nursing Research:** Focuses on establishing a scientific basis for the care of individuals throughout their lives.

▲ **National Library of Medicine:** Collects, organizes, and makes available biomedical science information to scientists, health professionals, and the public.

The Centers for Disease Control and Prevention (CDC) is part of the Department of Health and Human Services (DHHS) which is responsible for protecting the health and safety of U.S. citizens. The CDC provides essential vital research services in the area of disease.

6.2.2 Academic Health Centers

Academic health centers (AHCs) have created an explosion of knowledge in both basic biomedical science and clinical research. AHCs are also where the next generation of physicians, nurses, pharmacists, and other health professionals are trained. In addition, they run the specialty and subspecialty training programs that create the practitioners of the most advanced medical care in the world. According to the Association of Academic Health Centers, AHCs vary in their organization and structure, but all centers include a medical school, at least one other health professional school or program, and one or more owned or affiliated teaching hospitals.

Before World War II, AHCs were relatively modest in scope, had a main emphasis on education and research, and by contemporary terms were modest clinical enterprises. In the 1930s and 1940s the scientific era of medicine began to flourish, with the discovery of insulin, the initial success of antibiotics, and new technologies such as blood transfusion. World War II catalyzed further advances in medicine and surgery, and it was logical to believe that more research

FOR EXAMPLE

Coordinating Research across Facilities

In addition to conducting research themselves, the various institutes comprising the National Institutes of Health also fund complementary research in other facilities. Take, for example, the National Cancer Institute (NCI), which has a five-year $144.3 million initiative for nanotechnology in cancer research (that is, researching cancer at the molecular level by using medical devices that are too small to be seen by the human eye). The NCI formed partnerships with 12 research centers across the country and awarded several millions of dollars to these centers, including Northeastern University in Boston; University of Michigan in Ann Arbor, Michigan; Roswell Park Cancer Institute in Buffalo, New York; and others. Through such efforts, independent research projects can be coordinated to achieve a common goal.

would produce effective treatments for cancer, heart disease, and other killers. Also, the success of the Manhattan Project, which led to the rapid development of the atomic bomb, suggested that combining world-class talent with modern facilities and generous financial support could lead to similar success in conquering disease.

After the war, the expansion of the NIH (see the preceding section) and further advances in medical science provided fertile soil for accelerated growth. In the 1960s, the creation of the Medicare program and its support for graduate medical education, coupled with the national mood of faith in science and technology that led to continued increases in funding for the NIH, created further support for specialty training and research and continued expansions of the clinical enterprise. AHCs began to develop such technologies as intensive care units, burn centers, heart transplant programs, and comprehensive cancer centers. Academic health physicians became household names and even celebrities—Denton Cooley, who performed the first human heart transplant and founded the Texas Heart Institute in 1962, and Michael De Bakey, a pioneering cardiovascular surgeon who, during WWII, was director of the Surgical Consultants' Division in the U.S. Army's Surgeon General's Office, is credited with creating Mobile Army Surgical Hospital (M.A.S.H.) units to serve the wounded—and the nation's AHCs enjoyed unparalleled prestige, power, and influence.

6.2.3 Private Research Facilities

These are facilities that are privately owned and operated and conduct research in a variety of medical areas. Although privately owned and operated, often these facilities are part of academic institutions or larger centers. The staff at these facilities are similar to staff at public research facilities in terms of experience and credentials and, when associated with an academic or public institution, share duties. Funding for private research facilities is raised through donations, foundations, and sometimes grants. Two examples of private research facilities are St. Jude Children's Research Hospital and the Walther Cancer Institute, a private, nonprofit research organization. Both have helped research and discover cancer treatments.

6.2.4 Core Facilities

Some research equipment, such as light and electron microscopes, are almost prohibitively expensive. Core facilities house this type of equipment and make it available on a fee-for-service basis to independent research centers that could not otherwise afford it.

All core facilities are governed by applicable local, state, and federal laws and regulations for the type of material that they offer. Depending on the type of facility, the equipment used in the facility, and the research conducted, appropriate regulations would be enforced. Core facilities can be owned by private individuals but are usually associated with or controlled by academic or public institutions.

An example of a core facility is the Wadsworth Center in New York which provides genotyping, DNA purification, and PCR (polymerase chain reaction) troubleshooting/optimization. PCR is a technique for amplifying DNA and is used by medical professionals, among other things, for diagnosing hereditary diseases, cloning genes, paternity testing, and DNA computing. These services would be prohibitively expensive to do on one's own.

SELF-CHECK

- Describe what the NIH is and list three of the institutes that comprise the NIH.
- Explain what academic health centers are.
- Who uses core facilities?

6.3 Funding Research: Knowing Where the Money Comes from

Medical research is very expensive, requiring that personnel, equipment, and facilities be devoted over an extended period of time to an endeavor whose outcome is far from certain. The benefits, however, greatly outweigh the costs.

Organizations take different approaches to funding research. Some organizations use private funds while others use public funds. Still, some organizations use a combination of each.

6.3.1 Public Funds

The role of public funding of health care in the United States has increasingly grown over the past century. However, the role of public funding of research has been declining as compared to private funding of research. Public funds available for medical research have declined due to a number of factors including political and budgetary (within the U.S. government), and the fact that many more private companies are stepping up and doing their own medical research. The current rate of movement from public to private seems to indicate that the trend will continue. Public organizations and companies take on more and more of the medical research segment. This allows the government to move monies in its budget to different areas while allowing private companies to conduct research without as many limited constraints.

Public funding of research includes monies from federal, state, and local governments and agencies. The NIH is the nation's largest public funding body for medical research. The process is complicated, but essentially involves applying for funding and going through a series of steps that are not limited to, but include specifying what the funding will be used for; outlining the accountability protocols; and articulating the research timelines, procedures, and assessment. Most funding also requires that the researchers explain that the research meets a rational need.

6.3.2 Private Donors or Benefactors

Privately funded research makes up a large percentage of funding dollars. Private monies come from several sources, including private donations (from individuals or corporations).

Private foundations provide money to fund research in which they have an interest. Sources like the Bill and Melinda Gates Foundation and the Rockefeller Foundation are two philanthropic organizations that provide money for medical research. Another example is St. Jude Research Hospital, which is a large health care organization or hospital that is funded by donations and private monies. This funding is targeted to researching childhood cancers and related diseases. Money comes into this hospital exclusively through private donations, and that money is used to operate the hospital and research facilities.

Private corporations also provide a large share of private funding to medical research. Pharmaceutical companies and other related health care companies fund their own private research or subcontract out research. For instance, a pharmaceutical company may be doing research into a new flu vaccine. It will use its own private funds for this research. The benefits of this research will serve the public good; however, it will also profit the drug company as well. Many private companies and organizations like pharmaceutical companies allocate a portion of their budget back into research. Another example of private companies using their own monies to pay for medical research is tobacco companies which spend hundreds of millions of dollars researching the effects of smoking on humans.

FOR EXAMPLE

Deciding Where the Money Goes

The deadliest disease in the world is malaria. It kills more people every year than any other disease. Those at greatest risk live in developing countries, and not surprisingly, children account for the majority of malarial deaths. Despite these statistics, malaria gets a relatively small piece of the funding pie. More money, relatively speaking, goes toward research of less virulent diseases that plague people in Western countries. A key issue in funding, then, is who decides where the money goes? The answer is the donating parties. Foundations and private donors, including companies, often will stipulate where and how their money is to be spent.

SELF-CHECK

- What is the largest public funding body for medical research in the United States?
- In private donations, who decides where the money goes?

6.4 Assessment and Challenges of Continuing Medical Advancement

Medical care in the United States has enjoyed almost unprecedented advances during the later part of the twentieth century. Medical technology, knowledge, and strategies have improved such that health care today is vastly different from health care just three decades ago. Nevertheless, as medical research continues and medical technology moves forward, the issues discussed in the following section have the potential to affect medical research in this nation.

6.4.1 The Shift from Public to Private Research Endeavors

The shift from public funding to private funding of medical research in the United States has drawn much criticism and has raised many red flags. The criticism stems from the issue of objective research. Private funding of research through companies and businesses almost always is driven by profit, which creates pressures on researchers and their findings. Private companies tend not to fund research that doesn't have the possibility of becoming profitable in the future. Because of this, many critics of private medical research funding contend that a number of diseases and medical conditions that are not viewed as profitable may lack funding and therefore cannot be researched. Additionally, when a company sponsors medical research relating to its business, research findings are always suspect as not being totally objective and true. When tobacco companies sponsored smoking research decades ago, for example, results of that research showed that cigarette smoking was not harmful—even though other studies showed that it was extremely harmful.

6.4.2 Issues regarding Research in General Internal Medicine

In 1975, there was little research performed in general internal medicine, nor was there much support for that research. Today, general internal medicine research is robust, a leader in many departments of medicine, and a source of departmental prestige. Despite these successes, overall research funding for general internists is still relatively modest, especially compared with funding for biomedical and traditional subspecialty research. General medicine research often involves studying chronic disease, and these types of studies often require years. Such research depends on collaborations across disciplines and requires a substantial infrastructure to support a collaborative group. Building such infrastructures is challenging and expensive.

Another threat to research in general internal medicine is the practice of hiring only clinicians or clinician-teachers rather than researchers in departments of medicine. Although increasing the recruitment of staff in academic medical centers increases the total size of academic departments, these centers lack the ranks of general internist researchers that are needed to continue the advancement of medical science.

6.4.3 The Impact on AHCs

By the early 1990s, health care costs had continued to rise and, in certain areas of the country, managed care growth had begun to affect the clinical operations of AHCs significantly (refer to Section 6.2 for general information about AHCs). For example, contracts for managed care patients were not as lucrative and limited AHCs' ability to subsidize teaching, research, and indigent care. Interest in primary care among medical students and faculty fell dramatically, and AHCs continued to expand their clinical programs to support the service requirements of expanding specialty training programs and to increase clinical revenue.

Ultimately and more disturbing for AHCs, however, was the gradual erosion of their place at the center of power and influence in health care. By training too many specialists (who in turn set up competing tertiary care programs; refer to Section 3.1 for information on tertiary care), AHCs lost their natural monopoly on specialty care. The growth of managed care created powerful new corporations in the health care arena—organizations with no special reverence for the products and the values intrinsic to AHCs. Many AHCs neglected community concerns and were viewed as arrogant and insular institutions. Finally, the dramatic growth of overall health care spending led to a continued ascension of economics, business, and politics over medicine.

6.4.4 Cost of Health Care

As research in health care grows, new and advanced methods of treating disease and health care related issues are discovered. Because the cost of research that goes into finding those advances is great, the cost of the new health care treatment is initially high. The new advanced treatment also tends to be in great demand as the medical community promotes the advanced treatment and uses it more and more, which tends to sustain the high cost of the treatment. As the treatment saturates the market and the "new" advancement is enhanced and further tweaked, and as the initial costs of bringing the treatment to market are spread out, the cost of service decreases. This cycle, from high cost, high

FOR EXAMPLE

Supporting Medical Research

According to Research!America, a nonprofit biomedical research advocacy group, Americans are all for medical research. The findings, based on multiple state and federal surveys given between 1996 and 2005, suggest that although Americans are not as happy with their overall health care, they are very committed to medical research. According to Research!America, 94 percent of Americans believe that medical research is important to the U.S. economy; 79 percent said the federal government should support research "even if it brings no immediate benefit," and 67 percent are willing to pay more in taxes to support even more medical research.

demand to market saturation and lower cost, can take months or even years to complete.

An example of this cycle in action is laser eye surgery. This advancement was discovered and perfected by one company, which bore the high cost of researching, inventing, and then bringing this procedure to market. As a result, the cost of the procedure was very high, up to $10,000. This price was sustainable because the company that developed the procedure was the only one that performed it; it had to recoup the expenses related to bringing the procedure to market, and there was enough of a market of people who wanted the high-cost procedure and could afford it. Then other companies began to develop their own laser eye procedures and the machines to do the work. At the same time, laser surgery was advancing the original technology. These two trends converged to bring down costs. As costs decreased, the procedure was being offered at more places to more people, spurring additional price drops. This procedure, which used to cost $10,000, now costs as little as $2,000.

SELF-CHECK

- Why is funding for medical research shifting from public to private funds?
- Why are advancements in treatment generally more expensive than the procedures they replace?

SUMMARY

Health care has changed significantly in the last couple of decades. Medical break-throughs, as well as the growing sophistication of medical data and communication tools, have profoundly altered the type of care given and the dissemination of that care. These breakthroughs are the result of years of study at both public and private research facilities around the United States. They would not have been possible without funding from both the public and private sectors. As profound an effect as these changes have made thus far, even more changes—and future challenges—are in store for the U.S. health care system.

KEY TERMS

Academic health centers (AHCs)	Run the specialty and subspecialty training programs that create the practitioners of the most advanced medical care in the world; vary in their organization and structure, but all centers include a medical school, at least one other health professional school or program, and one or more owned or affiliated teaching hospitals.
Disease agent	A pathogen, or, an agent that causes disease, especially a living microorganism such as a bacterium, virus, or fungus.
National Institutes of Health (NIH)	Part of the U.S. Department of Health and Human Services. Conducts and supports medical research and is composed of twenty seven institutes and centers.
Scientific method	A process of scientific testing that relies on the following five steps: observation, inquiry, hypothesis, experimentation, and theory
Theory	A judgment, concept, or formula that is considered true or accurate based on experimental evidence and generalizations of fact, but not yet accepted as a law.
Arthroscope	A specific type of endoscope that is inserted into a joint through a tiny incision to examine, record, and treat.
Arthroscopic surgery	Type of surgery in which a small scope is inserted into a tiny incision to examine and repair an area.
Fluoroscope	A real-time imaging system used to see and record what is happening inside a patient utilizing X-rays, fluorescnet screens, and CCD cameras.

ASSESS YOUR UNDERSTANDING

Go to www.wiley.com/college/pointer to evaluate your knowledge of the medical and technological breakthroughs in the U.S. health care system.
Measure your learning by comparing pre-test and post-test results.

Summary Questions

1. To more effectively combat diseases, scientists have to know
   (a) how the human body is affected by environmental, biological, and psychological conditions.
   (b) how disease agents function.
   (c) how the body responds to treatment.
   (d) all of the above.

2. In addition to being better able to diagnose disease, what key change has occurred in the field of diagnosis?
   (a) diagnostic tools are less expensive
   (b) diagnostic tools can now predict the course a disease will take in an individual
   (c) diagnostic tools can now predict a predisposition toward a condition
   (d) all of the above

3. Which of the following statements is *true* about today's drugs?
   (a) they can replace existing treatments
   (b) they are more plentiful and less expensive
   (c) because of their effectiveness, they represent a relatively small portion of health care expenditures
   (d) all of the above

4. Define *telemedicine*.
   (a) the ability for physicians and patients to communicate via technology (phone, email, and so forth) rather than face-to-face
   (b) the ability to access health care long distance
   (c) a method by which people in health profession shortage areas can access medical care
   (d) all of the above

5. Twenty-seven centers comprise the National Institutes of Health. In the following, match the center to its focus.

Center	Focus
A. National Cancer Institute	**a.** How environmental exposures, genetic susceptibility, and age interact to affect a person's health
B. National Eye Institute	**b.** The design, development, and assessment of technological capabilities enabling images to be made of internal organs and tissues
C. National Human Genome Research Institute	**c.** Basic biomedical research not targeted to specific diseases
D. National Institute of Allergy and Infectious Diseases	**d.** Understanding and treating infectious, immunologic, and allergic diseases
E. National Institute of Biomedical Imaging and Bioengineering	**e.** The NIH contribution to the worldwide project of mapping human DNA
F. National Institute of Environmental Health Sciences	**f.** Cancer prevention, diagnosis, and treatment
G. National Institute of General Medical Sciences	**g.** To collect, organize, and make available biomedical science information to scientists, health professionals, and the public
H. National Institute of Nursing Research	**h.** Prevention and treatment of eye disease and other disorders
I. National Library of Medicine	**i.** Establishing a scientific basis for the care of individuals throughout their lives

6. An academic health center is
   (a) a teaching facility where medical personnel are trained.
   (b) a research facility.
   (c) one or more teaching hospitals.
   (d) all of the above.
7. The primary purpose of private research facilities, which are owned by corporations, is to find medical breakthroughs that can be sold for a profit. True or False?

8. Core research facilities are research facilities housing equipment that other research firms would not otherwise have access to. True or False?

9. Where do public funds come from?
   (a) tax dollars
   (b) federal, state, and local governments
   (c) private donations
   (d) a and b

10. Both corporations and private citizens fund private research. True or False?

11. New medical procedures, because they are generally less invasive, tend to cost less than the procedure they replace. True or False?

Review Questions

1. Identify which of the following represents an advancement in minimally invasive procedures, gene therapy, or xeno-transplantation.
   (a) using porcine (pig) neural cells to alleviate the symptoms of Parkinson's disease in human patients
   (b) Drano-like drugs clearing clogged arteries (minimally invasive procedure)
   (c) using replacement genes to a muscle protein missing in people with Duchenne muscular dystrophy

2. In what way are communication technologies potentially revolutionary in health care?
   (a) they allow for more effective data collection and dissemination
   (b) they enable medical personnel to conduct more sophisticated analysis of information in less time
   (c) they make it possible for people to access health care from a distance
   (d) all of the above

3. What three functions do academic health centers combine?

4. What event(s) led to the environment that fostered the expansion in both scope and prestige of academic health centers?

5. Define *core facility*, and provide an example.

6. Why has public funding of health care grown over the past century?

7. List three things that bring down the high cost of new medical procedures.

Applying This Chapter

1. Consider this scenario: **(1)** Following an unusually heavy rainy season, a malaria epidemic struck a village. As more and more people fell ill, residents began to avoid crowded places; health care workers refused to care for the sick. **(2)** To allay fears and better deal with the outbreak, researchers stepped in to discover how malaria spread. **(3)** They noticed that people who cared for malarial patients were sometimes infected and sometimes not; they also noticed that not all cases were the result of someone coming into contact with a sick person. In fact, there was no overriding similarity between the infected people except for their environment: The largest population of the sick were in the low country, which was hotter and more humid than the high country. **(4)** Based on what they had seen, the researchers came to believe that the disease was transmitted through insect bites. Some researchers thought the culprit was the fly. Others thought it was the mosquito. **(5)** The researchers quarantined healthy volunteers. One set of volunteers was exposed to flies; the other set was exposed to mosquitoes. **(6)** None of the fly-exposed volunteers fell ill. Several of the mosquito-exposed volunteers. **(7)** After verifying this result, the researchers sent word to local health authorities: Malaria is spread through contact with an infected mosquito.

   Identify which step of the scientific method each of the preceding numbered sections applies to:

   (a) Section 1

   (b) Section 2

   (c) Section 3

   (d) Section 4

   (e) Section 5

   (f) Section 6

   (g) Section 7

2. Indicate what type of medical advancement (in knowledge, in diagnostic techniques, in treatment, in pharmaceuticals, in technology) each of the following represent:

   (a) creating a 3-D image of the internal organs for a patient who complains of abdominal pain and lethargy

   (b) prescribing medication to alleviate depression

   (c) implanting genes into cells to reduce the symptoms of Parkinson's disease

(d) Understanding how the body's immune system reacts to disease agents

(e) Combining patient records in a central computer file that can be accessed by all caregivers

3. To apply for funding from the NIH, what types of information would your proposal have to include?

4. As a researcher interested in chronic diseases, what challenges do you face?

Understanding Medical Research

Of all the individual advances in health care, the single, overriding result has been that health care is less intrusive today than in years (and centuries) past. Explain how each area of advancement (refer to Section 6.1) has made care less intrusive.

Research Facilities

The United States does not have a single research program, meaning that various research facilities can (and often do) tackle the same issues independently. Do you think this overlap of endeavors is beneficial or not? Explain your answer.

Funding Research: Knowing Where the Money Comes from

Private funds are distributed according to the wishes of the donor rather than to the research areas of greatest need. Evaluate whether, and in what ways, the allocation of public funds is influenced by the desires of the public.

Assessment and Challenges of Continuing Medical Advancement

Evaluate how the profit motive of private research facilities impacts the type and reliability of research conducted.

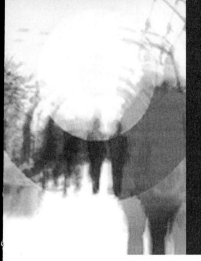

7

HOSPITALS IN THE UNITED STATES

The History and Health of American Hospitals

Starting Point

Go to www.wiley.com/college/pointer to assess your knowledge of U.S. hospitals. *Determine where you need to concentrate your effort.*

What You'll Learn in This Chapter

▲ How U.S. hospitals have evolved into the modern care centers of today
▲ Characteristics of hospitals during the various evolutionary phases
▲ The interrelated components of the modern hospital
▲ The factors impacting rising hospital expenditures
▲ Characteristics of the different types of hospitals
▲ Why care continues to evolve from acute care hospitals to outpatient settings

After Studying This Chapter, You'll Be Able To

▲ Diagram the stages of hospital evolution
▲ Describe how power shifted during the evolutionary stages
▲ Analyze the reasons hospital care costs are increasing
▲ Illustrate the relationship between the various hospital components
▲ Compare hospitals according to their classifications
▲ Analyze the factors fostering the competitive environment in health care

Goals and Outcomes

▲ Trace the evolution of American hospitals
▲ Differentiate between types of hospital
▲ Explain how a hospital's classification determines its patient base and the type of care provided
▲ Trace the impact that shorter hospital stays have on other aspects of U.S. health care
▲ Compare the roles and impact of the various hospital components on patient care
▲ Extrapolate the positive and negative impacts on patient care in each of the evolutionary eras
▲ Analyze the impact of outpatient and specialty care clinics of the financial health of traditional hospitals

INTRODUCTION

Hospitals have traditionally been at the center of the U.S. health care system. They have evolved from warehouses for the ill and infirm to modern medical centers. These centers employ hundreds of thousands of people and account for a large portion of U.S. health dollars. American hospitals also include a variety of institutions that serve a multitude of purposes and populations. The American hospital continues to change as economic factors force it to become a more efficient provider and a more competitive institution.

7.1 The Evolution of Hospitals in the United States

Years ago, medical shows on television centered around physicians: *Marcus Welby, M.D., Trapper John M.D., Dr. Kildare.* In today's medical shows and medical shows of the not-too-distant past, hospitals are the main characters: *St. Elsewhere, Chicago Hope, E.R.* The shift is revealing. Although individual care is still dispensed by doctors and nurses (refer to Chapter 5), the organization—in this case, the hospital—is also a pivotal player in how health care is provided.

The country's first hospital opened its doors in 1756. Over the past 250 years, hospitals have undergone many profound changes. Each stage of change—refuge, physician workshop, business, and system—entailed its own challenges, and the group best equipped to deal with them exercised the greatest power. Table 7-1 summarizes the main characteristics and power players of each stage.

7.1.1 Forming Hospitals: The Refuge Stage

The **refuge stage** was a period of institution building. Hospitals were new types of organizations with missions different from that of almshouses (warehouses for the poor, aged, and infirm), from which they evolved. The refuge stage lasted approximately 170 years, from the mid-1700s to the late 1920s.

Pennsylvania Hospital, the nation's first, opened in 1756; New York Hospital, the second, was founded in 1776. By the mid-1850s there were no more than a handful of organizations devoted to providing inpatient health care. A survey conducted in 1873 identified only 178 hospitals.

These early hospitals were very different from hospitals today. Then, medical knowledge was primitive and physicians could do little of value; treatments were primarily supportive rather than curative (alleviating pain, for example, rather than promoting a cure), and many were harmful (the reliance on leeching, for example, for nearly every ailment under the sun). The fact was, in this era, hospitals were dangerous places to be because of the risk of infection, due to the lack of sanitation and the primitive understanding of disease transmission. Patients who were able to pay received private care in their homes, leaving only the less fortunate to the fate of hospitalization.

Table 7-1: Evolution of U.S. Hospitals

Stage	Era	Challenge	Goal	Greatest power or influence
Refuge	Mid-eighteenth century to early twentieth century	Create institutions and raise funds	Provide care	Board members and/or trustees
Physician workshop	1930s to 1960s	Achieve efficacy; expand capacities and competencies	Produce cures	Physicians
Business	Mid-1960s to 1980s	Improve organizational effectiveness and efficiency	Manage growth and increase operational efficiency	Professional health care management personnel
System	Mid-1980s to present day	Improve organizational competitiveness	Combine and integrate health care organizations into self-sustaining health systems	Sharing and collaboration among board, management, insurers, and physicians

Nearly all hospitals were charitable organizations, and the money needed to create and operate them was donated. To survive, hospitals depended on gaining community acceptance and raising funds. Hospital boards, composed of a community's social and financial elite, were the only groups capable of fostering this acceptance (often in the name of religious duty or social obligation to help the less fortunate) and raising the money needed for the hospital's functioning. Consequently, board members possessed power and exercised influence that is hard to imagine today, since they had no one but themselves to answer to and because they, alone, could determine the direction and mission of the hospitals they served.

Despite the problems inherent during this stage, the number of hospitals in America grew from the handful in the late eighteenth century to more than 7000 by 1923. This growth, plus dramatic advances in biomedical science, precipitated the next stage and significantly altered the center of power in hospitals.

FOR EXAMPLE

The Pennsylvania Hospital, 1751–1841

America's first hospital, Pennsylvania Hospital, was founded by Dr. Thomas Bond, a Quaker, and Benjamin Franklin, a founding father, to care for Philadelphia's sick-poor and insane. The hospital contains a 13,000-volume library and America's first surgical amphitheater. In its time, it treated soldiers from every American war, beginning with the Revolutionary War. The hospital seal shows the image of the Good Samaritan and contains these words: "Take care of him and I will repay thee." Today, the hospital is a museum.

7.1.2 Hospitals as the Center of Health Care: Physician Workshop Stage

In the **physician workshop stage,** hospitals sought better and more effective diagnostic tools and treatment strategies. During this stage, the power transferred from the governing boards to the physicians. This stage began in the early 1930s and ended in the 1960s. With the task of institution building complete (refer to Section 7.1.1), hospitals turned toward improving their clinical effectiveness. The reason for the power shift was that physicians, because of their expertise, controlled the knowledge, skills, and technologies that transformed hospitals from offering supportive care to producing cures.

Basic biomedical knowledge, accumulating throughout the middle and late 1800s, reached critical mass in the first decades of the twentieth century, and hospitals were revolutionized in three ways:

▲ Because infections could be partially controlled, hospitals became much safer places.

▲ Treatments were developed that could alter the course of disease.

▲ Thanks to the development of anesthesia, surgery could be safely and effectively performed.

The late John Knowles, MD, former chief executive officer (CEO) of Massachusetts General Hospital, observed, "It was not until about 1915 that the average patient with a common disease entering the average hospital, being treated by the typical physician had a better than 50/50 chance of benefiting from the experience." Because of the improvement in hospital care, those who were able to pay began seeking care in hospitals.

Physicians controlled the knowledge base and flow of patients on which hospitals relied. Accordingly, hospital success became far more dependent on physicians than on trustees. Boards and administrators established the setting and resources employed by physicians, but the hospitals themselves became doctors' workshops. And because all but the simplest cases were treated by them, hospitals became the center of America's health care system.

7.1.3 Becoming More Business Oriented: The Business Stage

In the **business stage,** hospitals had to become more business oriented to provide physicians what they required to practice. As a consequence, far better managerial talent and systems were needed. The business stage ran from the mid-1960s through the 1980s.

Two factors played a large part in spurring the evolution from the physician workshop stage (explained in Section 7.1.2) to the business stage:

▲ Exponentially expanding medical knowledge and skills increased the hospital's size, scope, and complexity. As medical practice became more specialized, the amount and sophistication of facilities, equipment, and support personnel increased dramatically.

▲ The growth of private health insurance, combined with enactment of Medicare and Medicaid in the mid-1960s, infused huge amounts of money into the industry and increased the regulations with which hospitals had to comply.

The most important challenges facing hospitals were managing growth and improving operational effectiveness and efficiency. Professional health care managers acquired power and influence in the process; they moved from being servants of the board (in the refuge stage) and lieutenants of the medical staff (in the physician workshop stage) to full-fledged executives responsible for directing the affairs of complex, multimillion-dollar organizations.

At the beginning of this stage, a little more than 5 percent of the nation's gross domestic product was spent on health care; by 1985 the figure was 10 percent. Health care was now big business.

7.1.4 Managing Complex Systems: The System Stage

The **system stage** focused on forming and managing a diverse array of enterprises and relationships that allow hospitals to compete in markets undergoing significant change. This challenge requires high levels of coordination among boards, between management teams and physicians, and across organizations. As a consequence, power and influence are increasingly shared. The system stage began in the mid-1980s and continues to the present day.

Three developments define the system stage:

▲ **Increasing consolidation:** Health care organizations consolidated. Many hospitals, for example, merged and then combined with physician practices, nursing homes, and health insurance plans. Health systems (refer to Chapter 1) were created.

▲ **Greater competition:** As the industry became far more competitive, not only did health systems and hospitals compete with each other, but they also began competing with their own medical staffs, insurance companies, and managed care organizations. (You can read more about the competition hospitals face in the later section "Care and Competition in the Twenty-First Century.")

▲ **Dramatic changes in the nature and form of payment:** As change occurred in how providers were paid (explained in Section 4.2), purchasers sought to control double-digit inflation in their health care expenditures. Throughout the 1960s and 1970s, hospitals were reimbursed on the basis of their charges or incurred costs; physicians received fees or customary charges. In the 1980s, hospitals started being paid rates that were set prospectively (irrespective of their incurred costs), assuming some of the financial risk associated with providing services. Additionally, doctors, hospitals, and other health care organizations had to cooperate in order to offer the full spectrum of services demanded by purchasers.

SELF-CHECK

- List the four evolutionary stages of hospitals in the U.S. health care system; identify the main goal of each period.
- Describe the main difference between the business stage and the system stage.

7.2 Components and Cost of American Hospitals

There are just under 6000 hospitals in the country with about 1 million hospital beds; they admit more than 34 million patients each year, and employ 6 million people. Although hospitals provide outpatient services just as many ambulatory health care centers do, they are unique in the health care system because of their focus on inpatient services. Hospitals are the only health care organizations equipped and staffed to serve patients who require at least an overnight stay; all other patients can be treated elsewhere. During their stay, patients receive intensive, round-the-clock nursing care.

7.2.1 Hospital Components

The typical hospital is composed of four distinct, but highly interdependent, components (shown in Figure 7-1):

Figure 7-1

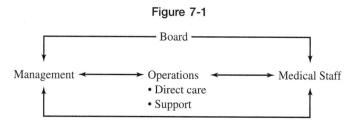

The interdependent components of the typical hospital.

▲ **The board:** The **board** is responsible for governing the hospital on behalf of its "owners"—the community in a nonprofit hospital, shareholders in a proprietary hospital, or constituents in a governmental hospital.

▲ **Management:** Management is accountable to the board for running the organization on a day-to-day basis—strategically, financially, and operationally. Typically, management is thought of as carrying out board directives. However, given the complexity of the contemporary hospital, executives are board partners in formulating an organization's vision and mission, goals, objectives, and policies.

▲ **Medical staff:** The medical staff provides, and directs provision of, clinical care within the hospital. Its members are physicians and sometimes other health care professionals (such as dentists and podiatrists) appointed by the board. In most hospitals, physicians are not employees. Rather, they are independent practitioners who use the hospital for the care of their patients. Go to Section 5.2 for information on the types of physicians and the organization of their work.

▲ **Operational staff:** The hospital's operational staff is responsible for performing nonmedical, clinical (for example, nursing), and support ("hotel" service, administrative, and technical) work. This component is directly accountable to management but influenced by members of the medical staff.

The interaction between these components becomes even more complex when you consider that many hospitals are affiliated with, or owned by, health care systems. For information on health systems, refer to Section 1.3.

7.2.2 Hospital Costs

Hospitals are the heavyweights of the health care industry. Expenditures for hospital care have increased from $9 billion in 1960 to more than $400 billion in 2000 (see Figure 7-2) and now account for about one-third of all health care expenditures.

Figure 7-2

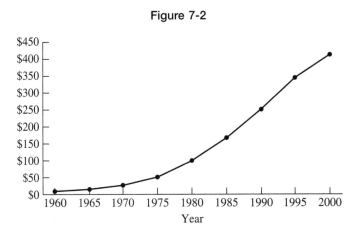

The rising costs of hospital care in billions of dollars.

The increasing costs are due to a host of factors:

▲ **Advancement of medical technologies and treatments;** These technologies enable hospitals to care and treat patients much more effectively; however, they are extremely expensive and the cost must be passed on to the patient.

▲ **Cost of prescription drugs:** Some experts believe that these costs, which also must be passed on to the patient, contribute as much as 20 percent to the overall increase of health care costs.

▲ **Aging population:** As a significant portion of the U.S. population gets older, more health care services are required. This causes a dramatic rise in the cost of hospital care.

▲ **Lifestyle choices:** Smoking, bad diet, lack of exercise, and other poor lifestyle choices increase the number of patients needing hospital treatment which also increase costs.

▲ **Increased governmental regulations and oversight:** Governmental and regulatory agency policies, laws, and regulations such as the Health Insurance Portability and Account Act (HIPPA) and others, are aimed at benefiting patients; however, they also increase overall health care costs because of the costs needed for health care organizations to comply.

SELF-CHECK

- Describe the four interdependent components of the modern hospital.
- Name two reasons why hospital costs are increasing.

7.3 Classifying Hospitals

When people think of hospitals, they generally think of their community hospitals: nongovernmental, short-term, acute care, general facilities. Certainly an organization of this kind is the mainstay of the nation's health system and one of a community's most important resources. The 5000 community hospitals in the United States provide a vast array of inpatient, outpatient, and emergency services; employ hundreds of people both full and part time; and manage budgets into the millions (see Table 7-2).

Table 7-2: Profile of the Community Hospital

Criterion	Total	Per hospital
Inpatient		
Beds	830,000	170
Admissions	32,359,000	6,500
Inpatient days	191,824,000	39,000
Average length of stay (days)	6	
Inpatient surgeries	9,540,000	1,900
Births	3,760,000	760
Outpatient		
Total outpatient visits	495,346,000	100,000
Emergency room visits	99,484,000	20,000
Outpatient surgeries	15,845,000	3,200
Personnel		
Total full time	3,298,000	670
Total part time	1,247,000	250
Financial statistics		
Gross revenue, inpatient	$436 billion	$88 million
Gross revenue, outpatient	$224 billion	$45 million
Total expenses	$335 billion	$68 million
Net margin	$16 billion	$3 million

The traditional community hospital, however, is not the only type of inpatient health care facility in the United States. In fact, many different types of hospitals exist, as the following sections explain.

Hospitals are typically classified by the following criteria:

▲ Length of stay.
▲ Type of service.
▲ Ownership.

Keep in mind that these designations are not exclusive. A single hospital can be a long-term, specialty care state hospital, for example.

7.3.1 Length of Stay: Short- and Long-Term Hospitals

Hospitals can be either short term or long term.

▲ **Short-term hospitals:** These hospitals treat individuals with acute problems requiring inpatient stays that average about five days; the typical community hospital is a short-stay facility.

The United States has nearly 6000 short-term hospitals that accommodate approximately 35 million inpatient visits and 85 million outpatient visits (see Table 7-3 for more statistics).

▲ **Long-term hospitals:** These facilities treat individuals with chronic conditions requiring stays that can range from a month to several years; examples are psychiatric, chronic disease, and rehabilitation facilities. See Table 7-4.

7.3.2 Type of Service: General and Specialty Hospitals

Hospitals can offer either general or specialty services. About 70 percent of the nation's hospitals are in the general category; the remainder are specialty hospitals.

Table 7-3: General, Short-Stay Hospital Statistics

Item	Amount
Organizations	5,800
Beds	1 million
Average beds occupied	66%
Average hospital size	170 beds
Annual inpatient admissions	35 million
Average inpatient stay	6.8 days
Annual outpatient visits	85 million
Annual emergency room visits	108 million
Annual expenditures	$412 billion

Table 7-4: General, Long-Stay Hospital Statistics

Item	Amount
Organizations	340 certified long-term-stay hospitals
Average beds occupied	31
Annual inpatient admissions	4.3 million
Average inpatient stay	61 days
Annual Medicare expenditures	2.8 billion

▲ **General hospitals:** Hospitals that offer an array of medical and surgical services.

▲ **Specialty hospitals:** Hospitals that treat a narrow range of patients— children, women, or those with a specific condition such as cancer or orthopedic problems.

Many of the nation's general hospitals are also public hospitals. As such, their bylaws or charters require that they accept patients regardless of their ability to pay. Many specialty hospitals, on the other hand, are privately owned and can limit their services to paying patients. The result is a large disparity between general and specialty hospitals in terms of their budgets, their expenditures, and the cost controls each must implement. The specialty hospital can focus on one or two areas of care and only take those patients who have the ability to pay; this strategy helps increase hospital profits.

The general hospital, on the other hand, typically covers the costs of its nonpaying and uninsured patients by passing on the cost to those patients who can pay and who seek care within the hospital's specialty areas, such as the orthopedics department or heart care clinic. For this reason, many general, public hospitals now deliver more specialized services both to compete with the specialty hospitals and as a way of off-setting the costs of caring for uninsured patients.

7.3.3 Ownership: Nonprofit, Proprietary, and Governmental

All hospitals—even state and federal hospitals—have an ownership designation. The people or entity owning the hospital determine the ownership classification. The major classifications are nonprofit, proprietary, federal government, and state or local government:

▲ **Nonprofit hospitals:** Typically referred to as voluntary hospitals, nonprofit hospitals are organized as 501(c)(3) tax-exempt corporations. They are "owned" by the community in which they operate, or by other charitable

FOR EXAMPLE

The Health of State Hospitals

Like many states, Alabama and Michigan have had to make the difficult decision to close state-run mental health hospitals. How well these closings go depend on what community resources and care facilities are in place to absorb the displaced residents and patients. When Michigan closed several of its hospitals between 1991 and 1999, the community-based system was not able to sufficiently address the needs of the patients. Alabama hopes to avoid that problem by creating new regional treatment areas that will retain a team of specializing physicians, nurses, psychiatrists, and dentists and by adding beds at two state psychiatric hospitals.

organizations such as religious congregations, fraternal organizations, and associations.

▲ **Proprietary hospitals:** Also called for-profit or investor-owned, these hospitals are operated for the purpose of producing a return for their investors. Throughout most of the twentieth century, the typical proprietary hospital was locally owned by an individual or a group of physicians. Beginning in the 1960s, many of these institutions were bought by commercial stock corporations, which, during the 1980s and1990s, increased the number of beds through building programs and by acquiring non-profit facilities.

▲ **Federal hospitals:** These hospitals, which include veteran's hospitals, are operated by the federal government and are paid for in part by tax dollars.

▲ **State or local hospitals:** These hospitals are run by state and local governments and are paid for by tax dollars. They can be specialty hospitals, such as mental health facilities or community hospitals.

SELF-CHECK

- List the criteria used to classify hospitals.
- Which type of hospitals is more common: general or specialty? Explain why.

7.4 Care and Competition in the Twenty-First Century

As discussed in Section 7.1, the American hospital has evolved from a repository for the poor with hopeless medical conditions to the site of our nation's most sophisticated diagnostic and therapeutic capabilities. The American hospital, however, has not reached its final iteration. The evolution of hospital care continues today, impacting patient care and fostering more intense competition among health care providers.

7.4.1 Hospital Care

The acute care hospital has been the base of the U.S. health care system for most of the last 100 years (refer to Section 7.1), yet the role of the acute care hospital is rapidly diminishing as more care is provided in outpatient settings. The escalating costs of hospitalization are partly responsible for this shift from hospital care to ambulatory and other sectors of care, even though these changes have not translated into cost savings. What this change has done, however, is produce a domino effect on the care of patients and the role of physicians:

- ▲ **Effect 1:** With the increasing shift of care to ambulatory settings and other types of health care organizations (such as home health agencies and long-term-care facilities), today's hospitals provide the most intense services to the sickest patients requiring the greatest amount of care.
- ▲ **Effect 2:** As the length of hospital stays has shortened (another cost-cutting measure), patients discharged from hospitals frequently need considerable medical and nursing care after discharge.
- ▲ **Effect 3:** As inpatient care has become more intensive and patients are discharged earlier, ambulatory care has become more demanding for two reasons: First, ambulatory care settings have to absorb the health care demands of patients whose illnesses no longer qualified for inpatient treatment. Second, they have to offer more intensive care to people who received inpatient care but were discharged sooner.
- ▲ **Effect 4:** The pressures of outpatient care have made it more difficult and less efficient for primary care physicians to remain involved with inpatient care. Whereas 20 years ago, many primary care physicians cared for up to 10 inpatients on any given day, that number has dropped to 1 or 2 today.
- ▲ **Effect 5:** As primary care physicians become less involved in inpatient care, this care is now increasingly being provided by dedicated hospital physicians, called *hospitalists*. (Some preliminary data suggest that hospitalist care may reduce lengths of stay and costs of hospitalization without compromising quality of care. For more information about hospitalists and their role in health care organizations, refer to Section 3.5.4.)

FOR EXAMPLE

Cost Savings?

As hospitals (and managed care organizations; see Section 12.2) try to contain costs by implementing shorter stays for inpatient procedures, some evidence suggests that the savings may not be that significant. According to a 2000 study, the savings of shorter length of stay is minimal. The reason? The first days in the hospital consume the most resources and therefore incur the most expenses. Thus, researchers suggest that a more effective cost-saving strategy would be one that addresses those first days in the hospital.

7.4.2 Competition in Health Care

Only a few decades ago, health care organizations didn't have much competition (or at least refused to acknowledge it). As the United States produced more and more physicians and created more and more hospital space—so much so, in fact, that there is now an overabundance of both—the competitive landscape in health care changed and health care costs began to rise. The result is a health care industry that is far more competitive today than in years past. Not only do health systems and hospitals compete against each other, but they also compete with their own medical staffs, insurance companies, and managed care organizations. Following are just a few of the pressures that health care organizations face:

▲ **Competition for insured patients' business:** Because insured patients now are more portable and are able and willing to receive services outside their immediate geographical area, health care organizations must work to attract these patients.

▲ **Technological advances:** The health systems with the latest technology attract the most affluent (in terms of ability to pay) patients. For this reason, hospitals strive to acquire the latest technology and promote its benefits to the communities that they serve.

▲ **Accountability:** With recent regulations and laws promoting accountability in health care, the health systems that are the most accountable may get more funding.

▲ **Marketing strategies:** Fierce marketing efforts have skyrocketed among health care organizations.

▲ **Availability of specialty services:** Specialty services have grown. The health care organizations that can provide these much-sought-after services are at an advantage.

▲ **Increase in outpatient clinics:** The growing number of outpatient clinics have taken business away from the traditional hospital, where these services were once given as a matter of course. Outpatient clinics, because of their easy access and their specialization, tend to attract paying patients away from hospital settings.

▲ **The growth of larger health systems:** Vertical integration of various health care organizations into larger systems (refer to Section 1.3) has contributed to the competitive atmosphere. What were once allied health care organizations are now competitors for the same business.

▲ **Staffing:** Health systems compete for physicians and support staff, particularly nurses, who are in short supply in many health care organizations.

This pervasive competition has had both a positive and a negative effect on health care. In some ways, the competition has driven down costs. Just as in any business, competition spurs an organization to deliver its product in more cost-efficient ways. The same is true for health organizations. Similarly, quality of care, to a degree, has increased because of the competition for better treatment technologies. Nevertheless, the competitive landscape in health care has also had negative implications: First, the bureaucracy of health care has grown as the systems, laws, and regulations become more complex. In addition, the increased presence and use of specialty hospitals by insured patients has caused some general nonprofit hospitals major financial problems and cost shifting has become more prevalent.

SELF-CHECK

- Trace the genesis of the hospitalist role to the intensity of outpatient care.
- Identify three pressures health care organizations face in today's competitive environment.

SUMMARY

Hospitals have long been the main providers of health care in the United States. Their evolution began in the mid-seventeenth century and continues today. To provide the care people have come to expect, hospitals rely on medical staff, operational staff, administrators, and boards of directors. American hospitals are classified by a number of criteria indicating the populations they serve, the type of care they provide, and the people or entity that owns them. As health care in the United States continues to evolve, so too does the American hospital.

KEY TERMS

Board	The entity responsible for governing the hospital on behalf of its "owners"—the community in a nonprofit hospital, shareholders in a proprietary hospital, or constituents in a governmental hospital.
Business stage	Evolutionary stage of hospital development in which hospitals became more business oriented to provide physicians what they required to practice.
Federal hospitals	Hospitals operated by the federal government and paid for in part by tax dollars.
General hospitals	Hospitals that offer an array of medical and surgical services.
Long-term hospitals	Hospitals that treat individuals with chronic conditions requiring stays that can range from a month to several years; examples are psychiatric, chronic disease, and rehabilitation facilities.
Nonprofit hospitals	Hospitals that are organized as 501(c)(3) tax-exempt corporations. They are "owned" by the community in which they operate, or by other charitable organizations such as religious congregations, fraternal organizations, and associations.
Physician workshop stage	Evolutionary stage of hospital development in which hospitals sought better and more effective diagnostic tools and treatment strategies.
Proprietary hospitals	Hospitals operated for the purpose of producing a return for their investors.
Refuge stage	Evolutionary stage of hospital development characterized by institution building.
Short-term hospitals	Hospitals that treat individuals with acute problems requiring inpatient stays that average about five days.
Specialty hospitals	Hospitals that treat a narrow range of patients—children, women, or those with a specific condition such as cancer or orthopedic problems.

State or local hospitals   Hospitals that are run by state and local govern-
                                      ments and are paid for by tax dollars. They can
                                      be specialty hospitals, such as mental health fa-
                                      cilities or community hospitals.

System stage   Evolutionary stage of hospital development
                                      characterized by a focus on forming and manag-
                                      ing a diverse array of enterprises and relation-
                                      ships that allow hospitals to compete in current
                                      markets.

ASSESS YOUR UNDERSTANDING

Go to www.wiley.com/college/pointer to evaluate your knowledge of U.S. hospitals. *Measure your learning by comparing pre-test and post-test results.*

Summary Questions

1. Which stage in hospital evolution was marked by profound medical breakthroughs?
   (a) refuge stage
   (b) physician workshop stage
   (c) business stage
   (d) system stage

2. Which stage in hospital evolution focused on growth and operational efficiency?
   (a) refuge stage
   (b) physician workshop stage
   (c) business stage
   (d) system stage

3. In what way are hospitals unique in the U.S. health care system?
   (a) they provide state-of-the-art medical care
   (b) they are private enterprises that perform public functions
   (c) they are the only facilities equipped to care for patients overnight
   (d) they are the only facilities equipped to provide emergency care around the clock

4. Identify which component—board, management, medical staff, or operational staff—each of the following represents:
   (a) surgical nurses
   (b) bill collection
   (c) director of operations
   (d) food service

5. Who owns governmental hospitals?
   (a) the board of directors
   (b) taxpayers
   (c) the government
   (d) physicians who work there

6. How does a specialty hospital differ from a general hospital?
   (a) it focuses on a particular health issue or a special population
   (b) it generally requires greater lengths of stay

(c) its staff is comprised solely of specialists

(d) all of the above

7. The next phase of hospital evolution shifts from hospital care to outpatient care. What is one of the reasons for this shift?

(a) overburdened hospital medical staff

(b) creation of independent emergency care facilities

(c) rising health costs

(d) falling numbers of community hospitals

8. How is the role of the acute care hospital changing?

(a) the role of hospitals is growing as more people seek medical care in the hospital setting

(b) the role of hospitals is diminishing as more people seek medical care in outpatient settings

(c) the role of hospitals is diminishing partly because of the expense of hospital care

(d) b and c

Review Questions

1. What stigma did early hospitals have to overcome?

(a) that they were staffed by incompetent physicians

(b) that they were unclean and primarily places for the poor

(c) that they offered little in the way of effective treatment

(d) b and c

(e) all of the above

2. In what way can the medical staff of a hospital be considered the most autonomous of the four components?

(a) they provide clinical care and therefore are indispensable to the hospital's functioning

(b) they are board appointed and therefore not answerable to management

(c) because the hospital doesn't employ them, they are independent practitioners

(d) all of the above

3. What influence does the hospital board have on management, medical staff, and operational staff?

4. Indicate what type of length of stay, service, and ownership designations each of the following hospitals would have:

(a) a mental health hospital run by the state

(b) a VA hospital

(c) an acute care community hospital that is owned by a health care maintenance organization and private stock holders

(d) a children's chronic and catastrophic care hospital run by a board of trustees

5. Offer a reason why the United States has more nonprofit hospitals than proprietary hospitals.

6. How has inpatient care changed during the last few years?

(a) because patients are sicker when admitted to the hospital, they require more intensive care

(b) hospital cost-cutting measures reduce length of stay, so patients leave the hospital before they are well

(c) hospitalists now deliver more inpatient care, whereas family doctors provide less care

(d) a and b

(e) all of the above

7. Which of the following is responsible for the increasing competition between health care organizations?

(a) overabundance of hospital space

(b) number of insured patients vs. uninsured patients

(c) increase in specialty services and outpatient clinics

(d) a and c

(e) all of the above

Applying This Chapter

1. Explain how hospitals overcame their reputations as dangerous places.
2. In what way is the medical staff influenced by other hospital components?
3. Argue both for and against shorter hospital stays.
4. Explain the relationship between the increasing number of outpatient and specialty services and the increasingly competitive environment in the health care field.

YOU TRY IT

The Evolution of Hospitals in the United States

Discuss what impact each evolutionary stage of hospital development has had on patient care. Which stage, in your opinion, has had the greatest positive impact? Negative impact? Explain your answers.

Components and Cost of American Hospitals

The United States is experiencing a backlash against managed care—specifically that nonmedical personnel (HMOs, hospital administrators, etc.) are having undue influence on medical decisions. What impact, if any, do you think this will have on future hospital power structures?

Classifying Hospitals

If hospitals take care of the sickest patients, how is it that outpatient centers are under more stress?

Care and Competition in the Twenty-First Century

In a health system in which patient choices regarding heatlh care providers are limited (insurers often determine which health care organization can provide care to their members, for example, or a smaller community may have only one hospital), explain why health care organizations engage in marketing compaigns.

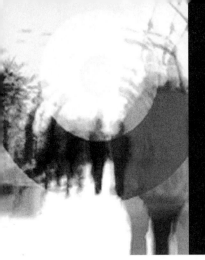

8

AMBULATORY CARE
Understanding Outpatient Health Services

Starting Point

Go to www.wiley.com/college/pointer to assess your knowledge of the basics of ambulatory care
Determine where you need to concentrate your effort.

What You'll Learn in This Chapter

▲ The definition of *ambulatory care*
▲ How ambulatory care services are accessed and paid for
▲ The accreditation process of ambulatory care facilities
▲ Who the ambulatory care providers are
▲ Characteristics of in-home ambulatory care

After Studying This Chapter, You'll Be Able To

▲ Differentiate ambulatory care from inpatient care
▲ Identify ambulatory care settings
▲ Recognize ambulatory care services and service providers
▲ Articulate the advantages and disadvantages of ambulatory care

Goals and Outcomes

▲ Master terminology relating to ambulatory care, care settings, and service providers
▲ Articulate the reasons for the growing importance of ambulatory care in U.S. health care
▲ Compare different types of ambulatory care settings
▲ Identify which ambulatory care settings are most appropriate for different health issues
▲ Explain the impact that the growing reliance on ambulatory care is having on inpatient and outpatient health services
▲ Evaluate ambulatory care as an alternative to inpatient care

INTRODUCTION

Ambulatory care is the backbone of the nation's personal health care system. As medical advances make diagnosis and treatments less invasive, and as rising costs of health care make inpatient care less cost effective, ambulatory care services have expanded. Most ambulatory care is provided in health care facilities such as hospitals, doctors' offices, and community health clinics. But, as home health care becomes more common, health professionals can also provide ambulatory care in patients' homes.

8.1 Understanding Ambulatory Care

Ambulatory care, despite its slightly misleading name, is an easy concept to grasp: It simply refers to any medical service—curative, investigative, and so on—provided to patients on an outpatient basis (that is, services that don't require admission to a hospital). Ambulatory care is the backbone of the U.S. personal health care system.

This type of care is important for several reasons:

▲ The vast majority of health care is provided on an ambulatory basis.
▲ An ambulatory care visit is the initial point of contact between patients and other system components.
▲ An increasing number of diagnostic and therapeutic procedures are now being carried out in ambulatory care settings.

To get an idea of the importance of ambulatory care in U.S. medicine, consider these facts about the primary ambulatory care setting—the doctor's office (the following information comes from a 2000 survey conducted by the National Center for Health Statistics):

▲ During the year, each person in the United States visited physicians an average of three times, totally 824 million physician visits.
▲ In 96 percent of these 824 million visits, patients were seen by physicians.
▲ Of the visits, most patients sought general health care (family practice, pediatrics, internal medicine, and so forth). The following table shows the distribution of these visits across specialty:

Area of Practice	Percentage of Visits
General and family practice	24
Internal medicine	15
Pediatrics	13

Area of Practice	Percentage of Visits
Obstetrics and gynecology	8
Orthopedic surgery	6
Ophthalmology	5
All others	29

▲ Sixty percent of patient–physician contacts were 1 to 15 minutes in length.

▲ About half of all visits were scheduled because of specific symptoms. Thirty-five percent of all visits were for acute problems (50 percent in patients under 15 years of age).

▲ At least one therapeutic or preventive service was ordered or provided during 35 percent of all visits.

▲ Sixty-six percent of visits resulted in prescription of pharmaceuticals.

8.1.1 The Growing Reliance on Ambulatory Care

Today, patients can receive in ambulatory care settings medical treatment that years ago had to be conducted in hospitals during an inpatient stay. In fact, not only *can* they receive complex treatment in ambulatory care settings, it is *expected* that they do so. The reasons for the reliance on ambulatory care settings to conduct ever more complex medical procedures include the following:

▲ **Dramatic advances in technology:** Advances in medical technology have created more effective and less intrusive diagnostic and treatment strategies. For example, many medical investigations that used to routinely require hospitalization, such as blood tests, X-rays, endoscopy, and even biopsies, can now be performed in outpatient settings. See Section 6.1 for more information on the impact of medical technological advances on the U.S. health care system.

▲ **Changes in financial incentives:** As health care costs skyrocket, insurers and providers look for ways to manage these increasing costs. Because ambulatory care is markedly less expensive than inpatient hospital care, significant savings can be realized by providing care—diagnostic, curative, and follow-up—in these settings. You can read more about the types of ambulatory services provided in Section 8.2.

▲ **Demands for greater patient convenience:** As the U.S. population has gone from accessing health care occasionally and for specific medical needs to accessing it regularly for preventive care, patients expect easier access to the services. Community health centers and physicians' offices, ample parking, and more accommodating scheduling are more likely in ambulatory settings than hospital settings.

8.1.2 Accessing Ambulatory Care

People access ambulatory care for a number of reasons. The most frequently cited reasons for visits (in order of magnitude) are:

- ▲ Follow-up care.
- ▲ Cough or throat conditions.
- ▲ Routine prenatal care.
- ▲ Postoperative care.
- ▲ Well-baby exams.
- ▲ Vision problems.
- ▲ Ear aches or infections.
- ▲ Back problems.
- ▲ Joint problems.
- ▲ Fever and skin rashes.

Despite the primacy of ambulatory care in dispensing health care services, access to and use of ambulatory care varies considerably with an individual's social, economic, and demographic characteristics. As Table 8-1 shows, a person's age, gender, race, and insurance status all impact whether he or she is more likely or not to take advantage of the health care resources in the United States.

8.1.3 Paying for Ambulatory Care

As you can see in Table 8-1, of all the factors, insurance status—not surprisingly—has the most profound impact on whether someone accesses health care. Consider these statistics:

- ▲ The source of payment for visits was private insurance (57 percent); Medicare (20 percent); Medicaid (9 percent); self-pay (9 percent); workers' compensation (2 percent); no charge (1 percent), or other (about 7 percent).
- ▲ Thirty percent of visits were by patients with some form of HMO coverage.
- ▲ One-third of physicians do not accept charity patients, 10 percent do not accept new Medicare patients, and 22 percent do not accept new Medicaid patients.

Furthermore, outpatient services delivered in ambulatory settings, as a rule, cost less than the same services delivered in hospital settings. In 2003, the Health and Human Services Office of the Inspector General recommended that set reimbursement rates be established for services, regardless of the setting, barring any compelling reason for the difference. If enacted, the OIG estimates that it could save $1.1 billion annually if it lowered the hospital reimbursement rates to the rates paid to ambulatory care settings.

Table 8-1: Adults (18–64) with No Regular Source of Care

Category	Percentage
All	18
Age	
18–24	27
25–44	20
45–54	12
55–64	9
Gender	
Male	24
Female	12
Race	
White	17
Black	19
Hispanic	31
Insurance status	
Insured	11
Uninsured	47

The implications of these facts are far-reaching, both in terms of health care costs and the health status of the U.S. population. To learn more about how the U.S. health care system is financed, refer to Section 4.2; Section 12.2 examines the financial challenges the U.S. health system will face in the coming years.

8.1.4 Ambulatory Care Accreditation

Like other health care organizations, ambulatory care organizations are subject to accreditation. Accreditation is a process in which an organization is able to measure quality and performance against national standards. Accreditation demonstrates to stakeholders that the health care organization has met certain standards and is performing well. Accrediting processes typically include a self-evaluation along with consultations and reviews by expert reviewers from the same field. These reviewers provide an outside viewpoint of an organization's performance. Accreditation is granted for a given time period and must be reviewed and renewed at regular intervals.

FOR EXAMPLE

Setting Ambulatory Care Quality Standards

In 2004, the Agency for Healthcare Research and Quality (AHRQ), America's Health Insurance Plans (AHIP), the American Academy of Family Physicians (AAFP), and the American College of Physicians (ACP) formed the Ambulatory Care Quality Alliance (AQA), a collaborative group whose mission was to create a set of standards against which ambulatory care providers could be measured. The subsequent performance measures, approved in April of 2005, include standards for preventive screening (for breast, colorectal, and cervical cancers, for example); management of chronic medical conditions such as heart disease, diabetes, asthma, and depression; and appropriate use of resources (for example, the overuse of antibiotics for childhood respiratory infections).

Several accrediting bodies exist that serve this function. Specifically for ambulatory organizations, the Accreditation Association for Ambulatory Health Care (AAAHC) is one of the major accrediting associations, setting standards across over 2500 organizations. The Joint Commission on Accreditation of Healthcare Organizations' (JCAHO) Ambulatory Care Accreditation program also accredits organizations on a national level.

SELF-CHECK

- Define **ambulatory care**.
- Name three reasons why more and more people seek ambulatory care.
- Identify the populations least likely to access or make use of ambulatory care.

8.2 Ambulatory Care Settings and Providers

A variety of health care providers provide ambulatory medical services. The following list includes several of the most common (go to Chapter 5 for more information about health care providers):

▲ Physicians.

▲ Physician assistants.

▲ Nurses.
▲ Dentists.
▲ Pharmacists.
▲ Chiropractors.
▲ Podiatrists.
▲ Physical therapists.
▲ Optometrists.
▲ Occupational therapists.
▲ Psychologists.
▲ Clinical social workers.

Patients receive ambulatory care in a number of settings: physicians' offices, urgent care facilities, same-day surgery centers, and so on. And, although the term itself refers to medical services that are provided on an outpatient basis, groups providing these services can also be housed in hospitals. (Remember, the key to ambulatory care isn't defined by the setting, but by the service provided.)

8.2.1 Physician Offices: Solo and Group Practices

The most common site of ambulatory care is the doctor's office. Ambulatory care provided by physicians isn't limited to general health care or general practitioners. Physicians from many specialties, including family medicine, internal medicine, obstetrics, gynecology, cardiology, gastroenterology, ophthalmology, and dermatology, deliver ambulatory care.

▲ **Solo practices:** physician practices consisting of an individual physician, generally assisted by several clinical and administrative personnel. Throughout most of the twentieth century, solo practice physicians provided most office-based ambulatory services. This trend, however, is changing as more physicians practice in groups rather than alone. Today more than two-thirds of all ambulatory care visits are to physicians engaged in some form of group practice.

▲ **Group practices** are the collective effort of three or more physicians, often complemented by other health care professionals, who share resources (facilities, personnel, systems), pool expenses and income, and collaborate in the care of patients.

The shift from solo to group practice is a result of

▲ The increasing complexity of medicine.
▲ The administrative burdens imposed by patient billing, filing insurance claims, and negotiating managed care contracts.
▲ The increasing cost of setting up and running a practice.

Figure 8-1

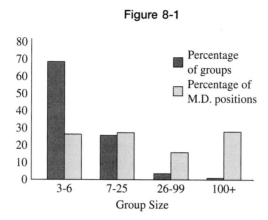

The size distribution of physician group practices.

Between 1969 and 1999, the number of physician groups grew from about 6000 to 21,000 (a threefold increase); during the same period the number of physicians participating in group practices increased from 40,000 to 214,000 (a fivefold increase).

Two principle types of group practices exist:

▲ **Single-specialty groups:** In these practices, physicians are members of the same medical or surgical specialty. These make up about 70 percent of physician groups.

▲ **Multispecialty groups:** These practices are composed of physicians representing various specialties.

As portrayed in Figure 8-1, groups vary considerably by size. Although 95 percent of physician groups have fewer than 25 members, 45 percent of the total number of physicians practicing in groups practice in groups with more than 25 members.

8.2.2 Emergency Rooms and Hospital Outpatient Departments

In addition to inpatient services, hospitals also offer many of the same ambulatory care services that independent group practices or community centers offer: same-day surgery and diagnoses, follow-up care, acute care, and so on. Often patients access these services through emergency room visits. (Remember: If the visit to the emergency room results in a hospital admission, then that visit is actually an emergency medicine visit, rather than ambulatory care.)

In a study conducted by researchers at the Johns Hopkins School of Public Health (published in 2000) comparing health care provided by physicians' offices, community health centers, and hospital outpatient departments, the researchers reached two interesting conclusions:

▲ Continuity of care was better in community health centers than in either physicians' offices or hospital outpatient departments.

▲ Patients who visited hospital outpatient departments underwent more imaging studies (MRIs) and minor surgeries, and were referred more often to specialists, than those seen in either physicians' offices or community health centers. The researchers speculate that, because people visit outpatient departments sporadically, continuity of care is more difficult to achieve. The result is that health care providers are often unfamiliar with their patients' health histories and so are forced to treat more aggressively.

This study brings into question whether hospital outpatient departments are suitable settings for providing adequate ambulatory care.

8.2.3 Urgent Care Facilities

Urgent care facilities evaluate and treat conditions that aren't severe enough to require an emergency room visit but that are serious enough to require treatment beyond normal physician office hours or before a physician appointment is available.

The Urgent Care Association of America (UCAOA) estimates that the nation has over 15,000 urgent care centers. These centers can treat many of the same problems that patients traditionally go to a primary care doctor for, but they include some services that primary care physicians, as a rule, don't offer, such as X-ray facilities and minor trauma rooms.

Like hospital emergency departments, urgent care centers don't "establish" patients as primary care physicians do because patients are seen on an episodic basis rather an ongoing basis. Essentially, urgent care centers are where patients go when they need medical attention (for an injury or an illness) but can't access their primary care provider either because the office is closed or a timely appointment can't be scheduled. In some instances, patients in this position go to the emergency room, but because these issues are not generally true emergencies, they are more suitably (and more economically) treated in urgent care centers.

8.2.4 Same-Day Surgery Centers

In the not-too-distant past, even common surgeries would often take hours, and recovery periods would often require a fairly lengthy hospital stay. Advances in surgical techniques and anesthetics, however, have changed that. Consider the following:

▲ Today, most surgical procedures can be performed in a little over an hour or less.

▲ Newer anesthetics have eliminated much of the nausea and grogginess of earlier drugs, allowing patients to more quickly and easily recover.

▲ The increasing use of minimally invasive techniques means that patients can recover more quickly, with less pain, discomfort, and scarring.

For these reasons, many surgeries are no longer performed in hospitals. Whereas 15 years ago, only one out of six operations was a same-day procedure, today two out of three are. Many of these same-day procedures are performed in surgery centers. Each center offers its own range of surgeries:

▲ **General surgery centers:** General surgery refers to most surgeries usually involving the abdomen and its contents. These centers perform general surgeries such as hernia, intestinal, and gall bladder surgeries, and so on.

▲ **Specialized surgery centers:** These centers perform more specialized surgeries such as orthopedic surgery, otolaryngological (ear, nose, throat) surgery, plastic surgery, and in some cases, obstetric and gynecological surgeries.

▲ **Combined surgery centers:** These centers offer a mix of general and specialized surgeries.

8.2.5 Community Health Centers or Clinics

Community health centers or clinics are organizations that provide health care services to poor or uninsured members of the community. These centers are community-based primary care facilities that provide medical care in medically underserved areas or to medically underserved populations (these designations are made by the U.S. Department of Health and Human Services). To qualify as a community health center (and to receive government funding), health organizations generally have to enter into a contractual agreement with the state (or local) department of health services. These agreements stipulate what services are provided and to whom they are made available. For example, many state governments require that their community health centers provide the following health services to their indigent patients:

▲ Prenatal care.

▲ Diagnostic services.

▲ Pharmacy services.

▲ Preventive health services.

▲ Preventive dental services.

▲ Emergency care.

In addition, the person receiving the health care generally has to meet one (or more) of the following criteria:

▲ Be a resident of the state.

▲ Be without medical insurance policy coverage.

▲ Be considered poor. Often this requirement is based on parameters set by the state. For example, in Arizona, a qualifying person must not have a family income of more than 200% of the federal poverty guidelines established by the U.S. Department of Health and Human Services.

▲ Not be eligible for state or federal indigent insurance programs.

8.2.6 Student Health Centers or Clinics

Student health centers or clinics are medical facilities located in university settings and designed to address the needs of students. The services provided at these clinics often include things such as

▲ Primary health care services (physical exams, preventive care, and so on).

▲ Diagnostic services (for example, laboratory and X-ray services).

▲ Mental health services and crisis consultation.

▲ First aid and urgent care.

▲ Medical recommendations for the campus (for example, disease prevention initiatives).

FOR EXAMPLE

Improving Quality of Care at Community Clinics

Ensuring that people in underserved areas receive the medical care they need can be challenging, particularly when you consider that there may be many obstacles to care, including language barriers, lack of information about prevalent health conditions, and lack of awareness that the care is available. Like health clinics around the country, Community Health Clinics in San Mateo Country, California, seek to address these issues through public health initiatives that improve both access and quality of care to their clients. The plan includes assigning all patients to primary care physicians, instituting community outreach and education programs, and helping patients tap into payor programs.

These services are available to students, as well as university faculty, staff, and, often, campus visitors.

8.2.7 Occupational Health Programs

Occupational health programs, located on employers' sites, deal with preserving the health of workers on the job and relate to a wide variety of on-the-job health issues:

▲ **Safety:** These issues relate to keeping employees safe on the job and include things like establishing a safe work environment to reduce the risk of injury to workers.

▲ **Occupational illnesses and conditions:** These issues address the conditions that can result from long-term exposure to a hazard, such as noise, hazardous materials, and so on.

▲ **Mental health:** Many employers offer mental health services (such as Employee Assistance Programs, or EAPs) for employees who need counseling.

▲ **On-site health services:** On-site health services are not uncommon in larger companies. They provide a fairly narrow range of services, including physical exams of prospective and existing employees, drug screening, and first aid.

SELF-CHECK

- What is the single, defining characteristic of ambulatory care settings?
- Identify three ambulatory care settings.
- Identify three ambulatory care providers.

8.3 Home Health and Visiting Nurse Agencies

Unlike the other ambulatory care settings that are housed in medical facilities, home health and visiting nurse agencies provide ambulatory care in patients' homes. This type of care is often necessary for those who are elderly or homebound, who have just been released from the hospital and are still recovering, or who have a chronic condition or illness that can be cared for at home.

Home health care agencies and visiting nurse agencies can provide the following services:

▲ **Skilled nursing:** Includes care by RNs and LVNs, as well as private duty nursing care. Refer to Section 5.4 for information about licensed nurses.

▲ **Home health aide care:** Services provided by individuals who follow doctors', nurses', or therapists' orders in providing care and are responsible for checking the patient's health status (pulse, temperature, etc.), dispensing medication, helping with general patient care (bathing, dressing, and grooming, for example), as well as general household chores (cleaning, laundry, meal planning and preparation, and so forth).

▲ **Physical therapy:** Includes preventing or alleviating a patient's physical disability and pain; restoring or enhancing motor function, and/or helping a patient adapt to a permanent disability.

▲ **Speech therapy:** Refers to corrective or rehabilitative treatment of physical or cognitive impairments resulting in difficulty with verbal communication. This difficulty can be related to speech (the formation of sounds) or language (the formation of meaning). Speech therapists often work with stroke victims, people with speech disorders (such as lisps or stutters), and those with other conditions, such as autism spectrum disorders, that impact both expressive and receptive language.

▲ **Occupational therapy:** Refers to helping people whose physical or mental health conditions affect their ability to engage in everyday, purposeful activities. Examples of these activities include bathing, dressing, using a phone, driving a care, managing a home and family, and returning to work or school. It differs from physical therapy in that physical therapy works on the ability to move, whereas occupational therapy focuses on using movement to achieve a purposeful end (or "occupation").

FOR EXAMPLE

Financial Issues for Home Health Care

Earning an average of $8 to $10 an hour, home health care aides are the lowest paid of the ambulatory care workforce, and current economic forces—specifically rising health care costs and rising fuel costs—are threatening to cut their wages even more. Home health aides, in general, travel from patient to patient and are expected to provide their own transportation. Although home health care agencies reimburse their employees for fuel costs, the reimbursements typically fall well below the national reimbursement rate of 48 cents per gallon. States, feeling the pinch of rising health care costs, are also seeking ways to cut expenses.

In addition, **medical social services,** provided by licensed social workers, intervene on the patient's behalf through the following interventions:

▲ **Community resource education and referral:** Provide information and education about, as well as referrals to, community resources available to meet the patient's needs.

▲ **Financial assistance information:** Provide information concerning financial assistance resources and assistance programs.

▲ **Continuity of care planning:** Work with medical team to identify patient needs for continued care and recovery and helps the patient and family develop strategies to meet the patient's ongoing needs.

▲ **Psychosocial assessment:** Assess the patient's illness, physical, mental, and cognitive functioning, mood, needs, education, and so on to assist in the development of the patient's treatment and discharge plans.

▲ **Psychosocial interventions:** Provide individual, family, and group counseling to increase understanding of an illness, as well as its treatment and the impact it can have on the patient and the patient's family; to help the patient and family adjust to the illness or disability; and to provide grief and loss counseling, as well as referrals to support groups.

▲ **Crisis interventions and trauma support:** Provide supportive counseling to patients and families facing a crisis or trauma situation.

SELF-CHECK

- Name three types of home health care providers.
- Identify three services that social workers provide to home health clients.

SUMMARY

Ambulatory care is a key component of the U.S. health care system. Ambulatory care services will continue to expand because of ongoing medical advancements and rising health care costs. Most patients receive ambulatory services in physicians' offices, community health centers or clinics, and hospitals. But homebound and recovering patients, who may not be able to travel to an outpatient care setting, can receive ambulatory care from home health and visiting nurse agencies.

KEY TERMS

Ambulatory care	Medical services provided to patients on an outpatient basis (that is, services that don't require an overnight stay in a hospital).
Group practices	Physician practices in which three or more physicians, often complemented by other health care professionals, share resources, pool expenses and income, and collaborate in the care of patients.
Medical social services	Services provided by licensed social workers, who intervene on the patient's behalf.
Solo practices	Physician practices consisting of an individual physician, generally assisted by several clinical and administrative personnel.

ASSESS YOUR UNDERSTANDING

Go to www.wiley.com/college/pointer to evaluate your knowledge of the basics of ambulatory care.

Measure your learning by comparing pre-test and post-test results.

Summary Questions

1. In what way has patient demand fostered the growth of ambulatory care?
   (a) patients demand greater convenience
   (b) patients' physicians are typically in solo or group practice and not associated with a hospital
   (c) patients desire less expensive health care
   (d) all of the above

2. Of age, gender, income, and insurance status, which is the biggest predictor of who does and doesn't receive ambulatory care?
   (a) age
   (b) income
   (c) gender
   (d) insurance status

3. What is the greatest source of payment for ambulatory care?
   (a) Medicare
   (b) Medicaid
   (c) private insurance
   (d) individual out-of-pocket

4. In which health care setting are the majority of ambulatory care services provided?
   (a) hospital outpatient departments
   (b) physicians' offices
   (c) community health centers or clinics
   (d) emergency rooms and urgent care clinics

5. General practitioners and family physicians are the primary providers of ambulatory care. True or False?

6. What kind of ambulatory care services do hospital emergency departments deliver?
   (a) specialized emergency care (required for sudden illnesses or injuries) only
   (b) the same kind of care that other outpatient settings do: same-day surgery, diagnosis, follow-up care, and so on

(c) care that leads to hospitalization

(d) hospital ERs do not offer ambulatory care

7. When are patients most likely to seek care from an urgent care facility?

(a) when their condition isn't serious enough to warrant a trip to the emergency room

(b) when they can't get in to see their family physician

(c) when they don't have insurance

(d) a and b

(e) all of the above

8. Which of the following characterizes same-day surgery centers?

(a) they can offer general surgery

(b) they can offer specialized surgery

(c) they are less costly than hospital surgeries

(d) a and c

(e) all of the above

9. What kind of ambulatory services do community health centers offer?

(a) general medical care

(b) emergency care

(c) prenatal care

(d) a and b

(e) all of the above

10. Home health and visiting nurses agencies are most likely to serve which patients?

(a) elderly and homebound patients

(b) those with chronic conditions

(c) those just released from the hospital

(d) a and c

(e) all of the above

11. Home health aides are responsible for

(a) implementing doctors' orders for their patients.

(b) helping patients bath, dress, groom, and so on.

(c) doing general household chores.

(d) a and b.

(e) all of the above.

Review Questions

1. Explain how hospitals, which excel at inpatient health care, can be ambulatory care providers.

2. In what way have medical advances fostered ambulatory care?
   (a) they've brought down the cost of health care
   (b) they've made diagnostic methods and treatments less invasive
   (c) they've made care options available to more people, regardless of insurance status
   (d) all of the above
3. What is the most common reason for accessing ambulatory care?
   (a) preventive care
   (b) symptoms of illness
   (c) obstetric care
   (d) follow-up care
4. Name a component of the accreditation process.
   (a) a peer review by other organizations in the same field
   (b) consultation and review by outside experts
   (c) a self-evaluation
   (d) b and c
   (e) all of the above
5. Explain how surgery can be considered an ambulatory care service.
6. In what way do hospital emergency departments not deliver optimum outpatient care?
   (a) they are less inclined to order further diagnostic studies for ER patients
   (b) they are less likely to refer ER patients to specialists
   (c) they don't deliver the same continuity of care that other outpatient settings deliver
   (d) all of the above
7. In what way are urgent care facilities like hospital emergency departments?
   (a) they can provide emergency services
   (b) by law, they must be open 24 hours a day and accept all who seek treatment, regardless of insurance status
   (c) he services they offer are as costly as those delivered in an emergency room
   (d) all of the above
8. Same-day surgery centers offer the same kind of care as which other ambulatory care facilities?
   (a) physicians' offices
   (b) hospital emergency departments

(c) urgent care facilities

(d) none of the above

9. Define the special role that community health centers have in providing ambulatory care.

10. Explain the difference between occupational and physical therapy.

11. Which home health caregiver would you need for the following tasks?

    (a) taking vital statistics

    (b) helping improve motor functioning

    (c) helping improve ability to perform everyday tasks

    (d) getting referrals for community resources

Applying This Chapter

1. Explain how rising health care costs have impacted ambulatory care.

2. Identify from which ambulatory care provider you would be likely to receive services from in the following situations:

    (a) as a first-year college student whose dorm houses a student who contracted meningitis

    (b) as a job applicant undergoing a drug screening

    (c) as a new mother receiving postnatal care

    (d) as an elderly person discharged from the hospital with a feeding tube

    (e) as a poor person who doesn't qualify for Medicare

3. Of the ambulatory care settings, which do you think is the least effective? Explain your answer.

Understanding Ambulatory Care

More and more complex diagnostic and treatment services are provided in ambulatory care settings because of cost savings and convenience. Identify the ways in which this reliance on ambulatory care is problematic. As a health officer, you're charged with seeing to the health needs of your community. Although you have adequate private health care facilities, you're particularly concerned about the large uninsured population in your community. Complicating matters is that the government is considering set reimbursement rates. Indicate the challenges you face and how you will likely address them.

Ambulatory Care Settings and Providers

If you were a generalist physician who had to decide on an ambulatory care setting, what factors would you look at as you made your decision.

Home Health and Visiting Nurse Agencies

You are a director of a community clinic and are looking for ways to cut costs and maintain quality of care. Your strategy is to hire social workers. Explain how this move will benefit your bottom line.

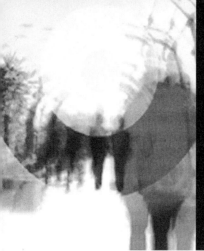

9

LONG-TERM CARE
Taking Care of Elderly, Injured, and Disabled Patients

Starting Point

Go to www.wiley.com/college/pointer to assess your knowledge of the basics of long-term care.
Determine where you need to concentrate your effort.

What You'll Learn in This Chapter

- ▲ The key characteristics of long-term care
- ▲ The different types of residential long-term-care facilities and their functions
- ▲ The purpose of home health care and community resources available to foster independent living
- ▲ The types of rehabilitation centers and their goals
- ▲ What hospice care is and how it differs from traditional health care

After Studying This Chapter, You'll Be Able To

- ▲ Examine the general goals of long-term care
- ▲ Categorize long-term-care facilities and services
- ▲ Describe the typical long-term-care patient
- ▲ Compare various personal care facilities
- ▲ Differentiate between types of rehabilitation facilities
- ▲ Examine hospice services and their purpose

Goals and Outcomes

- ▲ Master terminology used in discussing long-term-care facilities, personnel, and clients
- ▲ Differentiate long-term-care facilities in terms of client-base and services provided
- ▲ Identify what community-based services are appropriate for different health care needs
- ▲ Identify the rehabilitation needs of patients with different health conditions
- ▲ Compare hospice with other long-term health services in terms of strategy, purpose, and patient involvement
- ▲ Make an argument about what impact the aging U.S. population is likely to have on long-term care

INTRODUCTION

Although many people associate long-term care with nursing homes, a variety of situations—injury, accident, chronic health condition, or old age—can lead people to seek long-term care. At its most basic level, long-term care helps people who have difficulty performing the activities of daily living. Many patients receive long-term care at residential facilities designed to meet their needs. Others, who can still remain in their homes, have to tap into home health care services and community resources. Those seeking addiction counseling or other rehabilitative services can find help at rehabilitation centers. Hospice, unique in the long-term-care programs, helps terminally ill patients deal with end-of-life issues.

9.1 Understanding Long-Term Care

People who require long-term care are generally not sick in the traditional sense, but are, for whatever reason—injury, accident, chronic health condition, or old age—unable to perform some of the basic activities of daily living such as dressing, bathing, eating, toileting, getting in and out of a bed or chair, and walking.

9.1.1 Typical Long-Term-Care Services

Conditions that require long-term care go well beyond a single source. In fact, depending on the nature and the degree or severity of the condition, long-term care is made up of an array of health care services, such as the following:

▲ **Ambulatory medical services:** Simply put, ambulatory services are outpatient services. But that means more than simply visits to a doctor's office. To find out about the various kinds of ambulatory services available, refer to Sections 8.2 and 8.3.

▲ **Inpatient medical services:** These are medical services requiring admission to a hospital.

▲ **Mental-behavioral services:** People needing long-term care often can benefit from counseling, medication for depression, and occupational, physical, or speech therapy.

▲ **Social services:** Because long-term-care plans are generally complex and touch on various aspects of a patient's life, many patients (and their families) require the help of medical social workers to tap into the health care and social services resources they need. (Refer to Section 8.3 for information about social health services.)

▲ **Daily living support services:** The nature of conditions that place people in long-term care impair their ability to live independently. Daily living support services are services—such as Meals on Wheels, home health aides, and so on—that provide help taking care of day-to-day tasks.

Both health care professionals and family members and friends can provide long-term care. Likewise, long-term care often requires a combination of ambulatory and inpatient services. The patient's health care needs, support systems, and resources determine what type of care is provided and by whom.

9.1.2 People Who Need Long-Term Care

The primary users of long-term care are people who fall into one of the following two categories:

▲ **Individuals with temporary disabilities:** People in this group have injuries or illnesses that impair their ability to function independently for a period of time but who will eventually recover. Examples are those suffering from stroke, trauma, and severe bone fractures.

▲ **Individuals with chronic health problems:** People in this group have progressively degenerative and nonreversible physical or mental conditions, such as spinal cord injury, Alzheimer's disease, and infirmity due to aging.

Although even very young people may require long-term care, as you may suspect, most long-term-care services are consumed by elderly people, a segment of the population that's growing dramatically as baby boomers age. In 1990, 13 percent of the U.S. population was over the age of 65; by 2030 this group will make up about 20 percent of the population. The aging of the U.S. population has major implications for the kind of health care needed.

As the population ages and medical technology provides more effective and efficient care of acute illnesses, the predominant burden of disease is shifting to chronic conditions. These chronic diseases are often the result of many factors, coexist with other chronic diseases, and require complex medical approaches,

---

FOR EXAMPLE

Long-Term-Care Insurance Policies

Neither Medicare nor Medicaid supplemental insurance, or traditional health insurance cover most long-term-care costs. For that reason, many people are buying (or considering buying) long-term-care insurance policies specifically to pay for long-term health care needs. One of the most important factors to consider when you choose a long-term-care policy is the **benefit triggers.** Simply put, your policy won't pay out benefits unless you meet the criteria for needing long-term care. For most policies, you must be unable to perform a certain number of **activities of daily living (ADLs)** for the benefits to kick in. Examples of ADLs include bathing, continence, dressing, eating, getting in and out of bed, and so on.

including disease management, **palliative care** (which eases the symptoms or discomfort of the condition but doesn't cure it), and a holistic approach to medicine (see Section 12.4.5 for information about medical models).

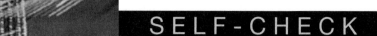

SELF-CHECK

- List the services that provide long-term health care.
- Describe the users of long-term health care.

9.2 Personal Care Facilities

Obviously, many people who need long-term care receive it in their own homes. The necessary health care team is assembled (or accessed) and community resources and family and friends are called upon to enable the patient to continue to live independently. For some people, however, staying at home is no longer an option. Either the necessary resources are not available (or affordable), or the patient's condition has progressed beyond what caregivers can adequately provide in the home setting. In these instances, patients receive care at **personal care facilities,** facilities for people who can no longer perform the functions of daily living without help and when staying at home is no longer possible. These facilities fall into several general categories, based on the care and services offered:

▲ **Assisted living facilities:** These facilities provide personal care services to people who need help with some activities of daily living, such as bathing, dressing, and eating.

▲ **Continuing care retirement communities:** These communities combine independent living, assisted living, nursing home and Alzheimer's/dementia services within a single large setting.

▲ **Congregate care facilities:** Congregate care facilities are very similar to continuing care retirement communities with one important difference: These facilities do not provide health care; residents must seek care elsewhere when it is needed.

▲ **Nursing homes:** Nursing homes provide care for people with medical needs that require daily attention from licensed nurses.

▲ **Alzheimer's/dementia facilities:** Sometimes housed within another facility, such as a nursing home, or independently, these facilities are designed for people with memory and other cognitive impairments that keep them from taking care of themselves and communicating normally.

The following sections describe these facilities in more detail.

9.2.1 Assisted Living Facilities

Assisted living facilities are long-term-care facilities for people who don't need skilled medical care but do need help with certain activities of daily living, such as bathing and dressing. Assisted living facilities may also offer some supervision of forgetful and easily confused residents, such as people in the early stages of Alzheimer's disease.

Residents typically live in private apartments or rooms and go to common areas for socializing, recreation, and planned activities. The purpose of the activities and common areas is to help residents avoid isolation and depression by coming into contact with others.

Assisted living facilities are staffed 24 hours a day and include registered nurses and nurse's aides. To provide security, these facilities often have controlled access—that is, people entering and leaving the building must do so through a common area such as a lobby or entrance way.

Other services these facilities may provide include shuttle service for errands, emergency monitoring systems, and in-room meals.

The traditional assisted living facility resembles, in many ways, a nursing home. The hospital-like setting, the round-the-clock staff, the secure entrances, and other features create an atmosphere—despite the personal touches—of a health care facility. For people who prefer more personalized environments and who don't need the services that come part and parcel with these settings, other assisted living arrangements may be suitable:

▲ **Board-and-care facilities:** Board-and-care facilities, sometimes called **personal care homes,** are smaller, less institutional assisted living facilities. They provide residents with a room, meals, housekeeping and cleaning services, personal care assistance, transportation, and some degree of supervision. They are not hospital-like, nor do they provide any medical, nursing, or rehabilitation care.

▲ **Adult foster care:** With adult foster care, a family takes in and looks after a dependent person. Social service agencies generally arrange adult foster care. The caregiving family provides meals, housekeeping services, help with personal tasks like bathing and dressing, and other activities of daily living.

Assisted living facilities are generally licensed by the state and undergo periodic reviews.

9.2.2 Continuing Care Retirement Communities (CCRCs)

Continuing care retirement communities (CCRCs), also called *life care facilities,* are self-sufficient communities designed for retirees. These complexes provide all levels of personal and medical services, from the least to the most intensive, with the expectation that residents will not have to move to other facilities as their long-term-care needs change.

In general, residents must pay a large, one-time entry fee, in addition to monthly maintenance fees. These fees buy residents the following:

▲ A living area, which can be a single-family home, condominium, apartment, or room, often with controlled access and safety features such as level walkways and grab bars.
▲ Health care services.
▲ Social services.
▲ Recreational facilities, such as swimming pools, game rooms, planned social activities, tours, and so on.

By offering independent living, assisted living, skilled nursing (nursing homes), and Alzheimer's/dementia care in a single setting, CCRCs give residents the freedom (and activities) associated with a retirement community with the security of long-term-care options.

In general, CCRCs generally accept only healthy seniors—that is, those who don't yet need help with activities of daily living. Once residents move in, however, they can access different levels of health care as they need it. CCRCs are licensed in accordance with laws governing nursing homes and assisted living facilities.

9.2.3 Congregate Care Facilities

Congregate care facilities are like CCRCs in most ways; however, in a congregate care facility, no health care services are provided. In a continuing care retirement community, the resident has the ability to utilize health care services from within. In a congregate care facility, residents must access health care services elsewhere. Congregate facilities focus on the instrumental activities of daily living (IADLs) such as preparing a meal, grocery shopping, housework, and medical appointments.

9.2.4 Nursing Homes

Nursing homes, also called skilled nursing facilities, provide a mix of intermediate-level nursing and personal services on a 24-hour basis to people who are either temporarily or permanently unable to care for themselves and require attention by a licensed nurse.

The United States has approximately 17,000 nursing homes. These homes can be either freestanding or a component of another organization (such as a hospital or retirement center). Here is a profile of these organizations:

▲ As a proportion of the $1.3 trillion spent on health in 2001, the largest expenditures for long-term care are nursing homes ($117 billion, or 9 percent of the total) and home health care ($39 billion, or 3 percent).

▲ Sixty-five percent of nursing homes are proprietary, 28 percent are non-profit, and 7 percent are governmental. Fifty-six percent of nursing homes are affiliated with a chain; 24 percent are independent.

▲ The number of beds per nursing home facility averages 107, and the occupancy rate is about 80 percent. During the year there are 2.4 million nursing home admissions; on a typical day, there are 1.6 million nursing home residents.

▲ The average charge for nursing home care is $3,900 per month. Overall, the source of a typical nursing home's revenue is 47 percent Medicaid; 12 percent Medicare; and 41 percent from private health insurance, out-of-pocket expenditures, and other.

▲ Not all patients in nursing homes are there for end-of-life care. In fact, nearly 41 percent of nursing home patients stay for a year or less.

All states require nursing homes, whether they are for-profit or nonprofit to be state licensed and regulated.

Nursing Home Staffing

Nursing homes may include the following staff positions:

▲ **Nurse's aides:** These aides provide much of the day-to-day care at nursing homes and perform tasks.

▲ **Social workers and case managers:** Social workers and case managers help seniors and their families with insurance issues and the coordination of care.

▲ **Dietitians, rehabilitation therapists, and other health professionals:** These people work to support and sustain seniors' physical and emotional well-being.

▲ **Administrative personnel:** The administrative personnel include the director, assistant director, clerical staff, and so on.

▲ **Licensed nurses:** Some nursing homes care for patients needing **subacute care** (for conditions that fall between **acute,** or sudden onset, and **chronic,** conditions that are long lasting or never changing). Treatment for subacute health issues typically requires frequent physician visits and intensive nursing. Those who breathe with ventilators, for example, need nursing supervision around the clock. These facilities have licensed registered nurses on staff to monitor and care for these patients. Other nursing home facilities, however, transfer patients requiring full-time care to long-term hospitals.

For-Profit and Nonprofit Nursing Homes

The earliest nursing homes were nineteenth-century government-run poorhouses for indigent and infirm people, many of whom were elderly. As the number of residents outgrew the capacity of these institutions, charitable and philanthropic organizations stepped in. The goal of these organizations was to create an environment where elderly people could live with dignity during their final years. At approximately the same time, other groups organized "benevolence societies," in which future residents could pay a weekly portion to receive elder care services in their later years. These organizations were nonprofit enterprises, meaning that their mission was to serve some philanthropic purpose; it was not to enrich the benefactors.

Just as many service sectors begin with nonprofit organizations and then eventually evolve to include for-profit entities, the health sector is no different. Today approximately 70 percent of nursing homes are for-profit organizations; many (nearly 40 percent) are part of a chain or nursing home franchise. Nonprofits now comprise less than 20 percent of the nursing homes in the United States, with the remaining nursing homes being government-run facilities.

Today, the question is what impact, if any, does the growing number of for-profit nursing homes have on nonprofit homes. In a study conducted by Will Mitchell and Aparna Venkatraman from Duke University and others, the data for several thousand nursing homes over the course of seven years was examined. Their report, published in 2004, reveals some interesting answers:

▲ Nonprofit nursing homes had fewer reported deficiencies on their annual inspection reports than did for-profit nursing homes. Nonprofits also had higher staffing levels, and therefore higher costs, than for-profit homes.

▲ Despite having higher costs than for-profits, nonprofit nursing homes tend to charge less for basic care than for-profit homes. (Nonprofits do charge more for skilled care, however.)

▲ Neither the dominance of for-profit nursing homes nor the competitive nature of health care seems to have an impact on the cost or quality of care provided by nonprofits.

▲ In those instances when for-profits acquire (or buy out) nonprofits, the quality of care at the acquired nursing home tends to fall and the prices tend to rise.

9.2.5 Alzheimer's/Dementia Facilities

Alzheimer's/dementia facilities can be independent units or a component of an assisted living facility or nursing home. These units care for people who cannot communicate normally or take care of themselves and provide the following services:

▲ **Constant supervision:** Well-designed units staffed with professionals trained to care for Alzheimer's and dementia patients are usually the safest environment for those prone to wandering.

FOR EXAMPLE

The Nursing Home Reform Act (NHRA)

In 1987, the federal government established comprehensive standards for nursing homes. Called the Nursing Home Reform Act, the NHRA covers a number of areas outlining nursing homes' obligation to residents, including:

▲ That nursing homes care for residents "in such a manner and in such an environment as will promote maintenance or enhancement of the quality of life of each resident."

▲ That patients be free from discrimination, physical or chemical restraints not required to treat the resident's medical symptoms, verbal, sexual, physical, and mental abuse, corporal punishment, and involuntary seclusion.

▲ That patients have access to all records pertaining to themselves and receive a written statement of fees, charges, and services.

▲ That nursing homes not deny residents the right to apply for Medicaid benefits, solicit money or a donation as a precondition of admission, or require that a friend or family member guarantee payment.

▲ **Help with activities of daily living and personalized care:** Staff members give patients as much mental and memory stimulation as possible.

Most states have licensing requirements for assisted living facilities, and all have licensing requirements for nursing homes, but none have requirements specifically for Alzheimer's/dementia units.

SELF-CHECK

• Identify and describe the four types of personal care facilities.

• Describe the type of licensing required by the following: (a) assisted living facilities, (b) continuing care retirement communities, (c) nursing homes, and (d) Alzheimer's/dementia facilities

9.3 Community-Based and Home Health Care

Many communities provide services and home health programs to help seniors and people with disabilities with a variety of personal activities. The goal of these services is to help clients remain independent, engaged, and healthy members of their communities. These services often overlap—for example, Meals on Wheels is a community-based service that is delivered in the home.

▲ **Home health care:** Supportive and curative care provided to patients in their homes. Services can range from simple (housekeeping and meals) to complex (skilled nursing; physical, respiratory, and intravenous therapies).

▲ **Community-based health care:** Care sponsored by the community, which is usually free or at low cost for qualifying individuals.

9.3.1 Receiving Care at Home

Most often, long-term care is rendered by family members and friends in the home, supplemented with ambulatory and inpatient services such as:

▲ Monitoring and care management provided in a doctor's office or clinic.

▲ Home visitors, including homemaker and personal care, visiting nursing, and Meals on Wheels.

▲ Respite care, to give caregivers a break.

▲ Hospice care, to help the family during the latter stages of a terminal illness.

During a typical year, 7 million people (3 percent of the population) use home health services provided by about 20,000 agencies. For additional information about in-home care, refer to Section 8.3.

Home health care agencies can fall into one of three types (refer to Section 7.3.3 for more on the types of ownership):

▲ **Voluntary nonprofit:** Private organizations that perform charitable functions or provide a community service.

▲ **Government:** State, local, or federal agencies.

▲ **Proprietary:** Private organizations that operate for a profit.

Agencies can either be freestanding or components of another type of organization (such as a health system, hospital, or nursing home), but the most important distinction among home health organizations (typically called agencies) is whether they are Medicare certified. Certified agencies must comply with conditions of participation specified by the Centers for Medicare and Medicaid Services (CMS), such as the following:

▲ Compliance with federal, state, and local laws.

▲ Proper organization of services and administration.

▲ Professional and properly credentialed personnel.

▲ Proper record-keeping.

▲ Evaluation and assessment of the program's performance.

Approximately 40 percent of all home health agencies are Medicare certified. (Of Medicare-certified agencies, 41 percent are freestanding proprietary and 30 percent are hospital based.)

The most common diagnoses of home health clients are diabetes, chronic hypertension (high blood pressure), heart failure, arthritis, cerebrovascular disease (damage to the blood vessels in the brain, resulting in a stroke), and chronic airway obstruction (emphysema or chronic bronchitis). The characteristics of people who use home health care services include:

▲ **Age:** Although many tend to think of home health care as care for elderly people, members of every age group receive home health care services.

- 34 percent of clients are under 65.
- 24 percent are 65 to 74.
- 42 percent are over 75.

▲ **Gender:** Sixty-four percent of clients are female, 36 percent male.

▲ **Race:** Sixty-three percent of clients are white, 8 percent are black, and the race or ethnicity of the remaining 29 percent is unspecified.

The charge for a home health visit averages about $90. That may not seem like a tremendous amount, until you consider that every year, $36 billion is spent on home care in the United States. Of this amount, Medicare finances 40 percent (in fact, 11 percent of Medicare beneficiaries use home health care during an average year, up from about 2 percent in 1974), Medicaid finances 15 percent, private insurance finances 11 percent, 22 percent is out-of-pocket, and 12 percent is other.

9.3.2 Taking Advantage of Community-Based Care

Community-based services often include the following:

▲ **Adult day care:** Adult day care services provide health, social, and recreational activities to adults who have functional and/or cognitive impairments that make it impossible for them to be left alone during the day, but who don't need 24-hour care. Some programs offer services in the evenings and on weekends, in addition to standard business hours. Medicaid may be available for adult day care provided that the patient is unable to afford the daily rates and that those rates are less than the daily cost of a nursing home. According to the 2000 census, the United States has nearly 3500 adult day care centers.

▲ **Respite care:** Respite care is temporary care provided to people with disabilities or chronic conditions so that their ordinary caregivers (generally families) can take a break from the physically and emotionally exhausting routine of their daily care. Some respite services are similar to day care or after-school programs, in which the individual participates for a period of time each day (adult day care is an example of this type of respite; see the preceding bullet). Other respite services involve overnight care for an extended period. Most respite services, however, are provided in the home, where the respite care worker sits or cares for the family member while the usual caregiver takes a break.

▲ **Senior centers:** Senior centers, located in many communities, provide a wide range of services, including nutrition, recreation, social and educational services, wellness and fitness activities, information and program referral services, and Internet training. Most of the services are provided free or at low cost to participants.

▲ **Transportation:** Some community-based care agencies offer door-to-door taxicab services, public bus transportation, or vans with wheelchair-accessible transportation.

▲ **Meals on Wheels:** Meals on Wheels is a nonprofit organization that fosters independent living by providing regular nutrition and personal contact on a daily basis. Clients receive two meals a day (lunch and dinner), and can specify a diet plan: regular, diabetic, low-fat, low-sodium, or mechanically soft (easy to chew).

▲ **Telephone reassurance:** People who live alone and have medical or other health needs often fear that they would not be able to call for help in an emergency. Several types of emergency telephone response systems address this concern. These systems use the telephone to check on a client on a regular basis.

Local organizations, called *Area Agencies on Aging,* coordinate these services.

FOR EXAMPLE

Continuing Services during Emergencies

Natural events around the world—hurricanes, earthquakes, and so on—have brought to light the need for, and difficulty with, providing services during times of crisis. Because elderly people and people with disabilities who receive in-home and community-based care are among the most vulnerable populations, many service providers are putting together contingency plans for disasters.

9.4 Rehabilitation Centers

Rehabilitation centers, commonly called simply *rehab centers,* are facilities that help patients recover and/or manage specific conditions, addictions, or impairments. Among the many types of rehabilitation services and centers, addiction rehab and medical rehab centers are the most common. Specialty rehab centers also exist. Examples include fitness facilities, orthopedic facilities, and mental health facilities. Rehab facilities can also further specialize between pediatrics and adults.

Rehabilitation centers can be stand-alone facilities, such as a drug rehab center, that offer all the necessary care independently of another health care organization. They can also be part of a larger health care organization or facility.

Some rehab centers are outpatient based; patients come in for rehabilitation during the day or evening. Other rehab centers are residential facilities; patients stay in rehab for days, weeks, or months until their rehabilitation is complete.

Because of the complex nature of many of the conditions that benefit from rehabilitative services, the care given at rehab centers is often multifaceted. Consider drug rehab, for example. This treatment often involves medical treatment

FOR EXAMPLE

Medical Rehabilitation Research

The federal government, through National Center for Medical Rehabilitation Research (NCMRR)—part of the National Institutes of Health (NIH)—promotes and supports rehabilitation research through funding research grants. The department's mission is to increase the effectiveness of medical rehabilitation practices by funding research in the following areas: improving mobility, promoting adaptation to functional impairments, studying the effectiveness of current medical rehabilitation therapies, creating technology to assist people with disabilities, understanding the effect of functional impairment on whole body systems, and more.

in addition to counseling and behavior modification strategies. In addition to medical services, orthopedic rehabilitation, for example, often includes mental health services, speech or occupational therapy services, and so on.

Each type of rehabilitation facility has specialized professional staff that are credentialed in the areas for which they practice. Additionally, rehab centers must meet certain certification criteria set fourth by a wide variety of credentialing organizations depending on the center's specialty.

SELF-CHECK

- • Define **rehabilitation center.**
- • List two types of rehabilitation centers.

9.5 Hospice Care

Hospice care is solely devoted to providing physical care and counseling to terminally ill patients and their families.

Both private companies or public agencies can provide hospice care, but in each case the goal is the same: to ease the end-of-life issues—fear, grief, and pain—that terminally ill patients face. It is *not* to provide a cure.

9.5.1 Hospice Service Providers

Hospice care is complex and highly integrated. It involves a care team that includes the following people, each providing assistance according to his or her area of expertise:

- ▲ **Medical personnel, including physicians, nurses, and hospice-certified nursing assistants:** These people help hospice patients manage pain and monitor their health. Although the hospice agency will provide a physician, patients can choose to use their physicians instead.
- ▲ **Social workers and counselors:** These people help hospice patients and their families come to grips with the idea of death and prepare for it. They also assess the living environment.
- ▲ **Clergy:** This person helps the patient and family deal with the spiritual and emotional issues surrounding the death, and helps the family during the grieving period after the death.
- ▲ **Therapists:** Generally physical and occupational therapists who help patients be as mobile and self-sufficient as they wish.

FOR EXAMPLE

The History of Hospice

The idea of hospice care isn't new—hospices have been around since medieval times. Centuries ago, hospices provided shelter for travelers as well as care for pregnant women, people recovering from an illness or injury, and the infirm. But then Cicely Saunders, an English nursing student during World War II, came to believe that the two most important things to people who were dying was to have their pain controlled and to die with dignity. This simple but profound realization resulted in the first modern hospice. Although most people today accept the role—and goals—of hospice, the idea of accepting and preparing for death had to be relearned. Past generations recognized death as part of life. Childhood illnesses, unchecked epidemics, ineffective medical practices, shorter life spans, and the fact that most people died at home made death familiar. During Saunders's time, however, medical breakthroughs, improved hygiene, better nutrition, and more sophisticated understanding of how disease is spread ushered in an era when most saw their parents reach old age, few witnessed the death of their childhood friends, and even horrible injuries and illnesses could be healed or cured through medical intervention. The conventional wisdom seemed to be that, if you could hold death at bay, you didn't need to deal with it. Saunders's hospice idea reintroduce the idea that death—always unavoidable—can be faced with dignity, without pain, at home, and surrounded by family.

▲ **Volunteers:** During the latter stages of the illness, patients always have someone with them. Because this can be a tremendous emotional and physical burden for family members, Hospice agencies provide volunteers who can stay with the patient so that family members can get a break and perform other support functions.

9.5.2 Hospice Services

After a person qualifies for hospice care, he or she can expect to receive the following services:

▲ **Assess patient needs:** Your hospice provider will assess your needs and put together an individualized care plan, recommending and making arrangements to obtain any necessary equipment, addressing the number of caregivers, and identifying the pain management plan.

▲ **Provide financial assistance:** One of the first things hospice does is assist families in finding out whether the patient is eligible for any coverage they may not be aware of. See Section 9.5.4 for more information about how hospice services are paid for.

▲ **Educate caregivers:** Hospice staff teach caregivers how to provide the necessary care (such as dispensing medication and monitoring the patient's condition) and visit regularly to see how things are going, provide support, and answer any medical questions the patient or his or her family has.

▲ **Provide support to caregivers:** Caring for a dying person is emotionally and physically draining. Not only do the health care needs become more intense, but patients often have someone there continuously (a common fear is dying alone). To help the primary caregivers during this difficult time, hospices provide volunteers to assist with errands and to stay temporarily with the patient so that the family can have time away.

▲ **Manage pain:** Hospice believes that emotional and spiritual pain are just as real and in need of attention as physical pain, so it can address each. Hospice nurses and doctors provide palliative care, that is, medications and devices for pain and symptom relief.

▲ **Provide physical or occupational therapy:** The purpose of this therapy is to assist patients to be as mobile and self-sufficient as they wish. Specialists schooled in music therapy, art therapy, massage, and diet counseling are also often involved.

▲ **Provide counseling:** Various counselors, including clergy, are available to assist family members as well as patients.

▲ **Provide support for the family after the patient dies:** Hospice provides continuing contact and support for caregivers for at least a year following the death of a loved one. Most hospices also sponsor bereavement groups and support for anyone in the community who has experienced a death of a family member, a friend, or similar losses.

9.5.3 Accessing Hospice Care

By law the decision to use hospice care has to be the patient's, but this is a decision that patients usually make in concert with their physicians. To qualify for hospice care, a patient must

▲ **Have a terminal illness that will result in the patient's death within six months:** One of the first things the hospice program will do is contact the patient's physician to make sure he or she agrees that hospice care is appropriate for this patient at this time.

▲ **Be willing to forgo all curative treatments:** In other words, the patient is willing to stop aggressive efforts to "beat" the disease.

▲ **Sign consent and insurance forms:** These are similar to the forms patients sign when they enter a hospital.

9.5.4 Financing Hospice Care

Hospice insurance coverage is widely available: Medicare provides it nationwide; Medicaid provides it in most states, and most private insurance providers cover it.

Medicare covers all services and supplies for the hospice patient related to the terminal illness. In some hospices, the patient may be required to pay a 5 percent or $5 "copayment" on medication and a 5 percent copayment for respite care.

Even if the patient doesn't have insurance coverage, most hospice programs provide for anyone who cannot pay using money raised from the community or from memorial or foundation gifts.

SELF-CHECK

- List types of hospice care providers.
- Define **hospice care** and explain how it differs from traditional health care.
- List three services hospice workers provide.

SUMMARY

As the U.S. population ages and chronic conditions take center stage in the U.S. population, long-term care is a growing health care concern. All people who need long-term care, despite the health issues that preceded their seeking such care, have one thing in common: They have difficulty performing everyday tasks and can no longer live independently. Various residential facilities are devoted to providing care and services to this population. Home health agencies and community resources are an option for those who can remain in their homes. Rehabilitation centers provide multiple types of rehabilitative services. Hospice programs provide palliative care and counseling services to terminally ill patients.

KEY TERMS

Activities of daily living (ADLs)	Fundamental activities of daily care that health care professionals use as a way to describe the functional status of a person. Examples of ADLs include bathing, continence, dressing, eating, getting in and out of bed, and so on.
Acute care	Care given for health conditions that happen suddenly and last for a finite period of time.

Alzheimer's/dementia facilities	Independent units or a component of an assisted living facility or nursing home; these units care for people who cannot communicate normally or take care of themselves and provide constant supervision and help with activities of daily living and personalized care.
Assisted living facilities	Long-term-care facilities for people who don't need skilled medical care but do need help with certain activities of daily living, or some degree of supervision.
Benefit triggers	Criteria for needing long-term care that must be met to generate payment of insurance benefits.
Chronic care	Care given for conditions that are long lasting or never changing.
Community-based health care	Care sponsored by the community, which are usually free or at low cost for qualifying individuals.
Congregate care facilities	Self-sufficient communities designed for retirees, which provide all levels of personal service *except* for health care services.
Continuing care retirement communities (CCRCs)	Self-sufficient communities designed for retirees, which provide all levels of personal and medical services, from the least to the most intensive.
Government agencies	Any state, local, or federal agencies.
Home health care	Supportive and curative care provided to patients in their homes.
Hospice care	Solely devoted to providing physical care and counseling to terminally ill patients and their families.
Nursing homes	Long-term-care facilities that provide a mix of intermediate-level nursing and personal services on a 24-hour basis to people who are either temporarily or permanently unable to care for themselves and require attention by a licensed nurse.
Palliative care	Care that eases the symptoms or discomfort of the condition but doesn't cure it.
Personal care facilities	Facilities for people who can no longer perform the functions of daily living without help.
Personal care homes	Smaller, less institutional assisted living facilities.

Proprietary health organizations	Private organizations that operate for a profit.
Rehabilitation centers	Facilities that help patients recover and/or manage specific conditions, addictions, or impairments. Also known as *rehab centers*.
Subacute care	Care for conditions that fall between acute, or sudden onset, and chronic, conditions that are long lasting or never changing).
Voluntary nonprofit health organizations	Private organizations that perform charitable functions or provide a community service.

ASSESS YOUR UNDERSTANDING

Go to www.wiley.com/college/pointer to evaluate your knowledge of the basics of long-term care.
Measure your learning by comparing pre-test and post-test results.

Summary Questions

1. Long-term care is health care provided only to those suffering from lengthy illnesses or disabling accidents. True or False?
2. Which of the following are long-term-care services?
    (a) inpatient and outpatient care
    (b) daily living support services
    (c) social services
    (d) a and b
    (e) all of the above
3. The primary users of long-term care are
    (a) those who are permanently disabled.
    (b) those recovering from temporary illnesses.
    (c) elderly people.
    (d) those with cognitive impairments.
4. When is residential long-term care necessary?
    (a) when patients must be on a ventilator or some other life-sustaining medical equipment
    (b) when patients can no longer receive adequate care at home
    (c) whenever patients state a preference for residential rather than at-home care
    (d) a and b
    (e) all of the above
5. Assisted living facilities offer what types of services?
    (a) skilled medical care
    (b) emergency care
    (c) help with certain activities of daily living
    (d) care for Alzheimer's/dementia patients
6. A potential resident of a continuing care retirement community must meet which of the following criteria?
    (a) be referred to the facility by a doctor
    (b) be healthy

(c) have no assets greater than an amount specified by the state in which the retirement community exists

(d) have private insurance

7. Nursing homes receive the most long-term health dollars. True or False?

8. Alzheimer's/dementia facilities are highly regulated by state health departments because of the vulnerability of the population they serve. True or False?

9. Which of the following describes in-home health care?

   (a) commonly provided by family members

   (b) often provided in conjunction with other ambulatory and inpatient services

   (c) majority of patients suffer from chronic health conditions

   (d) all of the above

10. Community-based services are coordinated by

    (a) social service agencies associated with local hospitals.

    (b) local Area Agencies on Aging.

    (c) local health departments.

    (d) all of the above.

11. The most common type of rehabilitation centers are

    (a) fitness facilities.

    (b) mental health facilities.

    (c) drug rehabilitation facilities.

    (d) none of the above.

12. Because of the complex nature of the conditions they treat, all rehabilitation centers are residential facilities. True or False?

13. Hospice care is end-of-life care for patients who are terminally ill. True or False?

14. The counseling component is a large part of hospice care. True or false?

15. When a hospice patient's illness goes into remission, what happens?

    (a) the length of stay in a hospice program is extended

    (b) he or she is no longer eligible for the hospice program

    (c) hospice care shifts to curative, rather than palliative, mode

    (d) there is no change in the care the patient receives

Review Questions

1. Long-term care addresses what health needs of its patients?

2. In what way is aging considered a chronic condition?

3. What is a substantive difference between the long-term care a person with a temporary health condition would receive compared to a person with a chronic health condition?
4. Identify which type of service is being provided in the following scenarios:
    (a) a social worker helps you fill out applications for assisted living
    (b) a health aide comes into your home to clean
    (c) you go to your primary care physician for pain management
    (d) a physical therapist comes to your home to help you with strengthening exercises
5. What care facility is a suitable alternative for a person who needs the care provided at an assisted living facility, but doesn't like the institutional settings at those facilities?
6. Differentiate between an assisted living community and a continuing care retirement community.
7. What long-term-care facilities would a person *not* approach to inquire about care for a spouse suffering from the early stages of Alzheimer's? Why?
8. What are home health agencies wanting Medicare certification required to do?
9. What is the profile of the person most likely to receive long-term health care at home?
10. Explain what it means for a home health care agency to be Medicare certified.
11. Despite the various types of community-based agencies, what one service do all the agencies provide?
12. Cite the features of rehabilitation centers.
13. What is the single significant difference between hospice care and care given by other long-term-care providers?

Applying This Chapter

1. Explain the impact that an aging population has on long-term health care.
2. In what ways are the various personal care facilities alike? In what significant ways are they different?
3. Indicate when home health care would be preferable to the other long-term-care options.
4. What type of rehab facility would you recommend to the following patients?
    (a) a 20-year-old who suffered a broken pelvis after a fall from a bike
    (b) a 5-year-old with autism
    (c) a senior citizen recovering from a heart attack

5. How does the composition of the hospice team reflect hospice goals?
6. Identify which type of long-term-care facility the following people would need:
   (a) an active, healthy elderly couple who want to prepare for the possibility of needing long-term care in the future
   (b) a homebound grandmother who needs help cleaning and preparing meals
   (c) a stroke victim who can no longer care for herself and needs nursing care around the clock
   (d) a man who has decided to stop chemotherapy for his end-stage liver cancer
   (e) a teenager with a drug addiction
7. Indicate what additional services you would recommend for an elderly patient recovering from a broken hip, who is receiving care at home, and who has no family in the area to help.

Understanding Long-Term Care

The focus of future health care is shifting from acute care to chronic care. Such a shift has profound implications for both the type of care provided and the way in which the care is provided. Explain the reason for this shift, how health care has to change as a result, and the way in which typical long-term services address these care issues.

Personal Care Facilities

As a director of a nursing home who is considering opening an Alzheimer's unit, what staffing issues would you have to address?

Rehabilitation Centers

In determining whether residential or outpatient rehabilitation were needed, what factors would you consider?

Hospice Care

As a hospice coordinator, indicate the types of questions you would ask a prospective client.

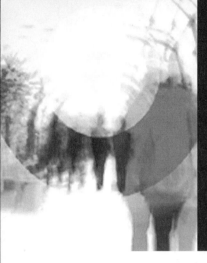

10

CARING FOR SPECIAL POPULATIONS
Mentally Ill, Homeless, Veteran, Immigrant, and Other Patients

Starting Point

Go to www.wiley.com/college/pointer to assess your knowledge of caring for special populations.
Determine where you need to concentrate your effort.

What You'll Learn in This Chapter

▲ The different populations with special health care challenges
▲ The health issues specific to certain populations
▲ Legal issues related to treating specific populations
▲ Types of mental health care available and sources of funding for mental health care

After Studying This Chapter, You'll Be Able To

▲ Compare legal issues impacting care of special populations
▲ Contrast the quality of ambulatory care and inpatient care
▲ Critique health care's current reliance on generalist medical care for mentally ill patients
▲ Examine the impact on quality of care when patients are unable to pay for health care

Goals and Outcomes

▲ Assess economic, social, and health issues as factors impacting special populations
▲ Propose potential strategies for overcoming obstacles to adequate health care for special populations

INTRODUCTION

Health care in the United States is comprised of a patchwork of health care providers, health care organizations, types of insurance and payment programs, and health care services. Navigating through this system is often overwhelming, and this is particularly true for people in certain populations who may have specific health care needs or who face particular health care challenges. This chapter defines these special populations, describes possible types and sources of care, explores challenges to receiving quality care, and examines legal issues related to treatment of mentally ill, homeless, veteran, immigrant, and other patient populations.

10.1 Caring for Mentally Ill Patients

Mental disease encompasses an array of psychological, biological, chemical, neurological, and behavioral disorders that impair cognitive, affective, and social functioning. Examples of these conditions include the following:

▲ Common mental illnesses, such as depression, anxiety, and phobias.
▲ Severe mental illness, such as psychosis, schizophrenia, and major depression.
▲ Behavioral problems such as obsessive-compulsive disorders.
▲ Mental retardation.
▲ Deterioration in brain function, such as Alzheimer's disease and dementia.
▲ Substance abuse.

Researchers estimate that approximately 40 percent of the people in the United States experience one or more psychiatric disorders requiring some form of care during their lifetime.

10.1.1 Providing Mental Health Services

In the first half of the twentieth century, most common mental disorders, such as depression and anxiety, went untreated primarily because they were not viewed as medical conditions that could be ameliorated but as immutable personality characteristics. People suffering from what today would be diagnosed as depression were simply sourpusses; people with anxiety were just "nervous types." In dealing with their illnesses, these people were dependent solely upon their own personal resources—"bucking up" or "chilling out"—and whatever support care their families could, or were willing to, provide. Individuals with major problems received care in local government psychiatric hospitals.

FOR EXAMPLE

Dorothea Dix

Dorothea Dix (1802–1887) was a social activist who spent her time and resources as an advocate for mentally ill individuals. During the early nineteenth century, people with mental illness were confined in almshouses (homes for the poor) or prisons, and treated accordingly. Dix, believing that mentally ill patients could be better served by being cared for in a family-like sanctuary removed from the pressures of daily living, successfully lobbied state legislatures to create asylums for those who were insane. In these asylums, Dix hoped, mentally ill patients could be humanely cared for. Unfortunately, these state-run mental hospitals failed to live up to Dix's vision and turned instead into huge "museums of madness" where mentally ill people were simply housed. For more about Dorothea Dix's life and accomplishments, review the biography offered by Dorothea Dix Hospital, Raleigh, NC (www.dhhs.state.nc.us/mhddsas/DIX).

Between the mid-1950s and the early 1980s, however, care of mentally ill patients changed dramatically:

▲ Researchers developed an array of effective psychotropic medications.
▲ Mental health facilities expanded ambulatory treatment alternatives.
▲ Society began to view mental and behavioral disabilities differently than it had in years past.

As a result of these changes, the inpatient population decreased significantly, and ambulatory care is now the norm for nearly all patients with mental and behavior disabilities. The United States has approximately 5,700 mental health facilities that offer either inpatient or outpatient care. Table 10-1 shows their distribution.

Ambulatory Care

Although mental health care is still provided in inpatient and outpatient facilities, the greatest volume of services, by far, is **ambulatory**, or delivered on an outpatient basis. Today, patients with mental and behavioral disorders receive care in settings such as:

▲ Primary care physician (PCP) offices.
▲ Psychiatrists' offices.
▲ Offices of mental health professionals (psychologists, clinical social workers, marriage and family counselors).
▲ Mental health centers.

Table 10-1: Inpatient and Outpatient Mental Health Facilities

Facilities	Number
Total	5722
State and county mental hospitals	229
Private psychiatric hospitals	348
Short-term general hospitals with designated psychiatric units	1707
Department of Veterans Affairs facilities, including VA neuropsychiatric hospitals, VA general hospital psychiatric services, and VA psychiatric outpatient units	145
Residential treatment facilities for emotionally disturbed children	461
Other, including freestanding psychiatric outpatient clinics, partial care organizations, and multi-service mental health facilities	2832

▲ General hospital outpatient departments and emergency rooms.
▲ Day care programs.
▲ Substance abuse centers.
▲ Psychiatric clinics.
▲ Focused programs such as Alcoholics Anonymous.
▲ Support groups.

Inpatient Care

Inpatient treatment is offered in the following settings:

▲ **Psychiatric units of short-term general hospitals:** These units, part of a larger general hospital, are aimed at short-term care of patients with mental health issues. Patients can be self-referred or referred by a PCP or a mental health professional. Patients utilizing these units are usually diagnosed with mental health conditions that are relatively temporary in nature and have a short-term treatment plan. Psychiatric units of general hospitals may also treat patients suffering from trauma, which calls for their mental health status to be examined.

▲ **Mental hospitals:** Mental hospitals focus exclusively on mental health issues and their related illnesses. Unlike a general hospital, the mental hospital specializes in mental health and is more likely to be equipped to handle the most difficult mental health patients. Patients in these facilities are usually referred by a physician, mental health care professional, or law enforcement agent. Patients in mental hospitals are usually admitted for longer terms than those cared for in psychiatric units of general hospitals. Mental hospitals also offer residential care to patients with the most extreme mental health issues.

▲ **Special purpose hospitals (such as substance abuse facilities or eating disorder clinics):** These are usually longer-term residential facilities. Patients in these kinds of hospitals are most often referred by other mental health professionals, physicians, or the legal system. Some special purpose hospitals also take self-referrals. In these facilities, the holistic approach is oftentimes the center of treatment.

For years, mental hospitals were seen (and indeed sometimes run) as prisons. Their primary purpose was to contain, rather than treat, mentally ill individuals. Psychiatric hospitals of years gone by were dark, scary, and misunderstood places. Fortunately, mental health care and facilities have advanced well beyond the care provided in these gloomy settings: Today's psychiatric hospitals are positive, caring facilities that focus on treatment of mental issues much like general hospitals focus on treating other kinds of illnesses. Nevertheless, these modern-day facilities continue to battle the legacy of the "insane asylums" of years past: the continuing misunderstanding of mental illness and the attendant reluctance of insurance providers to adequately fund mental health services.

10.1.2 Paying for Mental Health Services

Funding for mental health is relatively low. Some estimates show mental health as receiving only one-third the funding of other health care services. In 1996, total mental expenditures were estimated to be $69 billion (up from $4 billion in 1969); 47 percent derived from private sources and 53 percent from the government. Table 10-2 shows the source of funding by type of payer.

The issue of mental health insurance parity with other types of health insurance is an important one. Despite the tremendous advances made in mental health care—from understanding its multiple causes (including physiological and well as environmental triggers) to treatment strategies—mental health services do not receive the funding that other health care issues do.

Traditionally, mental health has been looked at as an extra in the health care system. Only a few decades ago, mental health issues were swept under the rug, and mental hospitals were seen as last-ditch places for society's lost citizens. Mental health professionals such as psychiatrists and psychologists and therapists

Table 10-2: Sources of Funding for Mental Health Services

Source	Percentage
Private	**47**
Private insurance	27
Out-of-pocket	17
Other	3
Public	**53**
Medicaid	19
State and local government	18
Medicare	14
Federal	2

were seen as second-class professionals. All of this has kept funding for mental health from reaching the same level as funding for other health issues. Even today, some insurance plans still refuse to pay for mental health–related services, and those that do reimburse patients still limit access to only a few visits to a therapist a year.

People with mental health issues are at particular risk when they are uninsured because their illnesses are not easily dealt with in emergency rooms or in urgent care centers. General public hospitals are required to take all patients regardless of illness or infirmity. This causes an undue burden on the health care system because traditional health care facilities have to deal with mentally ill patients and their list of related ailments (imagined or otherwise) when they may be unequipped to do so. This also takes time and resources away from other areas of the health care system.

10.1.3 Challenges to Accessing and Providing Care for Mentally Ill Patients

Health care for individuals with mental and behavioral disabilities has improved dramatically over the centuries. Some of the most dramatic changes, however, have occurred in the last few decades. The advent of effective psychiatric drugs has fostered an era in which psychiatric and behavioral disorders are being routinely treated and managed. This, combined with studies leading to greater understanding of the causes of mental and behavioral issues, has gone a long way toward reducing the stigma attached to such conditions.

Despite these advances, however, mental and behavioral health care faces some continuing challenges.

Displaced Populations

The cost crunch that the health care industry is facing is having a dramatic effect on mental health care. Many mental hospitals have closed their doors because of skyrocketing operating costs. It's simply not financially viable in most areas of the country to operate fully functioning mental hospitals.

Some claim that the short-term cost savings of not treating mental patients justifies shutting down these facilities; the reality, however, is that the costs have simply been shifted: to other health care facilities which are often ill-equipped to adequately deal with this special population; to community support services that are buckling under the strain of serving this new population with resources limited by their own budget cuts; to mentally ill patients themselves who, because of the nature of their illnesses, are most vulnerable.

Reliance on Outpatient Care

Outpatient care is a major trend in health care. It is no different in the mental health field. The trend to treat mental health issues on an outpatient basis seems, at first, to make sense in terms of cost and time. In fact, this is one of the rationales used to justify closing state mental hospitals. However, given the nature of many mental health–related issues and conditions, effectively dealing with mental health issues in 50-minute intervals is quite difficult. Many mental health conditions require extensive and intensive treatment that can be accomplished only in a longer-term facility.

Quality of Care

Because of the trend toward reducing mental health funding and relying solely on outpatient treatment, many people with mental health issues receive substandard treatment. First, in most communities that oversaw the shutting down of public mental health hospitals, no comprehensive mental health system was put in place to replace the hospital services. Instead, mental health in the United States relies on a patchwork of facilities and care providers that, in most instances, are not universally coordinated to provide ongoing, comprehensive care. Without the specialized care provided by mental health hospitals, general hospitals and small residential facilities must pick up the balance of care for many mental patients. Not only does this situation increase the overall costs of these fall-back providers, but it also negatively impacts the health care for the displaced populations.

In addition, some prematurely discharged patients receive no follow-up care because the communities in which they live have no mental health resources or resources that are difficult to access. In these instances, patients (and their families, if they are involved) are left to piece together care however they can. Many within this group go without. Obviously, the most severely mentally ill individuals in our society are at the greatest disadvantage, but they are not the only ones who are harmed by the lack of coordinated care. As more and more people receive ambulatory care for mental health problems, attention has shifted to the quality of care provided. Findings suggest the following:

▲ Generalists are not as skillful as psychiatrists at recognizing and treating depression, and they frequently miss clues to suicidal intent.

▲ Inpatients with depression received better management of the psychological aspects of their illnesses (although worse management of the medical aspects) when cared for in psychiatric wards.

▲ Psychiatrists' patients had better functional outcomes, largely as a result of more frequent counseling, more appropriate dosing of antidepressants, and less use of potentially harmful minor tranquilizers.

▲ Even when primary care providers were given diagnostic scales and treatment algorithms, fewer than half of the patients they identified with depression actually received treatment. The reasons for this lack of treatment are unclear, but researchers attribute it to any of the following possibilities:

  • Patient reluctance to take medicines.

  • Physicians' pessimism regarding the effectiveness of treatments.

  • The fact that generalists see a higher percentage of mildly depressed and less-motivated patients in whom the use of antidepressants may not be as effective.

  • The fact that adequately treating anxiety and depression is time and labor intensive, and reimbursement incentives encourage psychiatrists to offer more frequent and longer office visits for counseling.

▲ Generalists are frequently unsuccessful in identifying alcohol and drug abuse. While brief, extensively validated screening tests with good sensitivity and specificity exist and are simple to use, most alcoholics go unrecognized, and, even when diagnosed, are untreated.

10.1.4 Legal Issues regarding Health Care for Mentally Ill Patients

There are several key legal issues pertaining to health care for mentally ill patients. These legal issues have developed over time as U.S. society has developed and changed.

Commitment Laws

Commitment laws are laws that enable family members, law enforcement, or health care professionals to commit a person to a care facility or to a treatment plan. There are two major types of commitment laws. First, there is **voluntary commitment,** which occurs when people voluntarily commits themselves to a care facility such as a psychiatric ward, hospital, institution, or treatment center.

Generally, with voluntary commitment, a person is free to leave whenever he or she decides to with given notice.

A second type of commitment law is more involved. **Involuntary commitment laws** allow for committing people against their wishes. The majority of states have laws and procedures that deal with involuntarily commitment. These laws generally involve a hearing where it must be proven that the person in question is either dangerous to self or others, or suffering from a mental illness or some other disorder. When people are involuntary committed, they are not free to leave or stop treatment when they desire.

A subtype of involuntary commitment law that has come to gain further attention in recent years is involuntary outpatient mental health treatment law. (An example of this is Kendra's Law in New York state.) These laws make provisions for court-mandated orders to force people to seek assisted outpatient treatment and/or take medication. The laws involve a hearing and have set procedures for noncompliance.

Involuntary commitment laws are controversial, and are opposed by groups that cite them as unconstitutional and force people into incarceration-type conditions. In 1975, the U.S. Supreme Court ruled that these types of laws were indeed supported by the Constitution and were thus legal.

Discriminatory Insurance Practices against Mentally Ill Patients

People with mental illness traditionally have been discriminated against when it comes to adequate health insurance coverage. For decades, insurers and state governments have viewed mental illness with, if not skepticism, caution when it comes to granting insurance coverage. This caused a great gap in terms of coverage for those with mental illnesses. It also created a vicious circle of sorts: A person couldn't afford to pay for mental health treatment, so the mental illness became worse or affected other parts of society. This helped contribute to the disenfranchisement of many people suffering from mental illness, and also contributed to the stigma attached to people who had the disease.

As the mental health profession has matured, so has society's view on the mentally ill and on the significance of mental illness. This has caused the push for mental health care parity at the local, state, and federal levels. State laws have been passed that require insurers doing business within the state to insure mental illness–related issues with the same equivalents as they do other health care issues. Most recently in 2006, New York state passed Timothy's Law which grants insurance parity to those suffering mental health issues.

Applying the Americans with Disabilities Act

The *Americans with Disabilities Act (ADA)* prohibits the discrimination of a person in public accommodations, transportation, and employment who has a physical or mental impairment that substantially limits one or more major life activities. At first, this was interpreted as including a wide variety of mental illnesses.

However, since the passage of the ADA, the U.S. Supreme Court has made several rulings that limit the scope of the ADA to take into account mitigating circumstances in both physical and mental disabilities. Again, this becomes an issue of parity. With tighter interpretation of the ADA, mental illness may not be completely represented and accounted for in the ADA. This means that persons with mental illness are not afforded the same ADA protections as someone with another physical disability. There has been litigation attempting to bring mental health disability in line with other physical disabilities in the eyes of the ADA, but mental illness, in many ways, retains second-tier status in terms of the ADA.

SELF-CHECK

- Identify and define **mental disease, ambulatory care,** and **commitment laws.**
- List the types of conditions that fall under the category of mental illnesses.
- Describe ambulatory care settings in which mental health services are provided.
- Compare the three inpatient care settings where mentally ill patients can receive care.
- Classify sources of funding for mental health services.
- Identify three major challenges for providing health care to mentally ill patients.
- Describe potential downsides to relying on generalist, ambulatory care for mentally ill patients.
- Contrast voluntary and involuntary commitment.
- Discuss the changing role of the ADA in treating mentally ill patients.

10.2 Homeless Patients

Historically, the U.S. homeless population has included primarily single men. Although they still make up the majority of population, women and children have joined their ranks. Today, according to the U.S. Department of Health and Human Services, 600,000 men, women, and children are homeless every night in the United States. According to the National Coalition on the Homeless, homelessness has increased over the past 20 years because of the growing shortage of affordable rental housing and, at the same time, an increase in poverty. The result is that more families and couples are now homeless than ever before.

10.2.1 Health Issues in the Homeless Population

Homeless people have all the same types of health problems as housed people, but at rates three to six times greater. Not only are they more vulnerable to the same diseases as housed people, but they are also more likely to have diseases associated with poverty and less likely to access medical care. Consider the following:

▲ People without shelter often suffer from serious health problems such as parasites, frostbite, infections, and violence.

▲ Some illnesses, such as tuberculosis, AIDS, malnutrition, and severe dental problems, are closely associated with poverty and are common in homeless populations.

▲ Some health problems, such as alcoholism, mental illnesses, and drug abuse, are prominent in homeless populations.

▲ Other health conditions, such as diabetes, hypertension, and physical disabilities, are exacerbated by exposure and lack of care.

▲ Homeless patients who do receive health care often have difficulty following through with treatments. Taking medication, recuperating from an illness or surgery, and so on, becomes extremely difficult—if not impossible—without a stable, safe environment.

10.2.2 Challenges in Providing Health Care to Homeless People

Many homeless people are in dire need of health care services. Accessing those services, however, is problematic:

▲ Most homeless people do not have health insurance or money to pay for services.

▲ Many are not near health care facilities and often lack the transportation or means to travel to a clinic.

FOR EXAMPLE

Health Care for Homeless People Project

To address the special health needs of the homeless population in Honolulu, the Kalihi-Palama Health Center (www.healthhawaii.org) integrates traditional outpatient care with programs devised specifically for homeless patients. The project supports several medical clinics housed in homeless shelters and offering a wide range of medical services, a Shelter + Care program designed to help physically or mentally disabled homeless people live independently, and community education programs focusing on issues relating to homelessness in the community. As communities across the nation grapple with the growing homeless population, such integrated efforts are likely to become more common.

▲ Many avoid health care treatment because of fear or unpleasant experiences with health care providers.

▲ Avoidance of treatment results in health conditions worsening which leads to more complex treatments and higher costs when health care services are accessed.

▲ Many are more concerned with surviving day-to-day—securing shelter, food, clothing, and safety—than with their long-term health.

▲ Some health care providers unfamiliar with health issues associated with homeless may result in misdiagnosis or improper treatment.

SELF-CHECK

- Describe the changing demographics of today's homeless population.
- Identify specific health problems associated with homelessness.
- List typical obstacles health care providers encounter when treating homeless individuals.
- Explain why many homeless people delay seeking health care.

10.3 Veterans

Veterans are people who serve (or served) in the U.S. armed forces. The **Veteran's Health Administration (VA)** was originally established to provide care for Civil War veterans. With the end of World War I, however, the VA began contracting on a large scale with hospitals to provide VA services as well as building hospitals exclusive to veterans. Today the VA has grown into one of largest health care systems in the nation. The VA coordinates and operates more than 170 medical centers, almost 400 clinics, and more than 120 nursing home facilities.

Health care coverage for veterans meeting eligibility is provided by the VA. Health care coverage for active-duty personnel is provided by the Military Health Services program of the U.S. Department of Defense. These two government health care programs combine to cover veterans, active-duty military service personnel, their families, and retirees.

10.3.1 Health Issues for Veterans

Veterans have the same health issues as everyone else such as alcohol and drug abuse, cancer, and heart disease; however, many often have service- or combat-related issues as well. These issues require special treatment and special knowledge.

FOR EXAMPLE

Evaluating Veteran's Hospitals

A chief complaint of many and concern for others appears to be the quality of health care provided at VA hospitals (www.va.gov). Although the Walter Reed Army Medical Center (www.wramc.amedd.army.mil) is one of the most renowned VA hospitals in the United States and is generally considered to provide the highest quality of health care, other VA hospitals have been characterized less favorably. Complaints include unnecessary delays in treatment or access, substandard care, insufficient numbers of health care providers, and so on. To find out what the Veteran's Health Administration is doing to respond to criticism and provide excellent health care at www.va.gov/healtheligibility/gettingcare/patient_rights_and_responsibilities.asp.

Veterans have special health care needs resulting from their service. Depending on the nature of the health issue, these services may be temporary or they may be long term and/or recurring. Some of these special needs include:

▲ **Rehabilitation services:** services that help restore skills lost with injury or illness. The goal of rehab is to regain normal or near-normal functioning so that the veteran can lead a quality life.
▲ **Mental health issues:** services that help the veteran deal with the emotional pressures and stress resulting from their service.
▲ **Toxic agent exposure services:** services that treat veterans for exposure to the various toxic agents used in warfare and conflicts. In World War II radiation caused many service personnel myriad health care problems. In the Vietnam War, Agent Orange (dioxin) caused nerve and urological disorders, skin diseases, and soft-tissue cancers in many service personnel. Veterans of the Gulf War have been many times more likely to experience high rates of Lou Gehrig's disease, memory loss, brain cancers, and fibromyalgia.

This is not an exhaustive list of health care needs specific to veterans but it does illustrate the unique nature of many of the issues facing providers of health care to veterans.

10.3.2 Challenges in Providing Health Care to Veterans

The VA health delivery system is well equipped to handle the host of military service–related health issues such as combat fatigue, posttraumatic stress syndrome, radiation exposure, Agent Orange exposure, Gulf War syndrome, and a variety of other mental and physical disabilities and rehabilitation care. Medical coverage of veterans includes a *Standard Enhanced Health Benefits Plan,* and each veteran is placed into one of eight priority groups that help determine coverage.

There are many laws that relate specifically to veterans and the health care of veterans, and they primarily deal with coverage, eligibility, and reimbursement/compensation. The 1999 *Veterans Millennium Health Care and Benefits Act* deserves mention because it was the most recent law to be passed that expands long-term care and emergency service care for veterans, as well as defining eligibility priority groups. As laws and acts are passed in the United States, often they have special provisions for veterans.

SELF-CHECK

- Identify and define **veteran** and **Veteran's Health Administration**.
- Describe the basic health care benefits guaranteed to veterans under the Veterans Millennium Health Care and Benefits Act.
- List three specific areas of health care services needed by veteran patients.

10.4 Immigrants

Immigrants are people who come to the United States with the intention of establishing permanent residency. **Legal immigrants** are those who enter the country after following the procedures outlined by the Bureau of U.S. Citizenship and Immigration Services. **Illegal immigrants,** also referred to as undocumented immigrants, enter the United States without following these procedures. Both documented and undocumented immigrants face hurdles in accessing health care in this country, although undocumented immigrants face greater challenges.

10.4.1 Challenges in Providing Health Care to Immigrants

There are several challenges that are common to immigrants, illegal or otherwise. These issues include:

▲ **Language barriers:** Health care facilities may not have interpreters available and therefore must diagnose and treat without the ability to communicate.

▲ **Poorer country of origin health care:** Some immigrants come from countries that have less advanced medical systems and therefore their medical condition is worse because of delay in care.

▲ **Cultural variables:** Many cultures around the world look at illness and indeed, medical care, differently than the United States. American hospitals and clinics expect a patient to fit into the health care culture here immediately upon access. This can be confusing and disorienting to many immigrants and often they may fail to communicate their health issue or condition, which may lead to misdiagnosis or extended treatments.

10.4.2 Legal Issues Regarding Health Care for Immigrants

Immigrant health care issues center around access to care and the duty to treat. Any immigrant, legal or illegal, is given basic treatment in the U.S. health system because of the **duty to treat.** The U.S. health system holds that any human being deserves basic care. Because of this, hospitals and clinics will treat immigrants regardless of their status. Many illegal immigrants falsify Social Security numbers and make up names. Since most clinics do not check immigration identification, they are able to receive treatment. Clinics in border communities especially receive the bulk of immigrant patients. Because fear exists in many illegal immigrants, they do not seek medical attention until absolutely necessary. By this time, their medical conditions are at their worst and require more advanced (and expensive) care.

Legal immigrants may be entitled to some benefits under law depending on the status on which they enter the country; however, as laws tighten, immigrants are increasingly being required to have **sponsors**—family members or others

---

FOR EXAMPLE

Denying Medical Care to Illegal Aliens

In 2004, a bill was introduced into the U.S. House of Representatives that would require hospital emergency rooms to deny medical care to illegal aliens while at the same time alerting the U.S. Citizenship and Immigration Services Bureau (www.uscis.gov) to the undocumented immigrant's whereabouts. Hispanic legislators led opposition to the bill and joined medical groups in claiming that the bill would effectively turn hospitals into law enforcement agencies. It would also, opponents argued, stop illegal residents from accessing life-saving treatment. The bill was defeated by a large majority. Find out about the current status of medical care (and dozens of other government services) for illegal aliens by visiting www.uscis.gov/graphics/lawsregs/index.htm.

who will, in a sense, cosign for any cost the immigrant incurs. Illegal immigrants, on the other hand, access health care and never repay the system or have benefits. Hospitals, especially in border communities, incur huge costs treating illegal immigrants.

SELF-CHECK

- Identify and define **immigrant** and **sponsor**.
- Explain the differences between illegal and legal immigrants.
- Describe how the U.S. duty to treat impacts the health care services provided to legal and illegal immigrants.
- List major issues related to immigrants receiving good health care.

10.5 Caring for Other Special Populations

In addition to the groups discussed in the previous sections, other groups also have special health care needs and face challenges in receiving appropriate medical care. Consider the following:

10.5.1 People with AIDS and HIV

For people with AIDS and HIV, the problem is not accessing health care as much as being provided adequate care. Two studies indicate that people infected with HIV or AIDS who receive care from generalists have higher odds of being hospitalized and significantly shorter survival than those cared for by AIDS specialists. Researchers suspect that the reasons behind these findings are twofold:

▲ Generalists may be inappropriately delaying initiation of anti-infective therapy.
▲ Specialists' expertise makes them better at detecting AIDS-related complications at an earlier stage or in managing complications on an outpatient basis.

In recent nationwide surveys, majorities of residents and primary care physicians (PCPs) expressed concerns about the adequacy of their training in AIDS ambulatory care, and more than 80 percent of PCPs believed they lacked information needed to care for patients with those illnesses seen in advanced HIV infection. In fact, generalists failed to discern common HIV-associated lesions when confronted with standardized patients. Even those generalists with more

FOR EXAMPLE

Health Consequences of Child Abuse

According to the CDC's National Center for Injury Prevention and Control (www.cdc.gov/ncipc), in 2002 nearly a million children in the United States were confirmed as being maltreated—that is, victims of abuse (physical, sexual, or emotional) or neglect. The health care needs of these children go beyond treating the direct effects of the abuse or neglect. Consider these findings:

▲ Children who are maltreated are at increased risk for health issues as adults, including smoking, alcoholism, drug abuse, eating disorders, depression, suicide, certain chronic diseases, and more.

▲ Abuse or neglect during infancy or early childhood can negatively affect brain development and result in physical, mental, and emotional problems.

▲ About 25 to 30 percent of children who are victims of shaken baby syndrome die from their injuries; those who survive may suffer from varying degrees of visual impairment or brain damage.

experience managing HIV had significant knowledge gaps surrounding the treatment of AIDS-related health issues.

10.5.2 Victims of Violence

Physicians frequently fail to identify victims of domestic violence, even though 10 to 30 percent of women who go to emergency departments for treatment are victims of domestic abuse. Even when physicians recognize abuse, they often provide no treatment, or they provide inappropriate or harmful treatment.

Despite mandatory reporting laws, physicians also underrecognize and underreport abuse of elderly people, which has been estimated to affect approximately 10 percent of Americans older than 65 years.

SELF-CHECK

• List the two reasons why AIDS/HIV patients tend to have better outcomes with specialists rather than generalists.

• Discuss obstacles that block victims of abuse from receiving treatment.

SUMMARY

U.S. health care organizations provide services to numerous special patient populations. Today, mentally ill patients receive both ambulatory care and inpatient care, which is funded by an array of private and public sources. The recently displaced nature of this population, combined with the current reliance on outpatient care provided by generalists and many related legal issues, makes treating mentally ill patients particularly challenging. Homeless patients suffer with a variety of conditions and diseases related to poverty and a lack of shelter and food; treating these individuals is especially difficult due to lack of follow-through for medical treatments. Veterans are provided health care services through the Veteran's Health Administration, but these services and facilities often lack adequate funding or up-to-date facilities and treatments. Immigrant patients—both legal and illegal—are guaranteed basic medical care under the U.S. duty to treat principle, but deciding who pays for these services is a major political and legal question. Other patient populations with special issues and obstacles include individuals with HIV/AIDS and victims of abuse.

KEY TERMS

Ambulatory care	Health care delivered on an outpatient basis.
Commitment laws	Laws that enable family members, law enforcement, or health care professionals to commit a person to a care facility or to a treatment plan.
Duty to treat	Principle of the U.S. health system that any human being deserves basic care.
Illegal immigrants	Immigrants who enter the United States without following procedures outlined by the Bureau of U.S. Citizenship and Immigration Services; also referred to as undocumented immigrants.
Immigrants	People who come to the United States with the intention of establishing permanent residency.
Involuntary commitment	A patient is committed against his or her wishes.
Legal immigrants	Immigrants who enter the United States after following the procedures outlined by the Bureau of U.S. Citizenship and Immigration Services.
Mental disease	Term for an array of psychological, biological, chemical, neurological, and behavioral disorders that impair cognitive, affective, and social functioning.

Sponsors	Family members or others who will cosign for any health care cost an immigrant incurs.
Veteran	A person who serves (or served) in the U.S. armed forces.
Veteran's Health Administration (VA)	U.S. governmental agency that provides hospitals and health care services for veterans.
Voluntary commitment	A person voluntarily commits to a care facility such as a psychiatric ward, hospital, institution, or treatment center. Generally the person is free to leave at will, with given notice.

ASSESS YOUR UNDERSTANDING

Go to www.wiley.com/college/pointer to evaluate your knowledge of the basics of caring for special populations.

Measure your learning by comparing pre-test and post-test results.

Summary Questions

1. Which of the following conditions is classified as a mental illness?
   (a) phobia
   (b) mental retardation
   (c) Alzheimer's disease
   (d) a, c, and d

2. What impact did the creation of more effective treatments for mental health have on inpatient care?
   (a) inpatient services increased
   (b) inpatient services declined
   (c) inpatient services remained the same

3. Most of the services provided to mentally ill patients take place in outpatient settings. True or False?

4. Mental disease can be classified as any illness that impairs cognitive, affective, and social functioning. True or False?

5. As knowledge about and treatment of mental illness advances, the stigma associated with mental health care has disappeared, putting mental health services on par with medical services provided for other types of illnesses. True or False?

6. Two decades ago, the U.S. homeless population was largely elderly people and males; today it includes a significant number of women and children. True or False?

7. Although all health care issues affect homeless patients, which diseases are especially significant within homeless populations?
   (a) tuberculosis
   (b) alcoholism
   (c) AIDS
   (d) all of the above

8. For many homeless patients, receiving basic health care is more important than satisfying basic needs such as shelter and food. True or False?

9. Established to provide care for Civil War veterans, the Veteran's Health Administration now provides financial reimbursement to any veteran for health care services at any U.S. public or private hospital. True or False?

10. In addition to physical conditions, veteran patients frequently deal with mental health–related conditions, including:

    (a) early onset Alzheimer's.

    (b) posttraumatic stress disorder.

    (c) schizophrenia.

    (d) all the above.

11. In the United States, the duty to treat principle means

    (a) all individuals deserve basic health care services.

    (b) doctors have a responsibility to treat any patient they encounter.

    (c) patients can seek health care from any medical professional.

    (d) any hospital or clinic must offer services to the insured.

12. While many illegal and legal immigrants come from nations with less advanced medical systems and consequently tend to delay care, illegal immigrants have the additional obstacle of fearing that they'll be sent to jail or returned to their native country. True or False?

13. Someone who essentially cosigns with an immigrant to cover any medical costs the immigrant incurs is known as a

    (a) legal guardian.

    (b) health advocate.

    (c) custodian.

    (d) sponsor.

14. Which of the following statements about treating patients with HIV/AIDS is true?

    (a) patient confidentially is the most significant problem

    (b) disease transmission to health care workers is the most significant problem

    (c) cost of care is the most significant problem

    (d) adequate care—not access to care—is the most significant problem

15. Domestic violence studies show that

    (a) 25 to 30 percent of children who are victims of shaken baby syndrome die from their injuries.

    (b) abuse affects 10 percent of Americans over age 65.

    (c) 10 to 30 percent of all female emergency room cases are from domestic abuse.

    (d) all of the above.

Review Questions

1. Compare the experiences of mentally ill patients in ambulatory care and inpatient care.

2. A family decides their son is at severe risk of hurting himself or others and places him in a temporary hospitalization program. Which type of commitment laws are the family invoking?

3. Although health care for mentally ill patients has improved dramatically in the last two decades, care is still often lacking. What are two major challenges specifically related to caring for mentally ill patients?

4. Follow-through of treatments is a major challenge for homeless patients. What sort of activities constitute follow-through?

5. What are some possible reasons that more people are homeless today than ever before?

6. What substances are included in toxic agent exposure services, which are guaranteed to veteran patients?

7. What law guarantees health care benefits to veterans?

8. Immigrants are often in very poor health when they finally seek medical attention. Why?

9. Why are people with AIDS/HIV more likely to receive better health care through a specialist rather than a generalist?

Applying This Chapter

1. One of your close friends appears to have been suffering from extreme depression for more than six months and wants to seek help. Your friend knows you have an interest in health care and asks your opinion of what he should do. You know your friend has limited financial resources but also wants to get the most appropriate effective mental health care possible. How might you help your friend choose between seeing a medical generalist or a psychiatrist?

2. As the director of a homeless shelter, you are asked to present a wish list of free health care services you'd like to see local hospitals provide to individuals at your shelter. In your presentation, which diseases, conditions, and illnesses would you highlight as most in need of medical attention?

3. After several years of working as a counselor at a private mental health care facility, Raul has decided to shift his career to a position within a Veteran's Health Administration, working with veteran patients on their mental health issues. What aspects of his mental health care background will serve Raul well in his new career? What aspects of mental health training will he need to focus on and perhaps gain new skills and understanding in?

4. As part of an upcoming immigration bill, the U.S. government wants to cut funding to health care providers along the U.S.-Mexican border. The city you work in is five miles from the Mexican border. Your organization's resources are already limited and the budget cuts would make it nearly impossible to continue offering health care resources to legal and illegal immigrants. Why should budget cuts to your community be spared?

5. As part of a community communication committee, you are challenged to dispel the myths of domestic violence. To highlight the fact that abuse can happen to anyone, regardless of gender, age, or income, which statistics will you highlight? What groups will you target your message for?

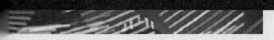
Caring for Mentally Ill Patients

In an effort to cut costs, many state-run mental health hospitals have been shut down in recent years. These individuals must continue to receive care, although now in different forms and often from multiple sources. As a member of an advisory panel, consider what you would recommend to four groups—your state and local government, health care insurers, families, and patients—if your state decided to close its mental health hospitals in the next six months.

Homeless Patients

Homeless patients often do not seek medical treatment because of a number of fears, including fear of being forced into social services, fear of mistreatment by medical staff, and fear of social stigmatization, among many others. What do you think are the top three fears that block homeless patients from seeking health care? In what way could an urban hospital or clinic address each of these fears directly and encourage homeless patients to seek medical help?

Veterans

Like most U.S. states, Colorado has set up a health care program for providing health care to the state's veterans at each of the current eight tiers, or "priority groups," of coverage. Review the Colorado plan at www. coloradomedicare.com/tricare/va_services_eligibility. asp. If you had an additional $50 million annually to spend in Colorado for veteran's care, how would you change the current benefits? If you had to cut $50 million for the current plan, what would you change?

Immigrants

For various reasons—including cultural, emotional, or financial—many immigrants wait until their medical conditions are at their worst before seeking health care. What are some innovative ways you can connect with immigrants and encourage them to access health care earlier and more frequently? Remember that health care doesn't have to be administered only in a hospital setting. What are some nontraditional ways immigrants can access health care information and services.

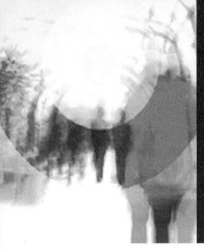

11

CARING FOR UNINSURED PATIENTS
Health Care for Patients without Insurance Coverage

Starting Point

Go to www.wiley.com/college/pointer to assess your knowledge of the health care issues impacting uninsured patients.
Determine where you need to concentrate your effort.

What You'll Learn in This Chapter

▲ The definitions of uninsured and underinsured patients
▲ Groups that typically comprise uninsured patients
▲ The severity of the U.S. health insurance crisis
▲ The types of health care facilities that treat uninsured patients
▲ The major challenges in treating uninsured patients
▲ Sources of funding for uninsured health care
▲ Laws that impact the care of uninsured patients

After Studying This Chapter, You'll Be Able To

▲ Categorize the types of patients who make up uninsured patients and underinsured patients
▲ Compare the services of health care facilities frequented by uninsured patients
▲ Critique current trends in emergency room usage by uninsured patients
▲ Contrast health-related and financial-related challenges associated with treating uninsured patients
▲ Examine cost-saving methods of health care organizations to deal with uninsured patients

Goals and Outcomes

▲ Assess the effectiveness of treating uninsured patients
▲ Recommend possible solutions for providing care in existing facilities frequented by uninsured patients
▲ Evaluate the effectiveness and ethics of various cost-saving methods related to treating uninsured patients in today's health care facilities

INTRODUCTION

More and more people in the United States are joining the ranks of uninsured patients, individuals who lack private health insurance coverage and who don't qualify for either Medicaid or Medicare (see Chapter 4). Uninsured patients, however, still receive medical services through community health centers, urgent care facilities, and emergency rooms. Not only do uninsured patients face challenges in maintaining adequate health care, but the institutions providing such care face challenges as well. The few existing laws have been unable to adequately address these issues.

11.1 Identifying Uninsured Patients

By definition, **uninsured patients** are those who lack any type of health insurance, including employer-provided insurance or privately purchased insurance, and who do not qualify for governmental insurance programs such as Medicaid and Medicare. In the U.S. health care system, which is based on a fee-for-service principle (that is, health care is a consumer product to be purchased) and which doesn't mandate universal health care for all citizens, people without health insurance are in a unique—and disadvantaged—situation.

The ranks of uninsured patients are populated by the working poor, the unemployed, and, increasingly, women and children. Middle-class workers whose employers do not provide insurance benefits and who do not earn enough to purchase private insurance are also a growing uninsured group.

As of 2005, 16 percent of the population in the United States was uninsured. The U.S. Census Bureau estimates that as many as 60 million people (approximately 25 percent of the population) will be without health insurance by 2007. More alarming projections indicate that by 2020 more than a third of all Americans will have no coverage.

These increasing numbers are the result of rising health care costs, which make insurance less affordable for both individuals and businesses; the increasing number of families falling into poverty, only half of whom qualify for Medicaid; and the decrease in the number of employers offering insurance plans to employees.

Some uninsured populations have very specific needs:

▲ **Mentally ill patients (see Section 10.1):** These patients need medical treatment and often are one of the least insured groups within the United States. Providing therapy and treatment for mental illness often requires

> ## FOR EXAMPLE
>
> ### Life without Health Insurance
>
> According to the Census Bureau, the number of uninsured is rising among the middle and upper-middle class. If you consider that the number of businesses offering insurance is declining while the cost of insurance coverage is rising (according to a 2005 Kaiser survey, the average annual cost of insurance for a family of four is $11,000, up 73 percent from 2000), this trend isn't so surprising. Nor is it particularly surprising that medical expenses are the second leading cause of bankruptcy in the United States. As more and more middle-class families land on the rolls of uninsured patients, health advocates say, Americans are less likely to see lack of health coverage as a problem impacting only the poor and the homeless. And *that,* they say, will lead to a renewed debate about how America's health care system is financed and functions.

repeat treatments and medications that are costly and hard to administer without proper conditions.

▲ **Homeless patients (see Section 10.2):** These patients frequently deal with health issues such as malnutrition and complications related to poor hygiene. Many diseases associated with homeless patients—including tuberculosis, typhus, skin diseases, and pneumonia—are not typically seen in most insured groups. These diseases require specific, often expensive, and regular treatments to be minimized or cured.

Also, because both mentally ill and homeless patients are not as stable in terms of employment, location, and income, administering treatment is much more difficult.

The United States also has a significant number of **underinsured** people. These groups, while having some insurance benefits, are lacking in the quality and scope of benefits that other insured groups enjoy. In the United States, children and elderly people have access to Medicaid and Medicare; however, these benefits are often not enough and places many of them in the underinsured category. Many of the underinsured have insurance coverage that limits access and treatment options. Although these people have some insurance coverage, they oftentimes are not able to pay the copays, deductibles, and prescription costs associated with their medical care. This causes the underinsured to face many of the same poor-health issues as uninsured patients.

SELF-CHECK

- Identify and define **uninsured** and **underinsured**.
- Describe the number and various types of individuals in the United States who now make up uninsured patients.
- Explain the specific needs of mentally ill and homeless patients, who are also uninsured.
- List challenges specific to underinsured patients.

11.2 Accessing Health Care When Uninsured

For the large number of uninsured, their only access to the health care system is through community health clinics, urgent care facilities, and emergency rooms.

11.2.1 Community Health Centers and Clinics

Community health centers and clinics are organizations that provide health care services to poor and uninsured people. Contractual agreements with the state or local department of health services determine what health care services these organizations provide and to whom they provide them. Typically, these health centers and clinics offer a wide range of diagnostic, pharmaceutical, prenatal, and preventive health services, as well as emergency care. To qualify for treatment at a community health center, patients generally have to meet certain criteria, such as be a resident of the state, be without medical insurance, be considered poor, and not be eligible for state or federal insurance programs.

Community health centers are usually located in inner-city areas. This location provides reasonable access for the poor and uninsured members of a particular community. Patients who qualify and go to these centers benefit in that they receive basic health care without having to travel to access a larger health care system. Since these centers are generally funded by public monies, however, the care received is not of the same quality as it might be in a larger or privately funded health center. Many of these centers do not have the latest equipment and have staffs that are overburdened and underpaid. Regardless, though, community health centers and clinics provide a needed function as first-responders to uninsured patients.

11.2.2 Urgent Care Facilities

Urgent care facilities evaluate and treat conditions that aren't severe enough to require an emergency room visit but that are serious enough to require treatment beyond normal physician office hours or before a physician appointment is available.

These facilities are usually located within a given community or within a certain geographical area not readily served by a hospital or a larger health care system. Many urgent care facilities are in the suburbs or in more rural areas and provide the ability for patients to receive care without having to travel to and access a larger medical facility such as a hospital in a central city. Some urgent care facilities are funded and operated as extensions of larger hospital systems. It's not uncommon to see a large urban hospital have urgent care centers on the outskirts of the city. Other urgent care centers are private companies that are funded privately.

Most urgent care facilities are accessed by insured, underinsured, and uninsured patients. For uninsured patients who have access to transportation, the benefits of going to an urgent care facility is that they are often much nicer in terms of facilities and may have better equipment than public-funded community health centers. The staffs at urgent care centers are usually less burdened and have more time to devote to each patient's medical issue.

When uninsured patients go to an urgent care facility, many times they must pay for services at the time of the visit. Some facilities operate with a fee structure so uninsured patients know what they will pay up-front. This can be beneficial to uninsured patients because they can pay for services on their own. However, it can be negative for uninsured patients because the fees for à la carte style medical care are usually priced high.

11.2.3 Emergency Rooms

Emergency rooms are designed and staffed to provide initial treatment for a broad range of illnesses and injuries, some of which may be life-threatening. Traditionally, patients seeking treatment at emergency rooms are examined, treated or stabilized, and then referred to other departments for continuing care or released. In these instances, emergency rooms function as triage or trauma wards.

Today, however, the role of the emergency room is changing as it becomes the safety net of the U.S. health care system for uninsured patients. Lacking access to routine care provided by independent practitioners, more and more uninsured go to the emergency room for such care. Because emergency rooms have operated under the policy of treating all who seek care, uninsured patients can still receive care. This is particularly the case if the community in which they live does not have a community health center or if the health center is not accessible.

Because patients without insurance typically enter the health system through hospital emergency rooms, the emergency rooms become de facto general family practices for first-time patients dealing with myriad basic health issues. This change in function may take the focus off traditional emergency room functions of triage and trauma.

FOR EXAMPLE

Screening Patients in the Emergency Room

Given the influx of uninsured patients in emergency rooms, health care institutions are looking for ways to protect their financial health. A controversial policy started by Denver Health Medical Center (www.denverhealth.org) and the University of Colorado Hospital (www.uch.edu) seeks to provide such a solution. Both hospitals screen emergency room patients prior to providing treating and turn away individuals who reside outside city boundaries or cannot pay. Although the policy stipulates that the turned-way patient must be stable and the condition cannot be life-threatening, Denver emergency rooms have denied treatment for such serious but non-life-threatening conditions as broken bones, infections, cancerous lumps, and detached retinas. Opponents of the policy say that although Denver's two largest hospitals may be acting in accordance with the law, the screenings are dangerous and unethical. The policy's defenders claim that, although the policy isn't ideal, it is better than the alternative: shutting down the emergency rooms altogether. Both hospitals receive federal dollars to care for uninsured patients.

For example, when we think of a traditional emergency room, we may think of a person having a heart attack or a car crash victim. The emergency room staff swings into action to help the heart attack patient or the victim. Perhaps surgery must be done immediately or perhaps some other form of trauma treatment must occur right there within the emergency room. Because of today's use of the emergency room by uninsured patients as first-response medical care, today's emergency rooms must also deal with medical issues as simple as the common cold, to broken fingers, to giving aspirin to children with slight fevers and a rash.

The trend of uninsured patients relying on emergency room services burdens the emergency room system within most hospitals and in some instances jeopardizes quality of care. Because of this trend, however, facilities with emergency rooms have begun prioritizing medical issues as patients come in. Those with life-threatening conditions are seen as first priority and get the emergency room staff's immediate attention. This causes those with non-life-threatening, but very real and often painful conditions to have to wait long hours for care. In medical systems that can afford it, some emergency rooms have begun to divide their emergency room facilities and/or increase staffs to recognize this trend. This enables reasonable quality and efficient operations in serving all patients coming into the emergency room.

11.3 Challenges in Providing Health Care to Uninsured Patients

The challenges of caring for uninsured patients are numerous but generally can be divided into two categories: health related and cost related.

11.3.1 Health-Related Challenges

The quality and effectiveness of health care that uninsured patients actually receive is problematic:

▲ **An uninsured person's health is typically worse than the health of the insured:** As a rule, most people who are uninsured do not receive preventive care and, therefore, do not benefit from regular health guidance and care that might help them avoid certain health conditions or find others in their early stages.

▲ **Illnesses are more advanced by the time treatment is sought:** Uninsured patients, because of the financial barrier in seeking care, generally do not seek medical care when the symptom or problem is manageable. Instead, they wait until things have gotten "bad enough" before seeing a doctor. Unfortunately, many chronic conditions, such as diabetes or glaucoma, and serious illnesses grow worse when left untreated.

▲ **Uninsured people are more likely to become progressively less healthy as time goes on simply because of the lack of care:** Uninsured people are unable to get treatment or can't afford it, therefore, what start out as minor medical issues become very large medical issues over time. Lack of preventive health care contributes to this decline in health status among uninsured patients. For example, a person who cuts the bottom of his foot and breaks two toes can easily be treated with antibiotics and a simple resetting of the toes. However, if the person is uninsured or unable to pay, the condition may go untreated. Over time, the toes may misalign and become crooked, making walking difficult. If the foot becomes infected, the person may stay off his feet and become sedentary, which causes him to gain weight and introduces a host of other health issues. While this is a simplified and extreme example, it illustrates how lack of access and ability to pay for health care can lead to consequences that would normally be easily preventable.

11.3.2 Financial-Related Challenges

Patients without insurance are often reluctant to seek medical attention simply because of their inability to pay. This delay in seeking treatment negatively impacts both the patient and the health care system because medical care, when it is received, is generally more involved and therefore more costly. Because uninsured patients seek treatment only after illnesses have advanced to the point that they can no longer live with the symptoms, more aggressive—and often more expensive—intervention is required. This places a burden on the health care system because it is now obligated to treat at a higher level of resources that cost considerably more.

Consider the example in Section 11.3.1. A patient with an untreated toe fracture may eventually be unable to walk and gangrene may set in. When the patient finally presents himself in an emergency room, physicians may determine that the toe must be removed, a process that requires a substantive amount of hospital resources, including inpatient time and attention, supplies, pharmaceuticals, physical therapy, monitoring, and medical equipment. A condition that could have been cured with simple antibiotics is now a major medical condition that must be treated and paid for by the hospital without the prospect of being reimbursed for time and costs.

In the United States, clinics and public hospitals have a duty to treat and provide basic medical and emergency services for anyone regardless of ability to pay. However, uninsured patients often end up paying more for health care in the long run when they enter the system through emergency rooms and urgent care facilities.

Typically, medical facilities have standard rates that they have negotiated with various insurance plans. These rates are often discounted and are lower than the medical facility's à la carte fees for the same services. Since uninsured patients lack the power of being part of these prenegotiated groups, they often are charged higher à la carte fees for services. Of course, the high charges are absurd because uninsured patients already can't afford high-price medical care and end up receiving even greater financial burden.

If the patient is unable to pay, the hospital typically ends up assuming some or all the costs of treatment. Often the hospital passes on these costs to paying patients and patients' insurance companies in the form of increased cost of services, which drives up insurance premiums.

Some institutions do provide for indigent care and have special funds set up to deal with patients who cannot afford to pay. Some states also provide for reimbursement to hospitals and health care facilities that care for indigent patients. These funds may come from:

▲ **Cost-shifting from other areas within the institutions:** This impacts the institution when precious financial resources are taken from one area to pay for services in another, thereby causing some areas to be less than fully financed.

▲ **Private sources:** Private sources include individual foundations, charitable foundations, and other entities. These private funds provide operating capital and/or subsidize clinics so they are able to treat patients who cannot afford it.

▲ **Public monies, such as grants:** Public sources of funding include special local, state, and federal taxes. Some local and state laws set up and allocate funds to be used specifically to treat uninsured patients. There are grants that are given at these three levels as well to establish, operate, and maintain medical services for specific segments of patients in specific areas. For example, several trust funds have been established to send up rural free clinics in an impoverished area of Appalachia.

Regardless of where funding comes from, there are always stipulations as to how and where the monies can be used. These criteria may be set by the health

FOR EXAMPLE

Bad Debt and Charity Care (BDCC) in New York

In New York, the Bad Debt and Charity Care law makes state funds available to nonprofit hospitals that provide care for uninsured and underinsured patients. In theory, hospitals provide charitable care to uninsured patients and then apply for BDCC funds to offset the cost of the care. The law has not been applied as intended, however. According to investigations by the New York Legal Aid Society and others, New York hospitals have access to these funds whether they provided indigent care or not. In fact, it was discovered that several hospitals that received BDCC funds did not have financial aid or charity care programs available for uninsured patients, didn't inform patients about such programs, and used aggressive collection tactics to recoup full payment from patients, even after they had received BDCC funds. The investigations go on and it is expected that the New York legislature will amend the law to close these loopholes. Visit www.legal-aid.org/Uploads/BDCCReport.pdf for a report of the effectiveness of New York's law.

care organization itself or the particular funding body. These organizations or funding bodies often set out some sort of formula that patients must meet in order to be eligible. These criteria can be health related or are more often income related. Responsibility of monitoring this falls on the funding body itself or its assignees. Many times, health care facilities are placed in charge of monitoring themselves in terms of how they use their monies. There are many local and state regulations and laws in place as well that deal with caring for indigent people.

SELF-CHECK

- List the health-related challenges of providing health care for uninsured patients.
- List the financial-related challenges of providing health care for uninsured patients.
- Describe the financial resources available to health care facilities to help pay for treating uninsured patients.

11.4 Legal Issues and Uninsured Patients

Legal issues surrounding uninsured patients are vast and varied depending on locality and state. Many localities and states have passed regulations, acts, and laws that govern how both uninsured patients and their services should be handled. One federal law, the **Emergency Medical Transfer and Active Labor Act (EMTALA)**, stipulates that all hospitals or health care facilities, when presented

FOR EXAMPLE

A Lack of Insurance Results in Poorer Care

In a landmark study published in 1992 in the *Journal of the American Medical Association*, Dr. Helen R. Burstin of the Harvard Medical School contended that there was a link between inferior treatment and insurance status and that uninsured patients often do not get the best treatment. They may receive basic treatment but, because they aren't able to pay for the latest technological diagnostic devices that an insurance plan may pay for, they may miss out on a diagnosis or treatment that would benefit them.

with a patient in the emergency room who has a legitimate medical emergency condition, must either:

▲ Treat or stabilize the condition within the staff and facilities available at the hospital for further medical examination and treatment.
▲ Transfer the individual to another medical facility in accordance with the act.

The EMTALA has been challenged in the court systems and continues to be challenged by both health care facilities and by patients who claim that the act infringes on their rights. Patient and other advocate groups have been vocal in support of this act, as well as in support of rights for uninsured patients.

SELF-CHECK

- Identify and define **Emergency Medical Transfer and Active Labor Act (EMTALA)**.

SUMMARY

The duty to treat principle in the United States inspires health care facilities to treat all patients, including those who are uninsured. The number and diversity of people who are uninsured or underinsured have been growing in the nation for many years—and appear to be on paths to continue growing. Uninsured patients receive health care in three primary ways: community health centers and clinics, urgent care facilities, and emergency rooms. The challenges to caring for uninsured patients are twofold: From a health-related perspective uninsured patients are usually in poor health and wait until conditions are quite severe to begin treatment. From a financial perspective, uninsured patients are typically more costly to treat and often cannot pay for services they receive. Federal, state, and local laws are frequently evaluated and redefined to provide health care to as many people as possible, while allowing for the financial security of health care facilities.

KEY TERMS

Community health center	Health care organization that provides health care services to poor and uninsured individuals.
Emergency room	Health care organization designed and staffed to provide initial treatment for a broad range of

	illnesses and injuries, some of which may be life-threatening.
Emergency Medical Transfer and Active Labor Act (EMTALA)	A federal law requiring that all health care facilities treat or transfer with a legitimate medical emergency.
Underinsured patient	Individual who has some insurance benefits but lacks the quality and scope of benefits that other insured groups enjoy.
Uninsured patient	Individual who lacks private health insurance coverage and who doesn't qualify for either Medicaid or Medicare.
Urgent care facility	A health care organization that evaluates and treats conditions that aren't severe enough to require an emergency room visit but that are serious enough to require treatment beyond normal physician office hours or before a physician appointment is available.

ASSESS YOUR UNDERSTANDING

Go to www.wiley.com/college/pointer to evaluate your knowledge of caring for uninsured patients.
Measure your learning by comparing pre-test and post-test results.

Summary Questions

1. Based on most estimates, the number of uninsured patients in the United States is likely to grow significantly in the next 10 years. True or False?

2. Individuals who have some insurance benefits but lack the quality and scope of benefits of others are considered
   (a) untreatable.
   (b) underinsured.
   (c) understaffed.
   (d) dependent.

3. Many special groups fill the ranks of uninsured patients. Significant groups include:
   (a) mentally ill patients and veterans
   (b) homeless and elderly patients
   (c) minorities and rural poor
   (d) homeless and mentally ill patients

4. Urgent care facilities typically provide prenatal, pharmaceutical, and preventive health care to uninsured patients because of contractual agreements with state and local health departments. True or False?

5. Today's emergency rooms end up treating uninsured patients while simultaneously continuing to respond to emergency medical conditions for all individuals. True or False?

6. Uninsured patients often seek and receive medical attention at
   (a) emergency rooms and mobile treatment units.
   (b) research hospitals and universities.
   (c) urgent care facilities and community health centers.
   (d) traditional doctors' offices and urgent care facilities.

7. Health care facilities that treat uninsured patients who are unable to pay for treatment often pass along costs for these services in increased fees to insurance companies and paying patients. True or False?

8. Private sources of funding for health care for uninsured patients include:
   (a) charitable foundations
   (b) nonprofit organizations

(c) donors

(d) all of the above

9. The Emergency Medical Transfer and Active Labor Act provides funding for all U.S. emergency care facilities, so they can better assess, treat, and provide health care for U.S. citizens. True or False?

Review Questions

1. What are some reasons for the increase in the number of uninsured people in the United States?
2. For uninsured patients, what are some benefits of utilizing the services of an urgent care facility?
3. What are three sources of funding for health care for uninsured patients?
4. Public monies and grants for providing health care to uninsured patients come from which three levels of government?
5. According to the EMTALA, all hospitals must do one of two things to any emergency room patient. What?

Applying This Chapter

1. You manage an emergency room facility in southern California. Although your hospital is located near an affluent suburb, the emergency room takes in a high number of uninsured and underinsured patients every day. You have been asked to give the board of directors a brief overview of the key uninsured and underinsured populations your facility treats. What populations will highlight your presentation?
2. Gina works on the communication staff of a large inner-city hospital. To help improve the ways in which uninsured patients access medical care—specifically community health centers, urgent care facilities, and emergency rooms—she is creating a wallet-size card that tells patients the pros and cons of various care options, and when it's most appropriate to visit a certain type of facility. What pros and cons should she list for each type of facility? When is it most appropriate to visit each type of facility?
3. As the chief financial officer of a major urban teaching hospital, you must make certain that your organization has enough money each year to cover all costs involved in treating both insured and uninsured patients. In the last five years, the number of uninsured patients using your emergency room facility has increased dramatically. Funding sources are available, including cost-shifting, cultivating private sources, and receiving public money through grants. What are the pros and cons of each option? How would you rank the importance of each funding resource for your facility?

YOU TRY IT

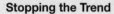

Stopping the Trend

The number of uninsured individuals in the United States has been rising for decades and is likely to continue rising. If you were given $100 million and asked to focus on just one of the top reasons for this increase—rising health care costs, increases in poverty, decreases in the number of employers offering health insurance to employees—which reason would you focus on? Why? How would you use your budget to improve factors related to your selected reason?

Setting ER Priorities

As uninsured patients increasingly rely on emergency rooms to access medical care, emergency rooms must still continue to perform their original duty—access and responding to severe and emergency medical conditions. If you were the manager of a suburban ER facility,

describe the way you'd evaluate patients and then attend to them based on finances (insured, uninsured, underinsured, and so on), medical condition, and any other factor you consider relevant.

Reconsidering the EMTALA

On first glance, the Emergency Medical Transfer and Active Labor Act (EMTALA) seems like an appropriate and essential federal law. However, consider the law if you work as an administrator at a private hospital, or a for-profit medical facility. In what ways might the law infringe on your organization's rights to operate as it sees fit? In what ways might the law negatively impact your financial responsibilities to investors? Can you think of some ways to comply with the law while still meeting your financial goals and responsibilities?

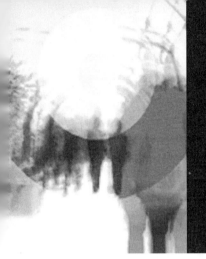

12

MANAGED CARE
Controlling Costs and Access to Health Services

Starting Point

Go to www.wiley.com/college/pointer to assess your knowledge of the basics of managed care.
Determine where you need to concentrate your effort.

What You'll Learn in This Chapter

▲ What indemnity plans are and their key characteristics
▲ What managed care plans are and their key characteristics
▲ The ways managed care tries to make health care more cost effective
▲ The different types of managed care plans
▲ How managed care cost-saving strategies affect quality of care

After Studying This Chapter, You'll Be Able To

▲ Differentiate between indemnity health plans and managed care plans
▲ Compare HMOs, PPOs, and POS plans in terms of features and cost-saving strategies
▲ Examine what changes managed care has influenced in how and by whom health care is provided
▲ Analyze the successes and failures of managed care to date

Goals and Outcomes

▲ Master terminology relating to managed care plans and organizations
▲ Explain the relationship between managed care plan features and regulations and cost-saving endeavors
▲ Assess the impact managed care has had on quality of care
▲ Evaluate managed care in terms of customer satisfaction, physician satisfaction, cost containment, and quality of care

INTRODUCTION

The steep incline of health care costs in the recent years has brought the idea of managed care to the forefront of U.S. health care. Similar to but significantly different from traditional insurance, managed care seeks to control health care costs by controlling access to care and negotiating fees for service. Although the three main types of managed care plans share important characteristics, such as reliance on primary care physicians (PCPs) and a network of health care providers, each offers significantly different arrangements to its members. How well the various managed care plans have been able to achieve the goal of cost-effective quality health care is still open for debate as physicians and patients alike have grown dissatisfied with the model.

12.1 Understanding Managed Care

Health care costs in the United States have been rising at an alarming rate for several years (refer to Section 4.1 for a discussion on the reasons for the sharp increases), and private health insurance companies started buckling under the strain. The goal became to make health care more cost effective and, at the same time, maintain—or improve—quality. In an effort to achieve this goal, managed care plans fundamentally restructured the way health care was delivered and underwritten.

12.1.1 Controlling Costs

Any effort to control health care costs must focus on two areas: controlling the volume of services accessed and controlling the prices associated with those services. Hence, the managed care system was born. Managed care attempts to make care more cost effective by doing the following:

▲ **Controlling access:** In any insurance plan, the person who receives medical care (the patient) isn't the one who pays for it. The result is a "consumer" who doesn't have to be concerned about the cost and who tends to access medical care without careful consideration of whether that care is actually necessary or, in some instances, even appropriate. To assume some control of when and how care is accessed, managed care plans set conditions regarding

- When patients can access care: Patients typically have to get a referral from their PCP (the gatekeeper) to see a specialist.
- What type of care they can access: Many managed care plans require that patients receive prior approval for a medical procedure before seeking treatment.
- Which providers they can seek medical care from: Managed care organizations enter into contractual agreements with a network of

health care providers. To be covered, plan members must see a health care provider in the plan's network.

▲ **Controlling price:** Managed care organizations negotiate set fees with the in-network providers. Essentially, the health care providers agree to accept what the managed care plan is willing to pay for any particular service and to assume the risk of financial loss if the cost of providing that service exceeds the negotiated amount. The benefit to providers is that they receive the fee whether a plan member requires the service or not and they receive referrals for new patients (plan members) from the managed care organization they're associated with.

Currently, some form of managed care has virtually replaced cost-based reimbursement to hospitals and fee-for-service medicine, both for people covered by employer-based insurance and for those on federally funded assistance programs. In fact, some kind of managed reimbursement now covers 75 percent of the U.S. population.

12.1.2 Ensuring Quality

On the premise that the health care individuals need is not so much the health care they think they want, but the care that is most effective, managed care restricts access to care and puts the decisions regarding what care is appropriate in the hands of the PCP or, in certain cases, in the hands of the plan administrators.

Ideally, these decisions should be made based on outcome-based health studies; for example, do women or babies who spend three days in the hospital after a normal delivery have better outcomes than those who are sent home after the first day? If medical research indicates that there is no measurable benefit to the extended stay, then, scientifically speaking, there is no medical reason justifying the extra days. Thus, a policy of discharging new mothers and their healthy infants after 24 hours is both medically sound and cost effective. The danger, however, is that the decisions regarding care are sometimes made without the backing of medical research but on the basis of cost reimbursement alone.

FOR EXAMPLE

Tobacco Policy as a Cost-Containment Issue

Managed care has come under scrutiny for promoting cost containment over quality of health care. But not all cost-containment initiatives make for bad medicine. Case in point: Many managed care organizations are looking into providing (or already provide) coverage to help members quit smoking. Their position is that spending money to get people to quit smoking is far less expensive than providing coverage for smoking-induced health problems—a position that makes sense medically *and* financially.

12.1.3 Understanding How Managed Care Works

In traditional health plans, called **indemnity plans,** patients are reimbursed for medical expenses they incur. After the patient meets a specified deductible, plan payments kick in and the patient and plan share responsibility for the expense, with each paying a portion of the total bill. In these plans, the health care provider is reimbursed for the cost of the service, and the patient can choose any provider he or she wishes.

In **managed care plans,** the plan member still has access to health services, but to receive full plan benefits must relinquish some control regarding when to seek medical care, what type of medical care to seek, and which health care provider to use. Typically, all managed care plans share these common features:

▲ **Utilization reviews:** Patients may be required to get approval from the managed care organization for certain services before receiving treatment.

▲ **Provider networks:** To be covered patients must use health care providers who have contracts with the managed care organization unless the plan offers out-of-network benefits (which are typically less comprehensive that in-network coverage).

▲ **Preventive care:** Managed care plans typically include comprehensive preventive coverage (for regular physicals and preventive screenings, for example), understanding that preventive care is both medically sound and financially beneficial (because it costs less than acute or palliative care).

▲ **Reduction of paperwork:** Members aren't required to fill out claim forms; however, plan members are the only ones who see a reduction in paperwork. Health care providers have an increased administrative burden when part of a managed care network; see Section 12.3.2 for details.

▲ **Copayments:** Members generally pay a flat fee (usually a nominal amount) at the time of service.

▲ **Gatekeeper:** To manage access to care, managed care plans require that members receive referrals from their PCP to see specialists or to access other health care services.

SELF-CHECK

- Define **indemnity plans** and **managed care plans.**
- Identify the two aspects of health care that managed care plans try to control in an effort to reduce health care costs.
- Name the features that all managed care plans share.

12.2 Types of Managed Care Organizations

Different types of managed care programs exist:

▲ Health maintenance organizations (HMOs).

▲ Preferred provider organizations (PPOs).

▲ Point-of-service (POS) plans.

Although they all share common characteristics, there are subtle but significant differences. The following sections explain the programs briefly.

12.2.1 Health Maintenance Organizations (HMOs)

A **health maintenance organization (HMO)** is a hybrid health care insurance and provider mechanism that offers a type of managed care plan. In its simplest form, an HMO links together (through contracts or ownership) a health plan, hospitals, and physicians into a provider network that consists of:

▲ A **health plan:** Contracts with purchasers, underwrites the financial risk of providing care, negotiates and manages relationships with providers, pays providers, and performs administrative functions.

▲ **Hospitals:** Provide inpatient health care services to beneficiaries and may include other entities such as nursing home, home health, rehabilitation, and mental or behavioral health facilities. HMOs can either contract with or own hospitals and other organizational providers, such as nursing homes. A contractual relationship is far more common than an ownership relationship. In addition, health plan hospitals can be either closed-staff or open-staff. In a **closed arrangement,** only physicians who are employees of, or have contracted with, the health plan are medical staff members. In an **open arrangement,** health plan and other physicians are admitted to the hospital's medical staff.

▲ **Physicians:** Provide primary and specialty medical services to beneficiaries and may include other professionals such as chiropractors, podiatrists, and psychologists. The HMO can secure professional services in three ways:

  • Contract with individual physicians, who remain independent and care for plan beneficiaries, as well as other patients, in their offices. This arrangement is called an **independent practice association (IPA) model HMO.**

  • Contract with organized groups of physicians, who either care for plan beneficiaries exclusively or do so in addition to other patients. This arrangement is called a **group model HMO.**

  • Hire physicians as employees. This arrangement is called a **staff model HMO.**

FOR EXAMPLE

Different Structure for Different HMOs

HMOs can vary in structure and employ multiple arrangements in providing health care. Although many contract with their care providers and others hire (or, in the case of health care facilities, buy) their providers, some HMOs take a dual approach. For example, an HMO can own the health plan and hospitals but contract with independent medical groups to provide professional services; it may employ PCPs and contract to provide specialty care; or it may own its hospitals and contract with a medical group but also have contracts with nonowned hospitals and independent physicians to provide some subspecialty services (for instance, cardiac surgery and transplants). The arrangement depends on the organization and its resources. For instance, in each of the regions in which it operates, Kaiser Foundation Health Plan (which operates its own hospitals) contracts with Kaiser Permanente Medical Group (an independent professional corporation).

HMOs can be either nonprofit or for-profit. They can also be independent organizations or components of a health plan (like BlueCross® BlueShield®), or owned and controlled by a separate corporation, hospital, or physician group.

In addition, HMOs share traits common to managed care plans:

▲ Members are required to see only providers within the network to have their health care paid for by the HMO. If the member receives care from a provider who isn't in the network, the HMO won't pay for care unless it was preauthorized by the HMO or deemed an emergency.

▲ Members select a PCP, often called a "gatekeeper" (refer to Section 12.1.3), who provides, arranges, coordinates and authorizes all aspects of the members' health care. PCPs are usually family doctors, internal medicine doctors, general practitioners and obstetricians/gynecologists.

▲ Members can see a specialist (for example, cardiologist, dermatologist, rheumatologist) only if the PCP authorized it. If the member sees a specialist without a referral, the HMO won't pay for the care.

HMOs are the most restrictive type of health plan because they give members the least choice in selecting a health care provider. However, HMOs typically provide members with a greater range of health benefits for the lowest out-of-pocket expenses, such as either no or a very low copayment (the amount of money a member is required to pay the provider in addition to what the HMO pays). It often must be paid prior to services being rendered.

HMOs rely on administration arrangements and economic incentives to increase clinical quality and efficiency, manage utilization of services, and control costs by

▲ Limiting the type of benefits and services available to those deemed clinically and cost effective.

▲ Restricting the use of nonplan providers.

▲ Paying set rates for services, irrespective of their actual cost.

▲ Providing health promotion and disease prevention services.

▲ Utilizing PCPs as gatekeepers who manage patients' use of hospital and specialist care.

▲ Authorizing services before they're provided.

12.2.2 Preferred Provider Organizations (PPOs)

Preferred provider organizations (PPOs) are similar to HMOs in that they enter into contractual arrangements with health care providers (such as physicians, hospitals, and other health care professionals) who together form a "provider network," but they don't use PCPs as gatekeepers.

PPOs differ from HMOs in the following ways:

▲ Members don't have a PCP that functions as a gatekeeper, nor do they have to use an in-network provider for their care. Although using in-network providers is not mandatory, PPOs do offer members more comprehensive, fuller benefits as financial incentives, such as lower deductibles, lower copayments, and higher reimbursements, to use network providers.

▲ PPO members typically don't have to get a referral to see a specialist. Again, most PPOs offer a financial incentive to use a specialist in the PPO's provider network.

▲ Although PPOs are less restrictive than HMOs in the choice of health care provider, they tend to require greater out-of-pocket payments from the members.

12.2.3 Point-of-Service (POS) plans

A **point-of-service (POS) plan,** often called an "open-ended" HMO, is essentially a combination of HMO and PPO (see Sections 12.2.1 and 12.2.2). POS plans offer both HMO and PPO services, and members choose which option— HMO or PPO—they'll use each time they seek health care.

Like HMOs and PPOs, a POS plan has a contracted provider network. Other characteristics of POS plans include the following:

▲ They encourage, but don't require, members to choose a PCP to act as a gatekeeper when making referrals.

▲ Members who choose not to use PCPs for referrals but still seek care from an in-network provider receive benefits but pay higher copays and/or deductibles than members who use their PCPs.

▲ POS plan members can opt to visit out-of-network providers, but if they do so, they pay substantially more in copayments and deductibles.

POS plans are becoming more popular because they offer more flexibility and freedom of choice than standard HMOs.

SELF-CHECK

- List and define the three types of managed care plans.
- Describe the three ways HMOs can secure the professional services of physicians.
- List the key characteristics of a PPO plan.
- List the key characteristics of a POS plan.

12.3 Assessing the Performance of Managed Care

As it has evolved over the last 20 years, managed care now more often involves managed reimbursement than managed care. In this new landscape, there has been intense economic competition among HMOs, PPOs, and POS programs. The essential elements of managed reimbursement have led to growing frustration on the part of physicians and patients alike.

12.3.1 Impact on Quality and Cost

The foundation of managed care plans is the reliance on PCPs. The expectation—that having a PCP to oversee general care and to act as a gatekeeper to other medical services would increase quality and reduce health care costs—has not been supported by evidence. Some studies note that primary care providers are not regularly superior in the delivery of secondary preventive services, and research continues to show that—not surprisingly—specialists are more current in their practices than PCPs.

In addition, patient and provider anger over gatekeeper arrangements, as well as highly publicized limitations on care in HMOs, has caused a managed care backlash. Consumers equate "quality" with "choice" and tend to see primary care as a barrier to quality, not as an enhancer.

Despite the hit on quality, managed care's use of discounts and the health insurance underwriting cycle succeeded in slowing the rate of health care cost increases in the mid- to late 1990s—an important object lesson suggesting that market forces can attack cost inflation.

12.3.2 Impact on Physicians and Health Care Providers

Managed care gets mixed reviews when it comes to assessing the impact it's had on physicians and health care providers. In some ways, the changes have been positive: They led to the creation and utilization of alternative provider positions to assume some of the burden (and reduce the cost of) primary care. In other ways, managed care's impact has been less positive. Physicians (and patients) are dissatisfied with the restrictions on care and the cost-containment policies that reduce revenue.

In important ways, managed care has changed the way health care is delivered. For example, managed care promoted the growth of nurse practitioner and physician assistant programs, both to enhance the productivity of physician practice and to offer a more cost-effective form of primary care itself. From 1992 to 1997, this group of health professionals doubled, and further growth is anticipated. In addition, managed care created the need for hospitals and medical groups to become more efficient in inpatient care, giving rise to the hospitalist movement (refer to Section 5.2.4).

Managed care has, overall, not been kind to U.S. physicians. Managed care's cost and utilization controls (refer to Section 12.1) have negatively impacted PCPs:

▲ On the whole, physicians receive less for their services than they used to while at the same time their expenses have gone up because of administrative chores associated with managed care authorization requirements.

▲ Physician professional satisfaction is falling. In 2000, the American Medical Association (AMA) published the result of a survey that examined the career plans for 300 U.S. physicians over 50. Its findings:

- 48 percent said they planned to either retire or change careers within the next one to three years.
- Only 18 percent foresaw no short-term professional changes.
- The remaining physicians said they planned to continue practicing medicine in a diminished capacity.
- Fifty-six percent said they would not choose a medical career again.
- Fifty-six percent cited managed care hassles as their biggest frustration.

> ## FOR EXAMPLE
>
> ### Antitrust Relief and Managed Care
>
> Most U.S. physicians have little or no bargaining power with health insurers, who present them with contracts on a take-it-or-leave-it basis. The AMA's position is that physicians should be allowed to negotiate contract terms and that they and their patients—and not insurers—should make decisions about health care needs. According to the AMA, the fact that many physicians feel forced to sign contracts that a reasonable business person would not accept indicates that new antitrust legislation is needed to allow physicians and other health care professionals to negotiate with health plans without fear of violating antitrust laws.

12.3.3 The Future of Managed Care

Managed care has become the "whipping boy" in U.S. health care. Despite its initial success in cost containment, a powerful backlash against managed care organizations has gathered momentum since the mid-1990s over such issues as "gag rules" for HMO physicians, denial of services, and "drive-through deliveries." It's already clear that managed care probably won't continue without major changes. Many HMOs, for example, are acceding to enrollees' demands for POS access to specialists, and less-effective cost containment appears inevitable.

It is important to recognize the distinction between managed care, described here, and managed reimbursement, which was mentioned earlier. Some managed care organizations, especially in the for-profit group, have focused on management of costs of care at the expense of quality of care, for the purpose of making profits for shareholders. Unfortunately, the many achievements toward cost-effective comprehensive care based on evidence-based outcomes, as exemplified by many nonprofit managed care organizations, are being unfairly included in the backlash. Indeed, some HMOs have been committed for up to 50 years to health promotion, preventive medicine, and a population-based approach to optimizing health care outcomes. It is unclear to what extent these efforts will continue.

SELF-CHECK

- Which two groups are least happy with managed care?
- What are the chief two complaints from each of these groups?

SUMMARY

Managed care, designed to address rising medical costs, is a key feature of health care in the United States. Unlike traditional insurance policies, managed care combines the provider and underwriting (insuring) function in one organization in an effort to control costs through utilization mandates and negotiated reimbursement rates. The three main types of managed care plans—health maintenance organizations (HMOs), preferred provider organizations (PPOs), and point-of-service (POS) plans—share managed care's goals with varying degrees of restrictions. Despite its promise, managed care has thus far not achieved one of its primary objectives—to maintain quality. How it evolves in the future remains to be seen.

KEY TERMS

Closed arrangement	A type of network in which only physicians who are employees of, or have contracted with, the health plan are medical staff members.
Copayment	Amount (generally a flat fee) members must pay at the time of service.
Gatekeeper	Primary care physician in managed care plans who provides general care to plan members and referrals to see specialists or to access other health care services.
Group model HMO	An HMO model in which the managed care organization contracts with organized groups of physicians, who either care for plan beneficiaries exclusively or do so in addition to other patients.
Health maintenance organization (HMO)	A managed care plan that combines into a single entity a health plan, hospitals, and physicians.
Indemnity plans	Traditional fee-for-service insurance plans in which patients are reimbursed for medical expenses they incur after having met a specified deductible.
Independent practice association (IPA) model HMO	An HMO model in which the managed care organization contracts with individual physicians, who remain independent and care for plan members, as well as other patients.
Managed care plans	The plan member still has access to health services, but to receive full plan benefits must relinquish some control regarding when to seek

	medical care, what type of medical care to seek, and which health care provider to use.
Open arrangement	A type of network in which independent physicians are admitted to the hospital's medical staff.
Point-of-service (POS) plan	A managed care plan that combines the characteristics of HMOs and PPOs. A POS plan offers both HMO and PPO services, and members choose which option they use at the each time they seek health care.
Preferred provider organization (PPO)	A managed care plan that includes a provider network but doesn't use primary care physicians as gatekeepers.
Provider networks	Network of care providers, including physicians, hospitals, and so on, that have a contractual agreement with the managed care plan to provide services for a negotiated rate.
Staff model HMO	An HMO model in which the managed care organization hires physicians as employees.
Utilization reviews	Managed care mandates requiring patients to get approval from the managed care organization for certain services before receiving treatment.

ASSESS YOUR UNDERSTANDING

Go to www.wiley.com/college/pointer to evaluate your knowledge of the basics of managed care.

Measure your learning by comparing pre-test and post-test results.

Summary Questions

1. Seventy-five percent of the insured in the United States have managed care health plans; the other 25 percent have private insurance. True or False?

2. How do managed care plans control when and how patients receive medical care?

    (a) by making patients get a referral from a PCP to see a specialist

    (b) by requiring preapproval for treatments

    (c) by limiting the pool of health care providers patients can see

    (d) all of the above

3. Define *utilization review.*

    (a) an evaluation of the health services to determine their effectiveness

    (b) a process by which the managed care organization preapproves treatment

    (c) a list of services reviewed to be effective and, therefore, allowable by the plan

    (d) none of the above

4. A closed arrangement is a managed care plan that is offered by an employer and available only to employees of the business. True or False?

5. Of the three types of managed care plans, which is the least restrictive?

    (a) health maintenance organizations (HMOs)

    (b) preferred provider organizations (PPOs)

    (c) point-of-service (POS) plans

6. The role of primary care physicians (PCPs), as providers of general patient care and gatekeepers to other care, has demonstrated that managed care plans can effectively control costs and at the same time ensure quality of care. True or False?

7. In what way have managed care plans had a positive effect on health care?

    (a) they have reduced the bureaucracy and burden of paperwork associated with traditional health plans

    (b) they have fostered the growth of alternative care providers, such as physician assistants and nurse practitioners, to relieve physicians of some of the burden of care

(c) by focusing on outcome-based studies, they have fundamentally changed patients' perception of quality

(d) all of the above

8. Why are physicians generally unhappy with managed care?

(a) the negotiated rates reduces their actual income

(b) the in-network referral system reduce the number of patients who are referred to them

(c) the growing number of alternative care providers is undermining their prestige and earning power

(d) all of the above

Review Questions

1. Describe the difference between managed care plans and indemnity health care plans.

2. Name three things that managed care plans require that traditional indemnity plans typically don't.

3. Identify the main points of difference between HMOs, PPOs, and POS plans.

4. In what way does the gatekeeper function control cost?

(a) it creates an additional step that patients have to take to access care and, as a result, dissuades some patients from entering the medical system

(b) it eliminates unnecessary tests and treatment by putting the decision regarding what care is necessary in the hands of the PCP

(c) it tracks the progress of a patient through the medical system to eliminate overlap of treatment or testing

(d) the primary function of the gatekeeper is not to control cost but to help patients access in-network care

5. How does a closed arrangement differ from an open arrangement in managed care?

(a) in a closed arrangement, the plan is available only to employees of the business

(b) in a closed arrangement, only other in-network physicians participate in the review of their peers

(c) in a closed arrangement, only physicians who have contracts with the health plan, or who are employed by it, are admitted to the hospital staff

(d) in a closed arrangement, the PCP can refer patients only to other in-network physicians

6. In all the cost-saving measures instituted by managed care plans, how is quality of care maintained?
   (a) by relying on outcome-based medical studies to decide where costs can be pared without compromising quality of care
   (b) by creating networks that include only the most highly reviewed physicians and care providers
   (c) by enforcing an annual review of all PCPs in the network and ranking them accordingly
   (d) by using the cost-savings to institute prevention initiatives such as antitobacco or fit-for-life programs

7. In what way are provider networks cost effective?
   (a) the physicians in the network have contracted with the managed care plan to offer services at a set rate
   (b) in-network providers, as employees of the managed care organization, receive salaries rather than fees for service
   (c) in-network referrals keep the income generated within the network
   (d) none of the above

8. How do PPOs and POS plans, which don't require members to use in-network physicians, control costs?
   (a) by reducing the number of approved procedures
   (b) by limiting their membership to those with no preexisting medical conditions
   (c) by offering financial incentives to members who use in-network physicians
   (d) by eliminating paperwork and other nonmedical expenses

9. What are the implications of the statement "Managed care now more often involves managed reimbursement than managed care"?
   (a) that managed care programs haven't adequately addressed quality issues
   (b) that managed care has been fairly successful as a reimbursement model
   (c) that managed care has thus far failed to meet its early promise
   (d) all of the above

10. Which of the following statements is *most* true?
    (a) managed care is likely to disappear as a health plan in the United States
    (b) managed care will likely continue only after major changes
    (c) managed care is stable and requires only some tweaking as it moves forward

Applying This Chapter

1. Describe how managed care plans achieve cost containment.

2. Identify whether an HMO, a PPO, or a POS plan would be best in each of the following situations. Explain your answers.

   (a) You have special health needs. Some of the physicians you work with are in the health plan's network; others are not.

   (b) You prefer to access specialty care as needed (to see your dermatologist, for example), without having to seek a referral from your family physician.

   (c) Money is tight and you want the least expensive plan available that offers the most comprehensive service.

3. In each of the following areas, give managed care a passing or failing grade and explain your answers.

   (a) quality

   (b) cost containment

   (c) physician satisfaction

   (d) delivery of care

YOU TRY IT

Understanding Managed Care

Imagine that you're a representative of a managed care company and you have to sell your plan to a physicians' group. List the objections you expect to encounter.

Types of Managed Care Organizations

You are the president of a small area hospital. A managed health network is moving to town and your hospital has become part of the plan's network. Indicate the impact this situation is likely to have on your hospital's financial health and workforce.

Assessing the Performance of Managed Care

Despite studies that new mothers discharged from hospitals after one day have the same outcomes as new mothers discharged after three days, some states have passed laws barring so-called drive-through deliveries. Explain the disconnect between the study results, which should have reassured new parents that the practice of early discharge was sound, and the legislation, which suggests that the practice was dangerous.

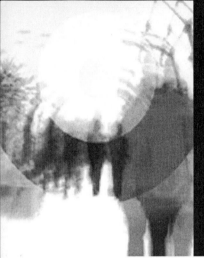

13

PROMOTING HEALTH AND PREVENTING DISEASE
Challenges Facing the U.S. Health Care System

Starting Point

Go to www.wiley.com/college/pointer to assess your knowledge of how the U.S. health care system is financed.
Determine where you need to concentrate your effort.

What You'll Learn in This Chapter

▲ The challenges impacting health systems and governing boards
▲ The funding crisis of Medicare and other health care financing challenges
▲ The reason for the increase in need for long-term care
▲ What changes will be required to address the health needs of an aging population
▲ Why primary care has not benefited from recent changes in health care
▲ The health crises facing populations in inner cities and rural areas
▲ The definition of underserved areas and strategies for addressing them

After Studying This Chapter, You'll Be Able To

▲ Articulate challenges facing private insurers and government programs such as Medicare
▲ Calculate the burden that an aging population places on U.S. health care.
▲ Assess the impact that managed care, the cult of specialty, and other forces have had on the number and job satisfaction of primary care physicians
▲ Analyze strategies for bolstering the availability of health care for underserved areas

Goals and Outcomes

▲ Identify long- and short-term strategies for addressing health professional shortage areas
▲ Explain the connection between rising health costs and health care funding strategies to reduce expenditures
▲ Analyze the connection between funding challenges and access challenges
▲ Extrapolate how the challenges facing primary care physicians correlate to the existence of underserved areas
▲ Formulate a theory on the overarching challenge facing U.S. health care

INTRODUCTION

As the U.S. health care system continues to evolve, it faces and must address a variety of challenges. Health systems have grown more complex, yet they've failed to produce the benefits expected, and governing boards are being held accountable for more than ever before. A key concern is how to finance health care without bankrupting company or congressional coffers. This concern occurs at the same time that many Americans will reach old age and require more care at greater cost. Complicating matters is that the United States does not have an adequate number of primary care providers. Another problem is the existence of underserved areas, where people are either too far from health care to access it or do not have the resources to do so. Strategies exist for eliminating these shortage areas, but implementing them requires a cogent, cohesive policy coordinated by medical educational institutions working with government health agencies.

13.1 Growing Complexity of the U.S. Health Care System

The U.S. health care system has, without question, grown more complex through the years. A large part of this complexity is the result of amazing advances in medical science and technology, as well as the evolving understanding of the human body and how its systems function and respond to treatment. As knowledge grows, so too does the opportunity for breakthroughs and the demand for treatment.

As important as the natural evolution of medical knowledge is in explaining the complexity, however, the changing relationship between Americans and the health care industry and the changing expectations about health care's role are also at play. Long gone are days when you saw a doctor only when you were ill and paid for the services from your own pocket or bartered for them with your own goods. Then, a doctor was essentially an emergency care provider. Today, a doctor—and the health care industry that's grown up around him or her—is part of a vast network whose goal is to keep you well. Your relationship with your doctor and the medical industry is more likely to be regular, ongoing, and—unless you're one of the more than 17 million Americans who are uninsured—paid for by insurance. In the best of all possible worlds, this relationship will help you maintain your good health or catch any problems that exist early enough to maximize the effectiveness of treatment. If not, then the physician becomes the field marshal, amassing and coordinating the health care resources and troops.

This shift, from reactive to proactive intervention, has had profound effect not only on the way that health care is accessed and provided, but also on how it is funded. The following sections touch briefly on the areas that are impacted by the growing complexity of the health care system.

13.1.1 The Effect on Governing Boards

As Chapter 2 explains, health care systems and organizations (such as hospitals) are governed by boards, which have four basic responsibilities:

▲ Formulating the organization's mission and developing strategies to accomplish the mission.

▲ Ensuring high-level management performance through selection and oversight of the organization's chief executive officer.

▲ Ensuring quality of patient care through staffing requirements and strategy planning.

▲ Ensuring financial health of the institution.

As the health care industry has grown more complex, so too has the involvement, decision making, and accountability of governance boards. The following are some of the changes that boards have to adapt to as they move their organizations through the twenty-first century.

▲ **Economic dynamics:** The health care industry's economic dynamics are changing, due in large part to the advent of managed care and the growing trend of traditional insurers to adopt some of managed care's strategies, such as negotiating fee rates and controlling access. In addition, most health care markets face increased competition. For these reasons, health care organizations' survival, let alone their "thrival," isn't ensured. Boards, which are responsible for the financial health of the institution, will be required to make crucial decisions that define the organization's future.

▲ **Burgeoning health care systems:** Health care organizations are becoming larger and more complex enterprises. As health systems grow (refer to Section 1.3), boards must oversee enterprises with revenues in the hundreds of millions or billions of dollars. As they shift costs to consumers, they must also deal with state governments that oppose their higher profits.

▲ **Higher expectations of accountability:** In the post-Enron era, the "cross bar" of governance responsibility and accountability has risen dramatically. The expectations are being defined by the following:

• New federal legislation such as the Sarbanes-Oxley Act (the most widely publicized provision requires CEOs and CFOs to attest to the accuracy of financial statements).

• Rules announced by the New York Stock Exchange, including those relating to the makeup of the board (specifically the number of independent directors; that is, those directors without a financial stake in the organization's earnings) and the purpose and makeup of certain mandatory committees, such as a Compensation Committee and an Audit Committee.

- Principles employed by large pension and trust funds and endorsed by the National Association of Corporate Directors.

Although presently these standards apply to commercial corporations only, most observers believe they will be extended to large nonprofit organizations. Even before then, however, these rules will increasingly affect what bond-rating agencies (such as Standard & Poor, which rates a company's bonds as "investment grade" or "junk"), insurers, regulators and accrediting bodies, state attorneys general, major donors and grant organizations, and the public expect of health care system governing boards.

13.1.2 The Challenge to Health Systems

During the 1980s and 1990s, health care organizations began to consolidate, vertically and horizontally, into health systems. The goal of horizontal combinations, particularly among hospitals, was to ensure that fixed overhead costs were spread across the organization (**economies of scale**) and increase the organization's share in local markets to have more negotiating power with health insurance plans. The goal of vertical combinations, where organizations with different functions are combined, was to create a continuum of services that would benefit both patients and managed care contractors. (You can read more about health systems in Section 1.3.)

The promise of such systems—that they can optimize care while simultaneously controlling costs—has for the most part not materialized:

▲ Mergers and acquisitions have produced large, complex, and unwieldy organizations.

▲ Cost reductions and economies of scale and scope have not been achieved.

▲ The purchase of physician practices and assumption of first-dollar risk on providing services (that is, moving into the health insurance business) have produced huge losses.

▲ The true integration of patient movement and clinical and management systems has been problematic.

As a result of these problems, the coming years may see fewer and fewer health care systems formed. Similarly, existing systems may decide to deintegrate, thus splitting into their component parts. Those systems that do survive will have to demonstrate added clinical, strategic, and operational value: In other words, they must overcome the preceding problems by providing better care, managing the care more efficiently, and controlling costs more effectively.

FOR EXAMPLE

Success Begetting Demand Begetting More Success

Cystic fibrosis is a life-threatening, genetic disorder that affects the respiratory, digestive, and reproductive systems. Although medical science has not been able to come up with a cure for the condition, researchers today have a better understanding of the condition's genetic basis, which has led to earlier detection and intervention. In addition, treatment has become more sophisticated and effective. Whereas years ago, the parents of children born with CF were told not to expect their children to live beyond their teens, today the average life span of a person with CF is 32. Although not wholly successful, the advances made in diagnosing and treating CF illustrate how advances in medical care and treatment options impact the health care system. Today, people with CF are living longer and more "normally"—many are even starting families of their own; a remarkable first—and as such are pushing the boundaries of what clinicians and researchers thought possible. As people with CF begin to expect to live longer and more comfortable lives, they will demand health care options that maximize their chances of doing so, and medical science, by keeping pace with the changing expectations, will only bolster these hopes until they become a reality.

SELF-CHECK

- List the three main challenges governing boards face.
- Identify two reasons that health systems have not been as successful as anticipated.

13.2 Financing Health Care

In 2003, Americans—public and private—spent approximately $1.6 trillion on medical expenses. In 2005, this amount is expected to increase by about 14 percent, to over $1.9 trillion. There are several reasons for the increase: general inflation, increased medical expense (as a component of the consumer price index, meaning that more money is going to medical expense than ever before), increasing population, and the demand and availability for more comprehensive and sophisticated services (you can read more about them in Section 6.1). The same factors that impacted health care costs in the past impact costs today. For that reason, experts agree that the cost of health care will continue to rise at a rate of

7.4 percent a year. The Centers for Medicare and Medicaid Services projects that, by 2010, health care costs will be $2.7 trillion, accounting for over 17 percent of the gross domestic product.

If burgeoning costs of health care don't present enough challenges in and of themselves, the issues are compounded by the growing number of people without any health insurance. The ranks of the uninsured has increased significantly since 1985. Today, 16 percent of people in America are not covered by health insurance. By 2007, that number is expected to increase to between 21 and 25 percent, due to rising health care costs, more families below the poverty level, and fewer employers providing insurance to employees. The link between the uninsured and rising health care costs is that people without insurance postpone seeking medical attention because of financial constraints. By the time they do enter the health care system, they are generally sicker and require more services—hence, the boost in cost.

The convergence of these two trends—rising health costs and the decreasing number of insured—is one of the biggest problems the nation faces, both in terms of economic security and public health.

13.2.1 Government Initiatives

During the early 1990s, the Clinton administration proposed major health care reform. The administration's efforts failed, and future legislative efforts are unlikely to succeed. In the foreseeable future, national health insurance will not be implemented, and no major programs to significantly expand federally mandated or financed health care benefits will be undertaken. The one exception, however, is Medicare, the federally funded insurance program for elderly people. Section 13.2.3 explains the financial challenges Medicare faces. (Read more about the program itself and how it differs from Medicaid in Section 4.6.)

FOR EXAMPLE

Universal Health Care

Although the United States spends more for medical care than any other industrialized nation, it's the only one that doesn't provide universal health coverage. Although Congress failed to pass the major medical reform proposed by the Clinton administration—which would have been a precursor to universal health care; no similar legislation has been introduced since—the idea of universal health care didn't die on the congressional floor. Several grassroots organizations continue to work toward a national health care system: Universal Health Care Action Network, American Health Care Reform.org, Physicians for a National Health Program, and American Medical Student Association are just a few.

Although unable (or unwilling) to advance a program for universal health care coverage, the government does address individual health care issues and concerns as they come up (and gains enough momentum to draw attention and scrutiny). So, in the coming years, expect continuous incremental change. Two areas that garner immediate attention include:

▲ Limiting federal government health care expenditures, either by changing eligibility requirements (to reduce the number of people in the program) or cutting benefits.
▲ Making health insurance plans (particularly HMOs) more accountable and patient-friendly.

13.2.2 Evolving Health Insurance and Health Plans

Over the last several decades, the biggest change in how health care services are purchased has been the rapid growth of managed care, particularly HMO plans. As Section 11.1 explains in more detail, the goal of managed care, in theory, is to provide optimum care for less cost. The mechanism through which it achieves this goal is to control, or manage, both access to health care and cost of services.

To manage access, these plans require people to use primary care physicians (PCPs) in the network and often stipulate when and how referrals to other service providers are made. To manage cost, these plans negotiate set fees for services, regardless of the cost to deliver those services. The reviews on how well managed care has achieved its goal are mixed: Physicians and other service providers aren't particularly happy, because they feel trapped by the low fees and added expense of processing managed care paperwork, and put out by the intrusion of a third party in the doctor–patient decision-making process. Many clients aren't happy because they fear lack of choice: If their preferred physician isn't "in-network," they have to forego insurance or pay a higher premium or deductible; if their provider recommends a procedure that the HMO denies, they have to assume the entire burden of the cost.

For these reasons—and despite its promising beginning—the managed care movement isn't considered the silver bullet that will slay rising health care costs, nor the silver lining that, in and of itself, can ensure that patients receive the best health care available. Although HMO enrollment will continue to grow and HMOs will continue to be dominant players, it will probably do so at a slower pace.

One outcome of the managed care movement has been that other insurance plans have adopted some of the managed care strategies. In the coming years, as costs of health care service continue to rise, expect these other plans to become more stringently "managed" in ways similar to HMOs: that is, these plans will assume more control over when and how health care is accessed (utilization) and how much it costs by negotiating fees.

Additionally, there will be a growth in **tiered health plans**. In these plans, hospitals, clinics, and doctors are placed in categories based on quality and cost. Plan members can choose which tier of care they want to receive and then pay accordingly. Those who choose the plan's preferred hospital pay little or nothing; use another hospital (one still in the plan but that charges more), and the out-of-pocket expenses increase. Tiered health plans, although not new (many insurance plans use tiered pricing for prescription drugs), have gained momentum as managed care plans try to respond to the criticism that they place too many restrictions on access to care.

13.2.3 Funding Medicare

Medicare is the industry's thousand-pound gorilla, the largest health plan and the biggest payer for hospital and physician services. Unfortunately, Medicare's financial structure is untenable. To be sustainable, the amount of money that goes in to the Medicare pot must equal or exceed the amount paid out to health care providers. In other words, the payroll tax contributions from employers and employees in addition to the premiums that Part B beneficiaries pay (refer to Section 4.6.1 to find out what a Part B beneficiary is) has to be enough to cover the programs expenditures.

If the forces—such as rising health care costs, the increasing number of uninsured, and the aging population—impacting health care coverage and expense continue as they are (and there's no reason to assume that they won't), the amount of money brought in will be less than the amount of money that goes out. This gap will widen, particularly after Medicare's prescription drug benefit goes into effect in 2006, and continue to grow bigger through 2010 and then increases dramatically each year thereafter.

Given this scenario, Congress and the president have only two alternatives. First, let Medicare go bankrupt. Obviously, this option is highly unlikely given the importance of this program to a large segment of the population and the amount of political capital at stake. Second, dramatically and fundamentally reconfigure Medicare, which would entail some, or all, of the following:

▲ Increasing age limits when benefits commence.
▲ Increasing employer and employee payroll taxes and contributions.
▲ Limiting coverage on the basis of need (implementing "means" tests to determine eligibility).
▲ Restricting benefits.
▲ Increasing coinsurance payments and deductibles.
▲ Further reducing payments to hospitals and physicians.

Any or all of these changes will have significant implications for health care organizations and professionals and the people who access their services.

13.3 Aging Population

One of the fundamental drivers of the challenges that our society in general and the health care industry in particular is facing is that the U.S. population is growing older. In 2010, baby boomers will begin to turn 65. In that year, the average life expectancy for males will be 76 and for females 86. Aging itself, as well as increased life expectancy, has an impact on the cost and demand for medical services. Just what this effect will be is unclear. Changing demographics is the health care industry's wild card. It will have a tremendous impact, but no one knows exactly what and how much. The following sections provide educated guesses.

13.3.1 Demand and Cost for Short-Term Care

Biological and physical-based disease and infirmity increase exponentially with age. This assertion alone may lead you to believe that demand for health care and health care costs will also rise exponentially. But it does not necessarily follow that just because more people are older, there will be greater demand for health care. How aging translates into demand for and cost of health care services is uncertain and depends on the following:

▲ **Changes in lifestyle:** People are, by and large, healthier today than they were years ago (the increasing life expectancy attests to the overall health of the U.S. population).

▲ **Biomedical and pharmacological technologies:** Advances in treatment strategies and drug technologies often mean better results and, in many cases, shorter recovery times. In other words, the cost of the advances may be offset by the less invasive or more effective treatment.

▲ **The way health care is provided:** As treatment shifts, for example, from inpatient to outpatient and home care, the cost for providing the service falls.

▲ **Financing priorities:** Insurance plans, managed care plans, and Medicare will likely try to control costs by rationing care for certain population groups or conditions.

13.3.2 Demand for Long-Term Care

Although no one can accurately predict what the impact of the aging population will have on short-term care, its impact on long-term care is less difficult to imagine. Essentially it will increase dramatically throughout the first half of the twenty-first century. There are two reasons for this increase:

▲ **An increase of chronic disease:** As population ages so does the incidence of chronic health conditions. Chronic diseases and conditions are long lasting and persistent. Examples include problems like diabetes, kidney disease, high blood pressure, cardiopulmonary disease, and so on.

▲ **Disappearance of nearby extended family:** The fact that fewer and fewer extended families stay in one area has an impact on the care options available for elderly people who need in-home care. Years ago, Grandma may have been able to recover from her hip surgery in her home or Grandpa could continue to live at home despite his increasing forgetfulness, because family was nearby to check in and help out. Today, however, for those without nearby family members, remaining at home is definitely more problematic and, often, impossible.

Whether this need translates into demand for nursing home and home health care depends on financing. Most people don't have long-term-care insurance, and private-pay nursing home care averages $50,000 per year, far beyond the means of all but the most well-to-do Americans. Medicare provides some long-term-care benefits, but only after a hospital stay and then with strict limitations. Medicaid covers nursing home care, but one must exhaust one's resources before being eligible and payments to providers are low.

FOR EXAMPLE

Smaller Is Sometimes Better

Traditional nursing homes are, without doubt, institutional settings. Formica floors, pale walls, fluorescent lighting, shared rooms, and an all-purpose cafeteria—many, despite their best efforts to look like home, are anything but. However, an interesting movement is under way in this country. Providers and patients alike are beginning to see the value of smaller home settings for elderly people. Often in smaller settings—sometimes even actual homes—these organizations offer group living arrangements designed to meet the needs of people who can't live independently, but don't require nursing home services. The idea is that more personal settings ease the transition for elderly people, while at the same time providing the care and oversight they need.

Expect a fast-growing gap between what people need and want—and are able to afford—and the scope of services the system is able to provide.

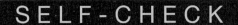

SELF-CHECK

- In terms of health care, how are elderly Americans better off today than years ago?
- Why are elderly people of today and tomorrow more likely to need long-term care?

13.4 Challenges for Primary Care

During the latter half of the twentieth century, primary care attracted a cadre of dedicated physicians drawn by the rewards of generalist practice: relationships with patients, families, and communities that endure over time; the intellectual breadth of comprehensive care; and the satisfaction of addressing fundamental human and clinical needs. Although the majority of medical school graduates pursued training in specialty fields, a solid foundation of primary care clinicians remained an essential piece of the system.

Yet doctors in the prime of their practice today face a very different (and far less hospitable) environment than when they entered practice. Confronted with restrictions on clinical autonomy due to management of care, their base of patients is increasingly determined and controlled by health plans; the amount of red tape and paperwork with which they must contend to receive payment for their services is overwhelming. Additionally, there is a growing oversupply of physicians, although their distribution remains uneven among states, urban and rural locales, and individual markets. There are approximately 570,000 active physicians, with another 170,000 in the pipeline (medical students and residents); 3 new physicians appear for every 1 who retires. Having little control over industrywide forces affecting them, many physicians feel disenfranchised. The following sections examine the problems besetting PCPs in the U.S. health care system.

13.4.1 The Cult of Specialization

Although specialty care has been responsible for remarkable medical achievements and advances, the United States has gone overboard in creating a cult of specialization. This situation has been shaped by four interrelated forces:

▲ **The public's acceptance of the biomedical model:** The idea that there is a pill or a surgical procedure for every human difficulty (see Section

13.4.5 for more about his model). This viewpoint heightens the value of specialty care and undervalues primary care's contributions of preventive services, management of the 80 to 90 percent of medical visits that involve common and not immediately life-threatening problems, and integration of care in a patient-centered or family-centered manner.

▲ **The financial structure of physician reimbursement:** This structure pays most specialists far more than PCPs for their time and their expertise. As a result, the average surgeon earns almost twice the income of the average family physician or pediatrician. And these income disparities are not shrinking.

▲ **The influence of specialist physicians:** Specialist physicians wield sufficient professional power to control the flow of resources into the health care sector; for example, as physicians often centered in hospitals, they received a free workplace from the federally funded Hill-Burton hospital construction program. PCPs, on the other hand, have to finance their own medical practices.

▲ **Lack of public policy regarding role of PCPs:** Unlike most nations, where regulations—administered by governmental health planning agencies—outline the central role of primary care through policies affecting physician payment, physician supply, and rules for obtaining specialty referrals, the United States lacks a formal publicly sanctioned role for primary care. Although managed care plans require a PCP, called a generalists to coordinate health care resources (and thus would seem to bolster the integral role of primary care doctors as an integral part of the health care team), the status of the PCP didn't rise as expected. (Refer to Section 11.1 for more about the role of the PCP in managed care health plans.)

Figure 13-1 illustrates the trend toward specialization and away from primary care practice. In 1931, 87 percent of physicians fell into the primary care category,

Figure 13-1

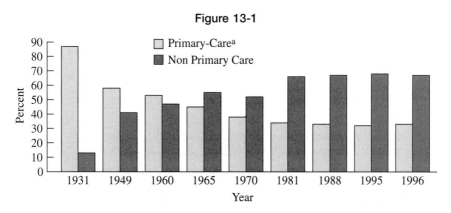

Percentage of primary-care and nonprimary care physicians.

which includes family physicians, general internists, and general pediatrics. By 1996, the majority of physicians (67 percent) were specialists.

13.4.2 Too Few Generalists; Too Many Specialists

A rational health care system must be based upon an infrastructure consisting of a majority of generalist physicians trained to provide quality primary care and an appropriate mix of other specialists to meet health care needs. Currently, however, the United States has too few generalists (family physicians, general internists, and general pediatricians) and too many specialists—a situation that will only be aggravated by the growing percentage of medical school graduates who plan to subspecialize. In addition to general practitioners, general surgeons are also in short supply. The lack of generalists is important for a number of reasons:

▲ **Access to health care:** Certain populations (rural and inner-city, specifically) don't have adequate access to health care primarily because there aren't enough PCPs to fill the health care voids in these areas and specialists tend to locate and practice in urban and upper-class areas.

▲ **Quality of primary care:** Although other specialists and subspecialists provide a significant amount of primary care, doctors who are trained, practice, and receive continuing education in the generalist disciplines provide more comprehensive and cost-effective care than nonprimary care specialists and subspecialists.

▲ **Care for elderly people:** Aging of the U.S. population will increase demand for surgical services, a growth that is likely to exceed the growth in the supply of general surgeons.

The solution to the lack of generalists isn't to train more doctors. Today, the current physician-to-population ratio in the nation is adequate. Simply increasing this ratio won't enhance public health or address the country's problems of access to health care. (Efforts to solve problems of access to health care by increasing the total physician supply haven't worked, and in fact, a growing physician oversupply is projected.) The solution is to produce more generalists and fewer specialists—a role for the medical schools.

13.4.3 The Unexpected Impact of Managed Care

The advent of managed care created expectations of a golden age of primary care, with primary care gatekeepers playing a commanding role in patient care and with managed care organizations demanding their services. For health policy futurists of the mid-1990s, the triumph of managed care was a virtual certainty. The supply of specialists was designated as excessive for a health system soon to be dominated by managed care plans. Medical students responded by briefly forsaking specialty careers and entering primary care in larger numbers.

Yet, reality was not so lustrous. PCPs were inundated with more patients than ever before, were expected to do far more for their patients than previously, were given new administrative tasks that consumed their time and increased overhead expenses, and saw little if any additional money to pay for these growing tasks. In California, a state with many patients enrolled in managed care plans, PCP satisfaction dropped from 48 percent in 1991 to 36 percent in 1996. As managed care plans pressured PCPs to limit specialty and ancillary services, some patients became disgruntled with their primary care gatekeepers.

Although managed care transformed much of the U.S. health care system into a primary care–based structure, it also created enormous expectations of primary caregivers and often placed intolerable stresses on them. Today, even as managed care declines, the public's high expectations of primary care continue. The gatekeeper role is abating, but the stresses are not. Most worrisome, at the same time that the large and demanding baby boomer generation ages, medical school graduates are less inclined to enter primary care.

As managed care faltered, specialty opportunities and incomes blossomed. Medical students began to flock back into coveted specialty residencies. The number of medical students choosing generalist careers fell from 40 percent in 1997 to 32 percent in 2000 and may continue to drop to the 20 percent levels of the early 1990s.

At the very time that U.S. medical school graduates are showing diminishing interest in primary care careers, the aging of the population guarantees that the demand for primary services will increase. In the year 2010, the first wave of baby boomers—Americans born between 1946 and 1964—will reach age 65. The 65-and-over population will swell from 35 million in 2000 to 39 million in 2010 and will then take off as the baby boomer population bulge fills the ranks of the elderly population. Some 53 million in 2020 and 70 million in 2030 will have reached or surpassed age 65, when chronic illness becomes common and begins to take its toll. From 2010 to 2030, the number of Americans 85 years and older will jump from 6 million to 9 million.

13.4.4 The Lack of Government Direction Regarding PCPs

The United States has no national physician workforce plan to meet the current and projected future health care needs of the American people. In addition, there is no coordinated financing strategy and integrated medical education system to implement such a plan. Instead, such critical policy issues as the physician supply and specialty mix are the result of a series of individual decisions make by the 126 allopathic and 15 osteopathic medical schools and nearly 1500 institutions and agencies that currently sponsor or affiliate with general medical education training programs.

In the absence of a national policy or directive, the nation's medical education system must be more responsive to public needs for more generalists

---

FOR EXAMPLE

Supply and Demand

In 2002, researchers at Dartmouth Medical School studied how frequently certain populations (elderly people and newborns) availed themselves of medical care and to what effect. Turns out that those who lived in areas with an abundance of medical services and facilities sought medical care disproportionately more than those in other areas and paid more for the care they received, even though their health was no better than their less-treated peers. Although more study needs to be done to ascertain actual cause and effect, it seems that supply drives demand.

(as well as underrepresented minority physicians and physicians for medically underserved rural and inner-city areas; see Section 13.5 for details on these challenges).

In the past 25 years, the U.S. system of undergraduate and graduate medical education has responded effectively to many of the country's health care needs, increasing the numbers of physicians, advancing biomedical research, and developing new medical technology. Today, the medical education system must respond to U.S. health care and physician workforce needs in the twenty-first century. These needs include

▲ More primary care research.
▲ Increased access to primary care, particularly in underserved rural and urban communities.

To achieve these goals, the medical education system will need to change the institutional mission, goals, admissions policies, curriculum, faculty composition and reward system, and the site for medical education and teaching.

13.4.5 Changing Medical Models

Physicians, as rule, fall into two groups: those who view disease as a physical aberration to be treated, and those who view disease as a biological state that is influenced by—and has impact upon—the patient's social, psychological, and behavioral aspects.

The first school of thought reflects the **biomedical model,** which is the model upon which traditional Western medicine is based. Biomedical dogma requires that all disease, including mental disease, be the result of underlying physical mechanisms gone awry. A tumor, for example, is the result of aberrant cells; depression is the result of faulty biochemical or neurophysiological processes. Ultimately, this model holds that disease is nothing more than a deviation from the norm and that all disease as well as any strange behavioral phenomena must be explained in terms of physicochemical principles; that is, the body is either physically abnormal or chemically imbalanced. As such, the biomedical model leaves no room within its framework for the social, psychological, and behavioral dimensions of illness.

Disenchantment with the biomedical approach is growing among physicians who are ready for a model that takes psychosocial issues into account. The charges against the biomedical model are

▲ It neglects the patient.
▲ It leads to unnecessary treatment and incomplete understanding of disease.
▲ It neglects the impact of nonbiological circumstances upon biological processes.

To provide a basis for understanding what causes a disease and to arrive at the appropriate treatments, the medical model must also take into account the patient, the social context in which he or she lives, and the role of the physician role and the health care system—in other words, a model that illuminates the impact of all aspects of a person's life that impact health and well-being.

The result is the **biopsychosocial model.** In this model, the doctor's task is to do the following:

1. Account for why the patient feels unwell and the symptoms that led to him or her seeking medical help.
2. Weigh the contributions that the person's social and psychological as well as of biological factors play in his or her feeling unwell.
3. Determine how much responsibility the patient takes to cooperate in his or her own health care.
4. Develop a rational program to treat the illness and restore and maintain the patient's help.

The boundaries between health and disease, between well and sick, are far from clear because they are diffused by cultural, social, and psychological considerations. The traditional biomedical view, that biological indicators are the basic criteria for defining disease, leads to the present paradox that some people with positive laboratory findings are told that they are in need of treatment when in fact they are feeling quite well, whereas others feeling sick are ensured that they have no disease. A biopsychosocial model that includes the patient as well as the illness would encompass both circumstances.

SELF-CHECK

- The United States is experiencing a shortage in what type of doctors?
- List three reasons why are PCPs are, as a group, unhappy with managed care.
- Define **biomedical model** and **biopsychosocial model**.

13.5 Examining the Underserved: Rural and Inner-City Areas

Health providers are not distributed adequately across the United States. Even though the 1990s have been marked by rapid expansion in the number of physicians to such a degree that the nation now faces an overabundance of doctors, substantial shortages of physicians have persisted in rural and inner-city areas. Consider that about 20 percent of the U.S. population—more than 50 million people—live in rural areas, but only 9 percent of the nation's physicians practice in rural communities.

Just as poverty and a lack of insurance have measurable consequences for the health of individuals, a medically underserved area has consequences for population health. People in underserved areas are sicker than residents of communities with sufficient doctors and health centers, and they tend to have a lower immunization rate, higher infant mortality, and other measurable deficits.

Access to primary care services is difficult in rural and inner-city areas because of the economic and social circumstances of rural and inner-city areas (medically underserved areas have a relatively high proportion of uninsured or inadequately insured patients), the shortage of minority and generalist physicians, and the distribution of practices between urban and rural areas. These factors are discussed in more detail in the following sections.

13.5.1 Lack of Racial and Ethnically Diverse Doctors

The racial and ethnic composition of U.S. physicians doesn't reflect the general population. Although African Americans, Hispanic Americans, and Native Americans constitute almost one-fourth of all Americans, they represent only 10 percent of practicing physicians and 3 percent of medical faculty. This lack of diversity contributes to access problems for underrepresented minorities because minority physicians are more likely than other physicians to serve inner-city populations.

13.5.2 Declining Numbers of General Practitioners

Like minority physicians, physicians in the three primary care specialties—family practice, general internal medicine, and general pediatrics—are more likely than their peers to serve underserved populations. But the shortage of general practitioners (refer to Section 13.4) means fewer doctors in these areas. The shortage is especially keen in two areas:

▲ **General surgery:** The decline in numbers of general surgeons entering rural practice is little recognized and has significant implications for access to trauma, obstetrical, and orthopedic services in rural settings and to the fiscal viability of rural hospitals.

▲ **Obstetrics:** Access to obstetrical care—or lack of it—has been in the national spotlight. Problems are greatest in rural and inner-city areas. Although the total number of obstetricians continues to increase, the proportion providing obstetrical services decreases dramatically with the number of years in practice. Less than 10 percent of obstetricians practice in rural settings. Consequently, family physicians historically provide the majority of rural obstetrical care. In recent years, however, the proportion of family physicians providing obstetrical services has also declined markedly. In other words, obstetrical care in rural areas is reaching crisis levels.

13.5.3 Location of Practices

Health care professionals tend to locate and practice in relatively affluent urban and suburban areas. In fact, only 2.6 percent of medical school graduates choose to practice in a small town or rural area, according to the Association of American Medical Colleges. Over the years, this has resulted in a lopsided scenario in which 51 million rural Americans—roughly 20 percent of the nation's population—are being cared for by less than 10 percent of the nation's practicing physicians. Poor inner-city neighborhoods are similarly underserved because of a scarcity of health care providers.

In addition, physician supply in rural areas is closely tied to the specialty mix of American physicians. Specialty has a powerful effect on physician location choice for each of the major specialty groups. Family physicians are the largest single source of physicians in rural areas. All other specialties are much more likely to settle in urban areas (see Figure 13-2).

Nothing affects the location decision of physicians more than specialty. The more highly specialized the physician, the less likely he or she will settle in a rural area. As a consequence, the growth of specialization is a major contributor to the geographic maldistribution of physicians. Many of the shortages in communities with fewer than 10,000 residents could have been reduced or

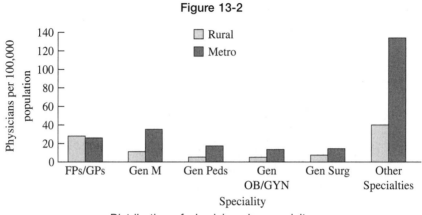

Distribution of physicians by specialty.

Source: Data provided by American Medical Association, 1997.

eliminated if even a small fraction of subspecialists produced over the past 15 years had chosen to become PCPs in rural or underserved areas.

13.5.4 Lack of Coordinated Effort to Address Shortage

Beyond the lack of ethnically diverse workforce, the shortage of general practitioners, or the preponderance of medical practices located in affluent, urban settings, another factor exacerbating the problem of underserved areas is the absence of a national plan to improve the geographic distribution of health care providers. Efforts to date have been largely piecemeal, with little coordination among government and private sector initiatives.

Historically, states have not, until recently anyway, paid much attention to their medically underserved areas. They often considered them a federal responsibility, similar to the provision of health insurance (Medicaid and Medicare), welfare, or

---

FOR EXAMPLE

Making Regular Health Care More Accessible

The Komed Health Center in Chicago, part of the federal government's community renewal initiative of 2000, provides health care to the largely African American community of Bronzeville. The center was created to make regular health care more accessible to residents of the area and to neighboring communities. The clinic offers pediatric, internal medicine, comprehensive obstetrics and gynecology services as well as dental services. It also provides regular follow-up to patients. Komed offers services on a sliding fee scale basis and provides care free of charge to uninsured patients.

housing support for the very poor. Although some states experimented with homegrown solutions, such as loan repayment and substitute doctor (*locum tenens*) programs to ease the economic and workload burden on providers, the majority simply clamored for more National Health Service Corps doctors, more federally funded clinics for poor and uninsured patients, and more federal response in general.

13.5.5 Role of Gender on Choice of Practice Location

Male generalist physicians far outnumber their female counterparts in rural areas across the United States. As the proportion of women in medical schools has increased (the number of female physicians in the United States more than quadrupled between 1970 and 1991 and has continued to rise), there have been concerns that the supply of rural physicians might dwindle if women continue to settle almost exclusively in urban areas and the largest rural cities.

Although the gap between male and female family physicians has narrowed dramatically for more recent graduates, women are still much less likely than their male counterparts to locate in rural areas. The continuing preference of women for urban practice—even though less pronounced than in earlier years—may still pose a problem for the future recruitment of rural physicians.

SELF-CHECK

- What two areas are most likely to have a shortage of physicians?
- List three reasons for the shortage of health care providers in these areas.
- In what two health care areas is the shortage of generalist physicians particularly keen?

13.6 Fixing the Problem of the Underserved

Reviving interest in family medicine and the other generalist disciplines is a major factor in addressing lack of health care providers in rural and inner-city areas. An improvement in the balance of generalists and specialists is a necessary precondition for eliminating rural and inner-city physician shortages. The following sections outline some possible solutions for drawing more physicians to underserved areas.

13.6.1 Bolstering an Ethnically Diverse Workforce

Increasing the percentage of underrepresented minorities in the medical profession is vital as a means of improving access to care and health status of these vulnerable and underserved populations. Minority physicians tend to practice more in minority or underserved areas, reduce language and cultural barriers to care, and provide much-needed community leadership.

Strategies to increase minority enrollment must emphasize increasing and strengthening the applicant pool, the acceptance rate from within this pool, and the student retention rate. These strategies must take into account disproportionately high rates of poverty, poor health status, poor schools, and a continued lack of access to educational and career opportunities. They must include both traditional short-term efforts and long-term strategies targeting younger students early in the education pipeline.

Consequently, more generalist physicians must be educated, and educational programs should specifically address skills needed in these settings. This must be accompanied by sufficient incentives to enter and remain in inner-city and rural practice and by the development of adequate health care systems in which they can practice.

13.6.2 Changing the Medical Education System

One of the most powerful ways to remedy problems of rural geographic maldistribution is to change the medical education system so that it selects, trains, and deploys more health care workers who choose to practice in rural areas. Much of the federal support incorporated within the **Title VII programs**—the major federal vehicle for generalist training—is based on the premise that this is an achievable goal. To do so requires accepting four basic "truths" about rural health:

▲ Students with rural origins are more likely to train in primary care and return to rural areas.
▲ Residents trained in rural areas are more likely to choose to practice in rural areas.
▲ Family medicine is the key discipline of rural health care.
▲ Residents practice close to where they train.

To the extent that these relationships are accurate—and evidence supports associations between these characteristics and the decision to practice in rural areas—modifying the training environment to incorporate these factors make sense.

Ample evidence exists that such an approach works. Publicly owned medical schools in rural states, particularly those that see their mission as training future family physicians, have high proportions of their graduating classes ultimately practicing in rural areas. By contrast, research-intensive private schools in metropolitan areas with no commitment to family medicine have virtually no rural graduates.

13.6.3 Changing Reimbursement Strategies of Medicare and Medicaid

A powerful mechanism to improve the flow of health professionals to rural and inner-city areas is the use of targeted incentives. Central to this approach is the belief that physicians and others act as rational economic beings. If some form of economic inducement enhances the reimbursement for rural services, then physicians are more likely to locate in these areas. This approach has been used with some success in Britain, Canada, and Australia, where a variety of bonuses increase reimbursement for selected rural practitioners.

13.6.4 Changing Existing Direct Federal and State Programs

When educational interventions and economic incentives fail to remedy geographic maldistribution, the solution often becomes creating programs that provide direct services to underserved areas. There are numerous examples of such programs, the largest of which are the community health centers (refer to Section 8.2.5) and the **National Health Service Corps (NHSC),** a federal program administered by the Department of Health and Human Services, which recruits physicians to practice in underserved areas. There is no question that these two federal programs remain the preeminent safety net programs for rural America.

Given the realities of the current system, future efforts should concentrate on the following:

▲ Improving the fit between need and services.
▲ Enhancing coordination—and reducing duplication—of services provided.
▲ Better identifying students to ultimately serve in the NHSC and state programs.
▲ Improving effectiveness and efficiency of government-sponsored health care services.

13.6.5 Relying on the Impact of Managed Care

Managed care is a major emerging influence on the delivery of rural health care. Although it has become dominant in many urban areas, its effect in rural areas is just beginning to be felt. More than 80 percent of all rural counties were in the service area of at least one health maintenance organization (HMO) by the end of 1995, although the percentage of the rural population enrolled in HMOs is estimated to be less than 8 percent. Managed care is not only a creature of the private sector; nationally, about a tenth of rural Medicaid recipients are enrolled in Medicaid HMOs and prepaid plans, and the number is increasing rapidly.

Managed care is a dual-edged sword, both with regard to geographic maldistribution and rural medical underservice. Although managed care networks

FOR EXAMPLE

Seeking Solutions in Technology

A challenge for those trying to address the health care problem in rural America is figuring out a way to most effectively provide health service in vast areas with few people. Some states are turning to technology. Kansas is experimenting with Telehealth, a education tool that, in addition to being a way to cost effectively provide training to dispersed health care providers, is also used to connect rural residents with providers in other areas of the state. Utah is trying Telepharmacy. Unable to afford hiring an on-site pharmacist, remote communities use an interactive video link to connect to pharmacists in more populated areas. As underserved areas continue to struggle with the provider shortage, expect more such innovativeness to enable rural residents to access the necessary health care.

have the potential to provide organizational vehicles for hiring and deploying physicians in areas that could not support independent physicians on their own, there are two potentially adverse effects of managed care systems on rural health:

▲ The loss of local control of health care systems: Most managed care systems are sponsored by large metropolitan organizations, and these entities may have little understanding of or empathy for isolated rural areas.

▲ The reluctance of private managed care systems to provide care to the uninsured. The presence of physicians hired through vertically integrated systems (refer to Section 1.3) may mean that the community has health professionals, but they may be of little use to the working poor who have neither Medicaid nor conventional health insurance.

The managed care industry is in rapid flux (see Section 13.2), and the extent to which managed care will ultimately dominate rural areas as it has dominated some urban ones is difficult to predict.

SELF-CHECK

- List three strategies for eliminating underserved areas.
- Define **National Health Service Corps (NHSC)**.

13.7 Other Challenges

The challenges mentioned previously are not the only issues facing the U.S. health care system. The following sections briefly discuss other factors that the system has to adapt to or address.

13.7.1 Advancing Technology

Major new medical technologies (devices, pharmaceuticals, and procedures) are being developed and introduced at a blistering pace. Many of these innovations are revolutionary and disruptive; that is, they will fundamentally alter, not just improve, clinical diagnostics and therapeutics.

Technologies likely to have the greatest impact include:

▲ Genetic testing, which employs maps of the human genome to identify predispositions for a host of diseases, conditions, and infirmities.
▲ Gene therapy, which uses site-specific gene "implants" to change the course of, or eliminate, diseases.
▲ Pharmaceuticals that will totally replace current forms of treatment, for example, "Drano-like" drugs that remove plaque from coronary arteries, to obviate implanting stints or doing bypass surgery.
▲ Xeno-transplantation, which uses animal cells, tissues, and organs as a source for human transplants.
▲ Minimally invasive procedures, accelerated development of devices and techniques that allow interventions to be performed without major surgery.

These and a host of other developments will change how health care services are organized, provided, and reimbursed.

In addition to the advances in medical technology are the dramatic developments in computer, Internet-based, and communications technologies that are sweeping across all sectors of the economy. In the health care industry, they will have a significant impact on how clinical and administrative information is collected, stored, analyzed, integrated, and used; on the effectiveness, efficiency, and timeliness of internal operating systems; and on how patients, purchasers, clinicians, and health care organizations interact with one another.

13.7.2 Shortage of Nurses

The nursing shortage is especially acute for hospitals. The nursing staff is the largest, and most important, professional component of the hospital workforce.

> ## FOR EXAMPLE
>
> ### Online Learning for Nurses
>
> Policy makers in Texas are trying to kill two birds with one online stone: In an attempt to address both the nursing shortage and the lack of health care professionals in rural areas, Texas offers online training for nurses. The program brings nursing school into students' homes. By studying at times that are convenient for them, these students can earn an associate's or bachelor's degree in nursing. All course work is offered online, and they can perform their clinical work in their communities. The hope is that these students will increase the ranks of nurses and, because some are likely to be rural residents themselves, stay in rural areas after graduation as health care providers.

Recruiting and keeping registered nurses (RNs) is a huge challenge, especially when you consider these factors:

▲ The average age of practicing RNs is 45 and increasing. More mature and experienced nurses are retiring, choosing to work part time or moving into outpatient settings where physical demands are less.

▲ Nurses bear most of the brunt of the "sicker-and-quicker" phenomenon, in which patients have shorter stays and require far more intense services—a result of increasingly stringent management of care and the shift of many procedures to ambulatory care settings (such as same-day surgery).

▲ Nursing school enrollment and graduation rates are flat because of a host of factors: a much expanded array of educational and employment opportunities for college-age women, changes in the structure of nursing education (toward a BSN as the degree required for entry into practice), and no growth in real-dollar nursing salaries over the past several decades.

13.7.3 Evolving Public Health Threats

HIV/AIDS, newly emerging viruses, antibiotic-resistant bacteria, increasing pollution of the environment, and threats of bioterrorism pose significant public health challenges. The public health system (actually a nonsystem) has been marginalized and is chronically underfunded, fragmented, overly bureaucratic, and focused on providing safety-net personal health care services. Absent a massive overhaul, the appropriateness and quality of public health services will continue to deteriorate.

13.7.4 Declining Financial Health of Hospitals

Thanks to alterations in the industry's fundamental economic structure and dynamics (refer to Section 4.1), the majority of general, short-stay hospitals now have margins from operations that are in the red. This degree of financial distress will continue and is likely to get worse. With minimal internally generated reserves and the inability to secure debt financing at reasonable rates, hospitals will find it increasingly difficult to modernize or replace facilities (whose half-life is eroding), mount or expand new programs and services, purchase and deploy innovative therapeutic and diagnostic technologies, and align wage rates for critical personnel with those in other industries.

SELF-CHECK

- List three challenges facing U.S. health care (beyond those outlined in Sections 13.1 through 13.6).
- What does it mean for a technology to be medically disruptive?
- Where is the nursing shortage greatest?

SUMMARY

A variety of challenges face the U.S. health care system. The system's complexity creates challenges for health systems and governing boards. The financial burden of health care overwhelms providers, private insurers, managed care programs, and government programs. The aging population creates issues of its own and exacerbates the other challenges U.S. health care faces. A key component of a viable health system is the PCP, but in the United States, PCPs are in short supply. Underserved areas in particular are most negatively impacted by the physician shortage. Strategies to attract physicians to these areas, if implemented, could address this problem. Without a coherent health policy, however, these issues will continue to be addressed piecemeal and with limited success.

KEY TERMS

Biomedical model	The medical model that views disease as nothing more than a deviation from the norm and that all disease as well as any strange behavioral phenomena must be explained in terms of physico-chemical principles; that is, the body is either physically abnormal or chemically imbalanced.
Biopsychosocial model	The medical model that, when dealing with health care, takes into account all aspects of a person's life—social, psychological, and behavioral—that impact health and well-being.

Economies of scale	The strategy of spreading overhead costs across an organization.
National Health Service Corps (NHSC)	A federal program administered by the Department of Health and Human Services, which recruits physicians to practice in underserved areas.
Tiered health plans	Health plans in which hospitals, clinics, and doctors are placed in categories based on quality and cost, which plan members can choose and pay for accordingly.
Title VII programs	The major federal vehicle for generalist training.

ASSESS YOUR UNDERSTANDING

Go to www.wiley.com/college/pointer to evaluate your knowledge of the challenges facing U.S. health care.
Measure your learning by comparing pre-test and post-test results.

Summary Questions

1. Which of the following is the primary reason health care in the United States has grown more complex?
   (a) the existence of more health organizations and health systems than in years past
   (b) the shift from viewing health care as a periodic necessity to address specific medical needs to ongoing intervention to maintain good health
   (c) the advent of managed care plans
   (d) the increasing number of medical specialties
2. What economic dynamics have put pressure on governing boards to make their organizations more cost effective?
   (a) the advent of managed care plans and increased competition with other health organizations
   (b) the higher rates demanded by doctors and other health care providers
   (c) the increasing federal regulations of health care organizations
   (d) all of the above
3. Define *economies of scale*.
   (a) reducing (scaling back) health costs to increase income
   (b) evaluating profit and loss across the various components or members of a health system
   (c) spreading cost evenly across the various components or members of a health system
   (d) none of the above
4. To deal with rising health care costs, the growing number of uninsured, and funding shortfalls for government health programs, the U.S. government is expected to initiate sweeping changes in the way health care is dispensed and paid for. True or False?
5. What is one strategy that managed care plans are implementing to address criticism regarding lack of patient choice?
   (a) abandoning the role of a gatekeeper for accessing services
   (b) making negotiated fees more generous to attract more providers into the plan's network

    (c) implementing tiered plans so that members can choose to pay more to receive higher quality of care

    (d) eliminating closed plans in which only network doctors can provide care

6. Medicare doesn't bring in enough money to sustain itself and is quickly going bankrupt. What are the sources of Medicare funding?

    (a) social security taxes

    (b) payroll taxes and premiums paid by beneficiaries

    (c) nonprofit contributions from charitable organizations

    (d) none of the above

7. What is the biggest demographic change the United States will see in the next two decades?

    (a) the increase in immigrants and foreign nationals

    (b) the aging of the U.S. population as baby boomers turn 65

    (c) the increasing numbers of low-income families

    (d) the decreasing size of the average family

8. As the U.S. population ages, demand for short-term health care and health care costs are likely to rise exponentially. True or False?

9. What type of health care are elderly Americans most likely to need in the coming decades?

    (a) short-term care

    (b) long-term care

    (c) preventative care

10. Because of the managed care model, which centers around the PCP, primary care has seen a boon in recent years that puts primary care practice almost on par with specialty practice. True or False?

11. In the United States, which organization or agency sets policy regarding the ratio of primary to specialty care physicians and the role that PCPs play?

    (a) the U.S. Department of Health and Human Services

    (b) the various state health departments

    (c) the medical schools themselves

    (d) no one

12. A medically underserved area is

    (a) one that lacks an adequate number of physicians to care for the population.

    (b) usually in rural or inner-city areas.

    (c) more likely than other areas to include poor and uninsured people.

    (d) all of the above.

13. What factor, more than any other, determines location of a practice?
    (a) physician gender
    (b) physician race or ethnicity
    (c) medical specialty
    (d) physician age

14. Traditionally, federal and state governments have worked closely together to address the needs of underserved populations. True or False?

15. Drawing physicians to family practice or other generalist specialties is one of the keys to eliminating underserved areas. True or False?

16. Of the following, who are more likely practice in rural areas?
    (a) students who grew up in rural areas
    (b) students who train in rural areas
    (c) students who study family medicine
    (d) b and c
    (e) all of the above

17. A pharmaceutical that replaces a current form of treatment—for example, a drug that cleans arteries and eliminates the need for surgery—is an example of a disruptive medical advancement. True or False?

18. Fewer candidates are studying nursing because
    (a) women have several more career opportunities today than in the past.
    (b) the educational requirements to become a nurse are greater now than they used to be.
    (c) nurses' salaries haven't increased in real dollars.
    (d) all of the above.

19. Despite the challenges hospitals face, most privately run hospitals are able to generate enough income to support their operations. True or False?

Review Questions

1. In what way has advancing medical knowledge and technology increased health care demands?

2. Why have health systems not been able to realize the cost and resource benefits they were designed to generate?

3. Managed care has not lived up to its early promise, yet it still has had a significant impact on financing health care. How has it influenced other types of insurance?

4. Tiered health plans address which criticisms of managed care?

5. Addressing the Medicare shortfall will require Congress to make significant changes to the program. These changes fall into two categories: increasing program funding and limiting program benefits. Identify which category each of the following changes falls into:

    (a) increasing age limits when benefits commence

    (b) increasing coinsurance payments and deductibles

    (c) increasing employer and employee payroll taxes and contributions

    (d) limiting coverage on the basis of need

6. Identify the factors affecting what impact aging will have on the demand for short-term care.

7. What factors may mitigate the high costs associated with caring for a large elderly population?

8. Is a generalist or a specialist most likely to implement the biopsychosocial health model?

9. Is a generalist or a specialist most likely to implement the biomedical model?

10. List three reasons that explain why more medical students are specializing rather than going into general care.

11. Which type of physicians are most likely to practice in underserved areas?

12. What effect does the preference of specialists to practice in urban or upscale areas have on the distribution of health care providers across the nation?

13. Of the strategies proposed for addressing medically underserved areas, which strategies address cultural obstacles to care and which address location obstacles to care?

14. In what way can increasing the ranks of minority and ethnically diverse doctors address underserved areas?

15. Name an example of how technology can help address health care in underserved populations.

16. In what way is computer technology affecting health care?

17. In what way is the nursing shortage in hospitals similar to the physician shortage in underserved areas?

18. In what way will the financial problems hospitals face today impact their performance in years to come?

Applying This Chapter

1. Explain the relationship between medical advancements and the high rates of uninsured people to the cost of health care.

2. Identify how HMOs, traditional insurance plans, and Medicare are evolving (or are likely to evolve) to address growing health care costs.

3. Why will the need for long-term-care facilities increase? Explain why this need may not result in additional facilities.

4. Describe how the advent of managed care failed to spur a golden age of the PCP.

5. Of the strategies offered for solving the problem of underserved areas (refer to Section 13.5), which three do you think are more likely to have a more profound impact in the short term? In the long term?

6. Taken together, all the topics in this chapter comprise the core challenge facing U.S. health care policy makers. Describe what this core challenge is.

YOU TRY IT

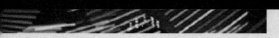

Growing Complexity of the U.S. Health Care System

What challenges discussed in the chapter have a direct impact on health organization governing boards?

Financing Health Care

What impact, if any, does managed care have on the shortage of generalists?

Aging Population

Explain what impact the growing elderly population will have on how health care is financed, the shortage of generalists, and the declining financial health of hospitals.

Challenges for Primary Care

Explain how America can have both an abundance of doctors and areas with health service shortages.

Address the proportion of PCPs to specialists and their distribution in your answer.

Examining the Underserved: Rural and Inner-City Areas

Explain how new technologies designed to improve care can be disruptive to a health system.

Fixing the Problem of the Underserved

Of the many strategies that can be used to address the shortage of physicians in underserved areas, indicate which you think would provide the most immediate benefit. Explain your answer.

Other Challenges

Of the challenges listed in Section 13.7, which do you consider to have the biggest impact on personal health care? Explain your answer:

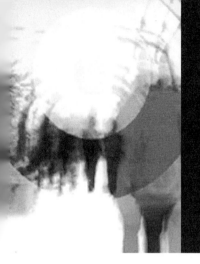

14

PUBLIC HEALTH POLICY
Understanding the Role of Government in the U.S. Health Care System

Starting Point

Go to www.wiley.com/college/pointer to assess your knowledge of public health policy.
Determine where you need to concentrate your effort.

What You'll Learn in This Chapter

▲ The key health functions of federal, state, and local governments
▲ Key laws defining and affecting U.S. health policy
▲ The critical policy issues that U.S. health policy still needs to address
▲ How the U.S. health care system compares to the health care system of other countries

After Studying This Chapter, You'll Be Able To

▲ Discuss the federal role in health policy in relation to state or local roles
▲ Analyze the key pieces of health care legislation and their impact on health care
▲ Identify critical policy issues
▲ Describe the U.S. health care system as it compares to other health systems
▲ Describe the difference between private and public health, and give examples of key historical public health events

Goals and Outcomes

▲ Describe the implication of critical policy issues on U.S. health care
▲ Describe the U.S. health care system as indicated by the system characteristics and type of practice
▲ Articulate succinctly how U.S. health policy differs from the U.S. health care system
▲ Assess the coherence of U.S. health policy, based on the role and function of government and characteristics of the U.S. health system
▲ Assess the impact of critical policy issues on the U.S. health care system
▲ Apply chapter ideas to defend or reject the idea that the United States has a coherent health policy
▲ Evaluate the effectiveness of U.S. health care policy in ensuring the health of its population

INTRODUCTION

Understanding the U.S. health care system requires that you be familiar with U.S. health policy and its components. Federal, state, and local governments each have important roles to play and vital functions to perform. Health care legislation is also a vital component of U.S. health policy. As the U.S. health care system continues to adapt, government must address critical policy issues. Comparing the U.S. health care system to the health systems of other nations is a helpful way of describing the U.S. system and evaluating the effectiveness of U.S. policy.

14.1 Public Health Services

Private health care deals with providing health services to individuals. **Public health care**, on the other hand, focuses on preventing disease and promoting health in populations. To understand the difference between the two, consider the polio outbreaks of the early and mid-twentieth century. Doctors who cared for patients stricken with the disease were practicing private health care; local government initiatives to close public pools and the work of the National Foundation for Infantile Paralysis (created in 1938 by Franklin Roosevelt to search for a cure for the disease) are examples of public health care.

Public health focuses on the health of a population or community, and has a "trickle-down" effect on the individual. Many significant public health contributions have helped shape the American climate as we now know it. As we look back at the history of public health, we see many key global events and discoveries that have contributed to the health and economy of the American individual:

▲ 1500–1700s: Plague, malaria, and smallpox take the lives of thousands in Europe, and then bring the diseases to the New World.

▲ 1796: Edward Jenner discovers a vaccination for smallpox.

▲ 1849: Dr. John Snow traces cholera to infected drinking water, leading to the linking of microorganism and disease.

▲ 1862: Louis Pasteur proposes germ theory regarding disease.

▲ 1872: American Public Health Association is founded.

▲ 1906: Pure Food and Drugs Act is implemented in the United States to regulate the food industry.

▲ 1965: Congress passes the Medicare and Medicaid bills.

Protection of the nation's public health is a government responsibility because doing so requires the ability to coordinate massive efforts across various agencies and contributors, as well as tremendous amounts of money. In 2000, for example, expenditures for public health were $44 billion. Such initiatives and expenditures are typically beyond the scope of personal or charitable organizations. Although private organizations and charities play an important role in public health (refer to Section 13.1.4), they lack the resources, manpower, and infrastructure to accomplish these things independently.

Public health agencies and institutions perform three core functions:

▲ **Assessment:** To fulfill its assessment obligation, government must understand community health needs, recognize health hazards, and understand their causes and impacts. To that end, government does the following:

1. Evaluates community health needs, for example, by examining health statistics such as infant mortality, virus frequency, and disease factors.

2. Investigates the occurrence of health hazards by establishing oversight agencies or departments to monitor these hazards. Public health departments, for example, have departments that specialize in inspecting dining establishments for example.

3. Analyzes the factors, such as industrial and environmental conditions and the community's health habits that produce and exacerbate public health problems

▲ **Policy development:** Government, by virtue of its legislative, or lawmaking, role, is the only entity responsible for creating public health policy. To that end, government must

1. Advocate and build constituencies. These constituencies include health care organizations, health care professional associations and boards, and private health care–related businesses such as insurance companies, med-tech companies, and so on.

2. Set priorities and simple goals and outcomes; for example, setting a goal to reduce infant mortality by 3 percent within two years. Infant mortality rate is an important statistic that can be used as an indicator of the quality of health care available to a population and potential health risks facing the population or subgroup. For example, in areas where access to health care is limited, infant mortality rates tend to be higher than in those where people typically have access to trained medical professionals.

3. Formulate plans and policies that get stakeholders to buy-in and to find legislative support for the legislative initiative.

▲ **Assurance:** Government, by virtue of its executive function—that is, executing or implementing policy directive—is also responsible for making sure that the public health policy is implemented. This function includes the following responsibilities:

1. Managing resources and developing organizational infrastructure by, for example, developing oversight departments, such as the National Institutes of Health.

2. Implementing programs by, for example, contracting programs out to various organizations and bodies that specialize in the types of programs needed.

3. Evaluating program outcomes by setting standards and success indicators. This evaluation usually takes place locally with the smaller implementing organization or body and is also evaluated at the higher level.

4. Informing and educating the public by publishing the findings and/or results and getting press for those findings.

These functions are performed through a complex set of relationships, as well as division of effort among federal, state, and local government public health agencies.

14.1.1 Federal Health Agencies

Federal responsibilities for public health are discharged primarily by the cabinet-level **Department of Health and Human Services (DHHS)**. The DHHS, through its various agencies, performs several major public health functions:

▲ **Data gathering and analysis, and surveillance and control:** The National Center for Health Statistics, and the **Centers for Disease Control and Prevention (CDC)**, the nation's primary public health agency, perform these functions. The CDC is the component of the DHHS that was founded in 1946 to help control malaria. The CDC now works to "prevent and control infectious and chronic diseases, injuries, workplace hazards, disabilities, and environmental health threats." They also conduct and apply research and respond to health emergencies (CDC.gov).

▲ **Conducting and sponsoring research:** The National Institutes of Health (NIH) is one of the sects that performs this function. This section of the DHHS is the primary federal agency for conducting and supporting medical research. It is supported by the American people and invests $28 billion in medical research. Examples of current research projects funded by the NIH include development of treatment and diagnosis of Parkinson's disease and Alzheimer's disease, and vaccines for diseases like HIV/AIDS, tuberculosis, malaria, and potential agents of bioterrorism, among many others.

▲ **Providing programmatic assistance to state and local governments:** The Health Resources and Services Administration performs this function.

▲ **Formulating objectives and policy:** The Office of the Assistant Secretary for Health performs this function.

▲ **Ensuring the safety of food and drugs:** The Food and Drug Administration (FDA) and the Agency for Toxic Substances and Disease Registry perform this function. The FDA was founded in 1906 and is responsible for regulating food, drugs, medical devices, biologics, animal feed and drugs, cosmetics, and radiation-emitting products. It also regulates the advertising and labeling of these products. The FDA is funded by the American people, with a cost to the taxpayer of about $3 per person (FDA.gov).

▲ **Ensuring access to health services by aged and poor people:** The Centers for Medicare and Medicaid Services (CMS) performs this function. Medicare is a national health insurance program enacted in 1965 for workers and their spouses 65 and older who are eligible for Social Security, persons with permanent kidney failure, or people with certain disabilities under the age of 65. These programs are funded by employers and employees contributing a certain percentage of their wages through the Social Security (FICA) tax. Medicaid is government-provided health insurance for poor people. Each state determines the eligibility requirements for this program. Federal and state governments fund this program.

▲ **Providing direct services to special populations:** The Indian Health Service is an agency that performs this function. In addition to directly managing federal health agencies, the federal government also contributes funding for state and local health programs.

14.1.2 State Health Agencies

The first state board (department) of public health was created by Massachusetts in 1855. Eventually, all other states (and territories) followed suit. Today, state departments or agencies perform several public health functions, such as the following:

▲ **Licensing health care professionals:** States set education and performance standards and issue licenses to health professionals, such as physicians, dentists, chiropractors, pharmacists, optometrists, nurses, and veterinarians, who intend to practice within the state.

▲ **Inspecting and licensing health care facilities:** Each state is responsible for licensing and inspecting health care facilities, such as hospitals and nursing homes, to ensure that these facilities meet state specifications regarding condition of the facility, qualification of the staff, record keeping, finances, and so on.

▲ **Collecting vital statistics:** States collect **vital statistics**, statistics related to births, deaths, marriages, health, and disease, for their populations. These vital statistics give us important data for the allocation of funds toward research and health service distribution.

▲ **Investigating and analyzing the epidemiology of disease:** To further public health goals, states investigate the **epidemiology** of diseases within their populations. Epidemiological studies include three factors:

- **Incidence: Incidence** is the number of times a health issue occurs. If someone is diagnosed with HIV, for example, that is considered an "incidence." The National Notifiable Disease Surveillance System is a national database that contains infectious disease incidence information. Each year, the CDC and the Council of State and Territorial Epidemiologists (CSTE) decide which diseases should be considered nationally notifiable. Each state then determines its own regulations for which diseases to report, and participation is voluntary. Reported diseases can also vary from year to year. The disease incidence data are then compiled and released to the public via a document titled the *Morbidity and Mortality Weekly Report (MMWR)*. As not all diseases are reported, this report is said to be a minimum estimation of the prevalence of disease in the United States. The most recent list of nationally notifiable diseases can be found at www.cdc.gov/epo/dphsi/infdis. htm (CDC.gov).

- **Distribution: Distribution** refers to the scope or spread of a disease or incidences. For example, it might be said that the distribution of incidences of cancer cases in a particular area are among 60 percent white females, 10 percent black females, and 20 percent Asian females. Distribution can also refer to geographical area. For example, 50 percent more cancer incidences have occurred in the communities within a five-mile radius of the steel factory than in the communities farther away from the steel factory.

- **Control: Control** simply refers to the health agencies' ability to manage incidences.

▲ **Observing and managing communicable diseases in the community:** Since the events of September 11, 2001, all states have in place a crisis management plan. These plans often include what is termed "outbreak" or communicable disease management. The plans address, among others issues, (1) how to identify an outbreak vs. incidences, (2) quarantine measures to curtail the spread, (3) response measures such as administration of vaccines and medicines, (4) setup of facilities to handle outbreak, and (5) surveillance and contact tracing (trail of exposure). These items along with outbreak and community-specific items make up the control function.

▲ **Registering disease and tumor information:** When incidences occur, those incidences must be recorded with the proper oversight or surveillance entity to ensure that the state health agency can track and research the disease in the best possible ways. In the case of communicable diseases, it's vital to report incidences to track exposure rates.

▲ **Providing laboratory services:** Many health departments and public health entities, including the state, have laboratory services that function to identify and survey incidences of disease within their own communities. These services can be open to the public to provide them with results of their health department–administered tests as well.

▲ **Formulating health policy and legislation:** These are political, sometimes grassroots-oriented, sometimes private-sector-oriented movements that present pertinent public health issues to legislative bodies for policy, regulation, and legal codifying. State legislators sometimes look to state and community boards of health and health agencies for advice and expertise on health policy matters.

▲ **Analyzing health policy or legislation's impact:** State health agencies assess at the state and local levels how well policy is working. This assessment helps form health policy at the state level.

▲ **Providing community health education:** For many state health agencies, educating the public is a key concern. By educating their citizens, states hope to minimize the spread of disease incidences and lessen the burden on the state public health systems.

In addition to directly managing state health agencies, the state government also contributes funding for local health programs.

14.1.3 Local Health Agencies

Most front-line public health services are provided locally. The United States has approximately 3,000 local public health agencies. Examples of the services local health agencies provide include the following:

▲ Food safety inspection.
▲ Sanitation services.
▲ Sewage disposal.
▲ Insect and pest control.
▲ Drinking water purification.
▲ Restaurant inspection and licensing.
▲ Communicable disease surveillance and immunization.
▲ Investigation and control of sexually transmitted diseases (STDs).
▲ Public health education.

Many regional health districts will be responsible for most of these community/public health services. Local agencies, in addition to their purely public health functions, also provide personal health services. In fact, approximately 40 million people annually receive some type of personal health care from local departments of public health. These services, such as those in the

Table 14-1: Sources of Funding for Local Public Health Agencies

Source	Percentage
Local government	44
State government	40
Federal government	3
Service reimbursement (billing insurance companies, Medicare and Medicaid for provision of covered personal health services)	19
Other	4

The distribution of local public health agencies are distributed across the United States accordingly.

following list, are typically for the poor and provided through city or county hospitals:

▲ Disease screening.
▲ Primary care.
▲ Mental health care.
▲ Maternal and child health.
▲ Family planning.
▲ Hospital care.

Local public health agencies spend about $13 billion per year. They receive their funds from the following:

Table 14-2: Distribution of Local Public Health Agencies

Jurisdiction	Percentage
County	60
Town or township	15
City	10
Multicounty	8
City county	7
Other	2

14.1.4 Private Initiatives in Public Health Policy

Private health care providers (such as hospitals, nursing homes, HMOs, physicians, and clinics) play a significant role in public health. As stated earlier, public health policies and initiatives involve multiple agencies and institutions. In addition to public contributors, public health policy also coordinates its efforts with private health care organizations. These organizations contribute to public health in the following ways:

▲ Engaging in surveillance and monitoring of diseases.

▲ Administering immunizations.

▲ Screening for communicable diseases.

▲ Offering patient education.

▲ Cooperating with state and local departments of public health by acquiring data.

▲ Coordinating the provision of private and public health services.

As well as working in conjunction with government agencies, some private organizations initiate and implement what would essentially be general health policies for their members. Many managed care organizations, for example, which are responsible for the care of a population of beneficiaries/members, often undertake large and sophisticated health promotion and disease prevention activities.

FOR EXAMPLE

Preparing for a Pandemic

The avian flu virus and the need to prepare for a potential pandemic represents a lesson in public health policy. The U.S. effort to forestall an epidemic here involves numerous agencies, all levels of government, and the private health sector. The federal government is formulating a plan that involves federal health agencies, the U.S. military, state and local health officials and policy makers, and private drug manufactures. The evolving federal blueprint involves state and local preparedness plans, involvement of the military to quarantine infected cities, ongoing research to develop a vaccine, work with drug manufacturers to develop a vaccine for the deadly strain and to increase production of current vaccines, and a study of how to most effectively use the limited number of immunizations already available.

SELF-CHECK

- Define **public health care** and distinguish it from **private health care.**
- Describe the role private initiatives play in public health.
- What federal department has the primary responsibility for public health and which agencies (list four) are associated with it?
- What health care services or providers are licensed by the states?
- Which level of government performs the bulk of front-line health policy and which services (give two) represent this role?

14.2 Federal and State Health Laws

Both the federal and state governments pass health care legislation. Although the purpose of these laws is to protect and promote the health of the U.S. population—and all health laws impact directly or indirectly, individual health—federal laws and state laws differ in important ways. Because preserving public health is a primary duty of the state, almost all specific health regulations and laws are state based. Federal health law, on the other hand, generally focuses on the activities of the U.S. Department of Health and Human Services (DHHS) and its constituent organizations, such as the FDA and the CDC.

14.2.1 Federal Statutes and Regulations

Title 21, also known as the "Federal Food, Drug, and Cosmetic Act," addresses, among other things, the labeling, sale, import/export, registering, and transportation of foods, drugs (particularly important in health care), and cosmetics. These acts were passed in order to protect the consumer and provide oversight. Before the formation of the FDA, consumers lived by the doctrine "let the buyer beware" which placed individuals at risk both financially and physically.

OSHA laws were enacted to, as the act states, "assure safe and healthful working conditions for working men and women." These laws are enforced by the Occupational Safety and Health Administration (OSHA) of the federal government. They govern various workplace practices, safety procedures, and training and ensure that employers provide a hazard-free work environment. They also govern how record-keeping pertaining to health and safety issues is to be conducted.

Some OSHA laws are particularly relevant to health care environments. Such laws particular are

▲ **The Hazard Communication Standard (HCS):** This standard involves ensuring that all hazardous chemicals are properly labeled, and that all employers and employees are informed of the risks associated with the use of those chemicals.

▲ **The Medical Waste Tracking Act:** This act was created in response to medical waste being washed ashore in New Jersey and Long Island. It involves a more structured approach to tracking medical waste and allocates funds to research regarding the effects of medical waste on health.

▲ **The Occupational Exposure to Bloodborne Pathogen Standard:** This set of regulations exists to protect those exposed to blood and other potentially infectious materials. These regulations involve protocols for handling and disposal of sharps, personal protection equipment, training, signs and labels, and so on.

These laws protect not only health care workers, but because of the uniqueness of the environment, they also protect patients as well.

The *Health Insurance Portability and Accountability Act (HIPAA)* is a large set of health care regulations and standards that basically deals with patient confidentiality and protection. Passed in 1996, HIPAA is broad in scope; covers a whole host of health care providers, facilities, and entities; and has had sweeping implications for the health care industry. Most people are familiar with HIPAA because, since the passage of the act, they have been required to sign forms (or something similar) pertaining to privacy of their medical records and information.

14.2.2 State Statutes and Regulations

States often pass laws and regulations to regulate health care within their state. Each state's laws address the health needs of its citizens as well as direct state policy on health care issues. As such, health care law differs significantly from state to state; a classic example of this is the difference in abortion laws from state to state. States vary dramatically on when, how, and what type of abortion

---

FOR EXAMPLE

Stem-Cell Research and Federal Regulations

Stem cells are embryonic cells that can be coaxed into developing into just about any type of cell found in the human body. With a little scientific nudge, a single stem cell can become a blood cell, a heart cell, a brain cell, or any other type of cell. The medical implications—that these cells can be used to treat or prevent disease—are astounding. The federal government has placed restrictions on stem-cell research funding. The regulation prohibits federal funding for research on human embryonic cells created after August 2001 and has effectively slowed stem-cell research in facilities that receive federal funding.

a woman can have. With recent Supreme Court appointments, states are grappling again with this explosive issue.

SELF-CHECK

- Define **federal health law** and distinguish it from state health law.
- Define **Title 21.**
- What main issue does HIPAA deal with?

14.3 Assessing U.S. Health Policy

The U.S. health system is vast, including various organizations, all levels of government, and numerous professionals and other health care providers. A **health policy** is an articulated health mission supported by laws and regulations and coordinated across all providers. Health policy requires enormous expenditures and is funded by various sources, and it addresses the health needs of communities and individuals alike.

U.S. health policy is, at best, a fragmented system of decisions on health care issues made by the legislative, judicial, and executive branches of the government. These decisions or principles are meant to serve a particular interest; however, they can, and usually do, serve specific stakeholders' interests as well. Stakeholders may be private or public entities and may or may not have the general public interests in mind. Because of these interests, the United States finds itself with a very loose and diverse set of policies concerning health care. Although there are politically stated national health care policies, one national umbrella, cohesive, and binding health care policy does not truly exist. In fact, it is argued that for the United States to have one cohesive health care policy would mean fundamental changes in the system of politics, stakeholder interest, and health care infrastructures.

Although the U.S. health care system lacks a coherent national health strategy, it is not entirely piecemeal. Health care policy in the United States is a product of a back-and-forth relationship between the health initiatives of different sectors: A legislative, public, or private entity sets forth a law or a principle. This law or principle fans out in many ways and generates a variety of health care responses and consequences—some intended, some unintended. These in turn spur other responses by other sectors, which themselves spur other responses, and so on and so forth. In this way, U.S. health policy is molded and further refined.

Consider, for example, the period during World War II when there was a national freeze on wages and a shortage of skilled employees. Employers, trying

---

FOR EXAMPLE

Combining Health and Foreign Policy

A 2001 report titled "Why Health Is Important to U.S. Foreign Policy," sponsored by the Council on Foreign Relations and the Milbank Memorial Fund, recommends that the United States add health policy to its foreign policy objectives. The report claims that addressing health issues in developing countries and countries in transition to democracy is not only the right thing to do, but also offers significant economic and social advantages—as well as national security benefits—to this country.

---

to attract applicants despite the wage freeze, decided to offer an alternative perk: employer-subsidized health insurance. Other businesses, completing for the same employees, did the same. Eventually, the employer-provided insurance plans became the norm. With so many people eventually covered by employer-sponsored plans (with no discernable negative impact of the financial health of businesses), this situation enabled the state and federal government to avoid addressing the universal provision of health care. As a result, the U.S. health care system of today is, in large part, dependent upon employer-sponsored health insurance, even though no national policy was set forth mandating that businesses provide health insurance. (Interestingly, as today's businesses struggle under the burden of rising health care costs, they may once again spur a fundamental change in the way insurance plans are subsidized.) Many changes in the way businesses handle health insurance can already be observed. Some individuals turn to state-funded health insurance programs in order to receive minimal health care services. Many businesses also restructure their staffing in order to limit the amount of employees receiving health insurance.

Medicare and Medicaid are two more examples of this dynamic. These programs came directly out of legislation and have affected health care policy in this country for over 30 years. The laws themselves directly spurred a whole host of implications, which in turn helped shape future policy on health care.

SELF-CHECK

- Define the term **health policy**.
- Identify U.S. health policy objectives.

14.4 Comparing U.S. Health Care to Health Care in Other Countries

The purpose of all health policy is to foster the health and well-being of the community. Assessing whether the policy is successful essentially comes down to whether or not the population as a whole is healthy, whether the health system functions effectively, and whether patients receive the type of care they need. In other words, health policy determines, to a large extent, how effective the **health system**—the infrastructure and all health care components that provide health services to a population—is in maximizing the health of its citizens.

14.4.1 Health Indicators

Health indicators, such as infant mortality rate, average life expectancy, number of people with chronic health conditions, and so on, are used to evaluate the health of a population. By studying these indicators, health officials can draw a picture of the overall health status of a community.

To evaluate the effectiveness of U.S. health policy, researchers have conducted surveys comparing the U.S. population to populations in other developed countries. These surveys indicate the following:

- ▲ **Cost:** The United States is the most expensive health care system in the world. Over 13 percent of the U.S. GDP goes toward health care.
- ▲ **Access:** This nation's health care system is one of only two developed countries that does not provide health care for all of its citizens.
- ▲ **Responsiveness:** The United States ranks number one in being responsive to patient needs and concerns.
- ▲ **Infant mortality:** The United States ranks in the middle of developed countries in terms of infant mortality rate.
- ▲ **Fairness of financing:** This country ranks as the lowest in terms of fairness of health care financing.

14.4.2 Characteristics of the Health System

Health systems are complex entities, and each country has its own health system. To classify a health system for comparison purposes, researchers look at a number of factors.

- ▲ **Degree of primary care regulation:** Regulated primary care implies that national policies influence the location of physician practice so that they are distributed throughout the population rather than concentrated in certain geographic areas. (Note: Public health centers are also assumed to represent the equitable distribution of physician resources.) Regulated primary care or public health centers are considered to be the highest commitment to primary care.

▲ **Type of financial access to health care:** A health system can be financed through national health insurance sponsored by government, national health insurance sponsored by nongovernmental agencies, or no national health insurance. Universal government-sponsored national health insurance or a national health entitlement is considered most conducive to access to primary care services. The absence of national health insurance is considered least conducive to access to primary care.

▲ **Whether the health system relies on generalists or specialists to provide primary care: Generalists** (family or general practitioners) are the ideal **primary care physicians (PCPs)** because their training is devoted exclusively to primary care practice. General pediatricians and general internists are considered intermediate primary care practitioners because their training has a major subspecialty focus (based on age). Other specialists are not considered PCPs because their training is focused on subspecialty issues.

14.4.3 Primary Care or Specialty Care Based System

The following factors indicate what type of practice—primary care or specialty care—is the foundation of a country's health system:

▲ **Extent to which the PCP acts as the point of entry into the system:** First contact implies that decisions about the need for specialty services are made after consulting the PCP. Requirements for access to specialists via referral from primary care are considered most consistent with the first-contact aspect of primary care. The ability of patients to self-refer to specialists is considered conducive to a specialty-oriented health system.

▲ **Extent to which the physician provides continuous care over time:** Continuity of care refers to the extent of the relationship between a patient and a practitioner or facility over time, regardless of the presence of specific types of health problems. An example of continuity of care would be when a patient enrolls with a physician as a primary care provider, with the expectation that that physician will provide all care that does not require a referral to a specialist.

▲ **Comprehensiveness of the care provided:** Comprehensiveness of care refers to the extent to which a full range of services is either directly provided by the PCP or specifically arranged for elsewhere.

▲ **Extent of coordination of services by the PCP:** Care is considered coordinated where there are formal guidelines for the transfer of information between PCPs and specialists.

Based on these factors, the U.S. health care system is a specialist-oriented system: No national policy exists regulating where physicians practice; a result is **health profession shortage areas (HPSAs)**, areas where there are too few physicians (see Chapter 3). The United States also has no universal health insurance plan, and no standard method of payment (see Chapter 4). Instead, U.S. health care is paid for through a combination of public monies (Medicare or Medicaid, for example), private insurance (employer-provided insurance or privately purchased insurance), and personal funds (out-of-pocket expenses). Finally, the U.S. health system is a specialist-oriented system. Many Americans receive primary care from specialists, and specialists outnumber generalists and dominate the medical field in terms of prestige and earnings.

SELF-CHECK

- Define the term **health system.**
- Compare the performance of the U.S. health system with the health systems of other countries in terms of these health indicators: (a) cost, (b) access, and (c) fairness of financing.
- To classify a health system for comparison purposes, researchers often look at three factors: (a) regulation of primary care, (b) type of financial access to health care, and (c) generalist or specialist based care. Identify the U.S. health system in relation to other countries' systems.

SUMMARY

Becoming familiar with U.S. health policy and its components is key to understanding the U.S. health care system. Formulating and implementing health care policy in this country requires complex coordination among all levels of government. Important health care legislation also has an impact. Despite governmental functions and the various laws affecting health care, critical policy issues still remain. Recognizing how this nation's health care system differs from health systems around the world offers a starting point for examining the overall effectiveness of U.S. health policy.

KEY TERMS

Centers for Disease Control and Prevention (CDC)	The nation's primary public health agency, under the auspices of the DHHS
Control	Health agencies' ability to manage incidences.
Department of Health and Human Services (DHHS)	Cabinet-level department responsible for public health through its various agencies
Distribution	The scope or spread of a disease or incidences.
Epidemiology	The field of study relating to the incidence, distribution, and control of a disease.
Generalists	Physicians whose training is not oriented in a specific medical specialty but instead covers a variety of medical problems; generalists are the key physicians in primary care systems
Health indicators	Indicators, such as infant mortality rate, average life expectancy, number of people with chronic health conditions, and so on, that researchers use to develop a comprehensive view of the overall health status of a community.
Health policy	An articulated health mission supported by law and regulations and coordinated across all health care providers.
Health profession shortage areas (HPSAs)	Areas recognized by the federal government as having too few physicians to meet the health care needs of the population. The bulk of HPSAs are in rural and inner city areas
Health system	The infrastructure and all health care components that provide health services to a population.
Incidence	The number of times a health issue occurs.
Private health care	Health care dealing with the provision of health services to individuals.
Primary care physician (PCP)	Physician who acts as the point of entry into the health care system, provides general medical care, and provides referrals for and coordinates specialty care
Public health care	Health care dealing with preventing disease and promoting health in populations.
Vital statistics	Statistics related to births, deaths, marriages, health, disease, and so on for a population.

ASSESS YOUR UNDERSTANDING

Go to www.wiley.com/college/pointer to evaluate your knowledge of public health policy.
Measure your learning by comparing pre-test and post-test results.

Summary Questions

1. Public health services focus on preventing disease and promoting health in populations. True or False?
2. Federal, state, and local governments are responsible for public health because private organizations lack the resources and infrastructure to perform functions associated with public health. True or False?
3. Which of the following is *not* one of the three core functions performed by public health agencies?
   (a) assessment
   (b) policy development
   (c) assurance
   (d) absorption
4. Identify the cabinet-level department responsible for most federal health initiatives.
5. Which agencies provide the majority of front-line public health services: federal agencies, state agencies, or local agencies?
6. Federal and state laws prohibit the participation of private health care agencies to perform public health functions. True or False?
7. Federal health law generally focuses on
   (a) specific regulations regarding delivery of health care to individuals.
   (b) the activities of the U.S. DHHS.
   (c) delivery of health care to veterans and members of the Armed Services.
   (d) embryonic stem-cell research.
8. The primary concern of OSHA laws is workplace safety. True or False?
9. States, in order to meet the requirements of federal regulations, often have the same health laws and regulations. True or False?
10. Which of the following are *true* about health policy in the United States?
   (a) it involves federal, state, and local governmental agencies
   (b) it includes health initiatives created and implemented by private health care agencies
   (c) it requires enormous expenditures and is funded by various sources

(d) a and c

(e) all of the above

11. The United States has no national health policy; all health policies are determined at the state level. True or False?

12. Who makes health policy in the United States?

(a) Congress

(b) state legislatures

(c) federal and state judiciary

(d) all of the above

13. Although this nation spends more on health care than any other industrialized country, it also has the highest ranking for all health indicators, including quality of care and infant mortality. True or False?

14. In the United States, how regulated is primary care?

(a) very regulated; health policy stipulates the number of primary care providers and their distribution throughout the country

(b) somewhat regulated; although the United States doesn't regulate distribution of primary care providers, it does mandate a certain primary-care-to-specialty-care ratio in communities

(c) not regulated; U.S. health care policy does not manage the number or distribution of PCPs, instead letting physician preference and the health market be the deciding factors

15. How is the U.S. health system financed?

(a) through national health insurance sponsored by the government

(b) through national health insurance sponsored by nongovernmental agencies

(c) through public and private funds

(d) a combination of b and c

16. The primary physician in the U.S. health system is the

(a) specialist.

(b) generalist.

(c) PCP.

(d) all of the above.

Review Questions

1. Public health focuses on promoting health and preventing disease in populations. Explain how government and private health organizations together address public health issues.

2. Federal, state, and local governments all have a role in public health. Which public health functions do the three levels of government share?

3. All states have state health departments. Which of the following is *not* a function of state health departments?

   (a) collecting vital statistics

   (b) observing and managing communicable diseases

   (c) inspecting food

   (d) providing laboratory services

4. Both state and federal governments pass laws regarding public health. How do federal health laws differ from state health laws?

5. Who is responsible for enforcing the provisions outlined in OSHA?

6. Name a function of Title 21.

7. Which sector is responsible for initiating health policy in the United States?

8. Researchers look at a variety of criteria to classify a health system. Which criteria would accurately describe the current U.S. health system?

Applying This Chapter

1. Identify whether the following are functions of the federal, state, or local government:

   (a) health policy formulation

   (b) professional staff licensing

   (c) insect and pest control

   (d) food and drug regulation

   (e) immunization

2. You've been asked to delegate the public health initiatives to the appropriate team. Each team is responsible for performing one of the three core public health functions—assessment, policy development, and assurance. Indicate, for each of the following, which team you'll assign the project to: Assessment team, Policy Development team, or Assurance team.

   (a) studying the effect of a recently passed health initiative

   (b) creating a commission to study the health needs of a growing immigrant community

   (c) encouraging involvement of private health organizations in public health endeavors

   (d) putting together a flow chart outlining first-responder responsibilities in the event of a natural disaster

   (e) passing laws regarding childhood immunizations and school enrollment

3. For each of the following, indicate the relevant federal law (Title 21, OSHA, or HIPAA):

   (a) the ability of one health care provider to fax medical records to another health care provider

   (b) the importing of prescription drugs from Canada

   (c) the safety features installed in a steel refinery

   (d) the transportation of oranges from Florida to the Midwest

4. Identify whether each of the following is a component of a health system or health policy:

   (a) a local health care organization providing immunizations to local school children

   (b) a state law requiring immunization of all children before entering elementary school

   (c) the goal of the DHHS to reduce the number of babies born with fetal alcohol syndrome

   (d) medical researchers at a private facility studying the effects of alcohol on unborn children

   (e) eliminating polio in the U.S. population

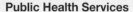
Public Health Services

Imagine that you've been charged with improving access to health care for all Americans. Although several factors make accessing medical care in the United States difficult, you decide to address proximity to medical care. Describe four health policy initiatives you would introduce to address this problem.

Federal and State Health Laws

As a health advocate for migrant workers, what federal health laws would you rely on in addressing the concerns of your clients? Explain.

Assessing U.S. Health Policy

Some American corporations are trying to offset health care costs by shifting more of the burden of the costs to their employees. Their strategy is to modify company-sponsored insurance plans that that have higher deductibles, requiring greater out-of-pocket contributions. At the same time, some politicians are advocating tax deferment for health savings accounts. Describe how this scenario potentially illustrates the evolution of national health policy in the United States.

Comparing U.S. Health Care to Health Care in Other Countries

Health policy and health systems are closely related. Explain that relationship and discuss what elements of the U.S. health system make achieving health policy goals more difficult.

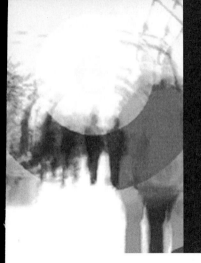

ENDNOTES

Chapter 1

1. Institute of Medicine, *To Err Is Human: Building a Safer Health System* (Washington, DC: National Academy of Sciences, 2000).
2. Smith, C., Cowan, C., Heffler, S., Catlin, A. et al., "National Health Spending in 2004: Recent Slowdown Led by Prescription Drug Spending," *Health Affairs* 25, no. 1 (January/February 2006):186–96.

Chapter 2

1. American Hospital Association, *Taking the Pulse: The State of America's Hospitals,* http://www.aha.org/aha/resource_center/statistics/statistics/html.
2. Magee, M., *Health Politics: Power, Populism and Health* (Bronxville, NY: Spencer, 2005).
3. Tyler, L., and Biggs, E., *Practical Governance* (Chicago: Health Administration Press, 2001).
4. Zuckerman, A. M., *Health Strategic Planning: Approaches for the 21st Century* (Chicago: Health Administration Press, 1998).

Chapter 3

1. Medicare Payment Advisory Commission (MedPAC), *Report to the Congress: Medicare Payment Policy* (Washington, DC: Author, March 2006), 15.
2. Kindig, D. A., and Movassaghi, H., "The Adequacy of Physician Supply in Small Rural Counties," *Health Affairs* 81 (1989):61–76.
3. Kindig, D. A., Movassaghi, H., Cross-Dunham, N., Zwick, D. I. et al., "Trends in Physician Availability in Ten Urban Areas from 1963 to 1980," *Inquiry* 24 (1987):136–46.

4. Grumbach, K., and Bodenheimer, T., "Reconstructing Primary Care for the Twenty-First Century," in *General Medicine and the US Health System,* ed. S. L. Isaacs and J. R. Knickman (San Francisco: Jossey-Bass, 2003).

5. MedPAC, "Report to the Congress," 15.

6. Grumbach and Bodenheimer, "Reconstructing Primary Care."

7. Starfield, B., "Primary Care: Is It Essential?" *Lancet* 344 (1994):1129–33.

8. Grumbach and Bodenheimer, "Reconstructing Primary Care."

9. Kaiser Family Foundation, *National Survey of Consumer Experiences with Health Plans* (Menlo Park, CA: Author, 2000).

10. Braddock, C. H., "Informed Decision Making in Outpatient Practice," *JAMA* 282 (1999): 2313–20.

11. MedPAC, "Report to the Congress," 6.

Chapter 4

1. MedPAC, "Report to the Congress," 13.

2. Ibid.

3. Smith, C. et al., "National Health Spending," 186–96.

4. MedPAC, "Report to the Congress," 13.

5. Rossiter, L., *Understanding Medical Managed Care* (Chicago: Health Administration Press, 2001).

6. Ibid., 345.

7. Ibid., 344.

8. MedPAC, "Report to the Congress."

9. The Heritage Foundation, *Medicare Trustees Report,* March 2004.

10. Kovner, A. R., and Knickman, J. R., *Jonas and Kovner's Health Care Delivery System,* 8th ed. (New York: Springer, 2005).

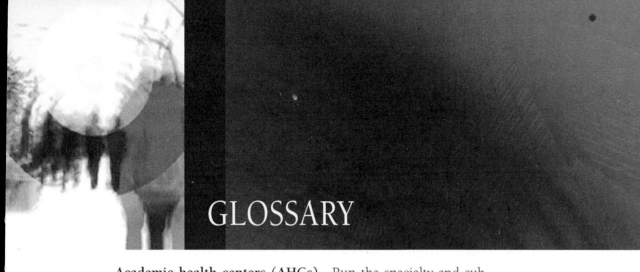

GLOSSARY

Academic health centers (AHCs) Run the specialty and sub-specialty training programs that create the practitioners of the most advanced medical care in the world; vary in their organization and structure, but all centers include a medical school, at least one other health professional school or program, and one or more owned or affiliated teaching hospitals.

Accessibility How easily a patient can obtain and make use of medical care from his or her physician, and how timely such access is.

Activities of daily living (ADLs) Fundamental activities of daily care that health care professionals use as a way to describe the functional status of a person. Examples of ADLs include bathing, continence, dressing, eating, getting in and out of bed, and so on.

Acute care Care given for health conditions that happen suddenly and last for a finite period of time.

Administrative personnel Administrative support staff and managers responsible for overseeing and managing the operation of a health care facility.

Allopathic physicians A medical designation for physicians who graduate from allopathic schools of medicine and focus on treating disease. Known as MDs.

Alzheimer's/dementia facilities Independent units or a component of an assisted living facility or nursing home; these units care for people who cannot communicate normally or take care of themselves and provide constant supervision and help with activities of daily living and personalized care

Ambulatory care   Medical services provided to patients on an out-patient basis (that is, services that don't require an overnight stay in a hospital).

Arthroscope   A specific type of endoscope that is inserted into a joint through a tiny incision to examine, record, and treat.

Arthroscopic surgery   Type of surgery in which a small scope is inserted into a tiny incision to examine and repair an area.

Assisted living facilities   Long-term-care facilities for people who don't need skilled medical care but do need help with certain activities of daily living, or some degree of supervision.

Audit committee   Standing committee responsible for ensuring that all necessary audits are conducted and reported to the board of directors.

Beneficiaries   Individuals receiving health care services.

Benefit triggers   Criteria for needing long-term care that must be met to generate payment of insurance benefits.

Biomedical model   The medical model that views disease as nothing more than a deviation from the norm and that all disease as well as any strange behavioral phenomena must be explained in terms of physicochemical principles; that is, the body is either physically abnormal or chemically imbalanced.

Biopsychosocial model   The medical model that, when dealing with health care, takes into account all aspects of a person's life—social, psychological, and behavioral—that impact health and well-being.

BlueCross BlueShield   Commonly called *Blues*, health insurance plans that are closely tied to the hospital industry and medical profession.

Board   The entity responsible for governing the hospital on behalf of its "owners"—the community in a nonprofit hospital, shareholders in a proprietary hospital, or constituents in a governmental hospital.

Board composition   The characteristics, knowledge, skills, perspectives, and experience of board members.

Board infrastructure   The resources and systems that support the performance of the board's work.

Board of directors   A group of people who oversee the affairs of a corporation.

Board structure   How the board is divided and coordinates the governance work within the organization, specifically relating to board size, the number and type of committees, and the number of boards and their relationships.

Board-certified   A physician who has passed the medical board specialty exam.

Board-eligible   To complete the course of specialty study but has not taken or passed the medical board specialty exam.

Business stage   Evolutionary stage of hospital development in which hospitals became more business oriented to provide physicians what they required to practice.

Centers for Disease Control and Prevention (CDC)   The nation's primary public health agency, under the auspices of the DHHS.

Chief executive officer (CEO)   The management executive responsible for the day-to-day operation of the facility or health system, who formulates strategies that support the goals outlined in an organization's mission statement.

Chiropractors   Medical professionals who diagnose and treat problems of the nervous, muscle, and skeletal systems, especially the spine, by adjusting and manipulating the musculoskeletal system.

Chronic care model   Health care model that uses evidence-based research to proactively address health concerns of people with chronic illnesses, such as diabetes and asthma.

Chronic care   Care given for conditions that are long lasting or never changing.

Clinical education   The last two years of medical training that takes place in patient care settings (hospitals and ambulatory care facilities) under the supervision of physician faculty members. During this phase of their education, future doctors learn to diagnose and treat patients and perform medical procedures.

Clinical nurse specialist   Registered nurse who, after receiving additional training and certification, is able to diagnose and treat health problems.

Closed arrangement   A type of network in which only physicians who are employees of, or have contracted with, the health plan are medical staff members.

Combined HMO model   HMO model that includes both independent physicians (the IPA model), as well as physicians or groups employed by the HMO or under exclusive contract to it (group model).

Commercial plan   Commercial health insurance plans can be either nonprofit or for-profit; some are owned by their policy holders; others are stock corporations.

Commitment laws   Laws that enable family members, law enforcement, or health care professionals to commit a person to a care facility or to a treatment plan.

Community health center   Health care organization that provides health care services to poor and uninsured individuals.

Community-based health care   Care sponsored by the community, which are usually free or at low cost for qualifying individuals.

Compensation committee   Standing committee that looks at performance issues in regard to salary, benefits, and bonuses.

Comprehensiveness of care   The breadth and depth of care that primary physicians provide directly to their patients (beyond the coordinating and referral function).

Congregate care facilities   Self-sufficient communities designed for retirees, which provide all levels of personal service *except* for health care services.

Continuing care retirement communities (CCRCs)   Self-sufficient communities designed for retirees, which provide all levels of personal and medical services, from the least to the most intensive.

Continuity of care   The systematic ability to have relevant information about previous episodes of care move with the patient among providers.

Control   Health agencies' ability to manage incidences.

Copayment   Amount (generally a flat fee) members must pay at the time of service.

Dentists   Medical professionals who prevent, diagnose, and treat diseases of the mouth, teeth, gums, and associated structures.

Department of Health and Human Services (DHHS)   Cabinet-level department responsible for public health through its various agencies.

Disease agent   A pathogen, or, an agent that causes disease, especially a living microorganism such as a bacterium, virus, or fungus.

Distribution   The scope or spread of a disease or incidences.

Duty to treat   Principle of the U.S. health system that any human being deserves basic care.

Economies of scale   The strategy of spreading overhead costs across an organization.

Emergency Medical Transfer and Active Labor Act (EMTALA)   A federal law requiring that all health care facilities treat or transfer with a legitimate medical emergency.

Emergency room   Health care organization designed and staffed to provide initial treatment for a broad range of illnesses and injuries, some of which may be life-threatening.

Enablers   Organizations that support and facilitate the provision of health services, such as trade and professional organizations and public interest groups.

Epidemiology   The field of study relating to the incidence, distribution, and control of a disease.

Evidence-based medicine   A medical movement that bases care decisions for individual patients on evidence from clinical studies.

Executive committee   Standing committee consisting of senior-level board members, which conducts the business of the board.

Federal hospitals   Hospitals operated by the federal government and paid for in part by tax dollars.

Finance committee   Standing committee that deals with budgeting guidelines and performance, long-range financial planning, and debt structure. Standing committee members typically include the treasurer, CFO (chief financial officer), and others.

Fluoroscope   A real-time imaging system used to see and record what is happening inside a patient utilizing X-rays, fluorescnet screens, and CCD cameras.

Gatekeeper   Primary care physician in managed care plans who provides general care to plan members and referrals to see specialists or to access other health care services.

General counsel   The chief attorney for a health care organization.

General hospitals   Hospitals that offer an array of medical and surgical services.

General practitioners   Doctors who focus their practice on primary care of individuals and families.

Generalists   Physicians whose training is not oriented in a specific medical specialty but instead covers a variety of medical problems; generalists are the key physicians in primary care systems.

Governing board   The entity charged with overseeing the affairs of a corporation.

Government agencies   Any state, local, or federal agencies.

Graduate medical education   Specialty training that includes some academic instruction, but mostly caring for patients under the supervision of experienced physician specialists.

Gross domestic product (GDP)   The total value of goods and services produced in the U.S.

Gross Goods   Medications and medical supplies.

Group model HMO   An HMO model in which the managed care organization contracts with organized groups of physicians, who either care for plan beneficiaries exclusively or do so in addition to other patients.

Group practices   Physician practices in which three or more physicians, often complemented by other health care professionals, share resources, pool expenses and income, and collaborate in the care of patients.

Health Care Quality Improvement Act (HCQIA) of 1986   Act established primarily to protect individuals and hospitals conducting medical peer review against legal action by physicians whose practice privileges were revoked.

Health indicators   Indicators, such as infant mortality rate, average life expectancy, number of people with chronic health conditions, and so on, that researchers use to develop a comprehensive view of the overall health status of a community.

Health maintenance organizations (HMOs)   Managed care plans that combine the insurance function (underwriting) with delivery of health services through an owned or contracted network of providers.

Health plans   The organizations that collect premiums, reimburse providers, and perform other administrative functions.

Health policy   An articulated health mission supported by law and regulations and coordinated across all health care providers.

Health profession shortage areas (HPSAs)   Areas recognized by the federal government as having too few physicians to meet the health care needs of the population. The bulk of HPSAs are in rural and inner city areas.

Health system   The infrastructure and all health care components that provide health services to a population.

Home health care   Supportive and curative care provided to patients in their homes.

Horizontal systems   Combine functionally similar organizations; can be composed of similar organizations in a particular market or those spread across a number of markets.

Hospice care   Solely devoted to providing physical care and counseling to terminally ill patients and their families.

Hospitalist   A hospital-based general physician who takes over the care of hospitalized patients in the place of their primary care physician.

Illegal immigrants   Immigrants who enter the United States without following procedures outlined by the Bureau of U.S. Citizenship and Immigration Services; also referred to as undocumented immigrants.

Immigrants   People who come to the United States with the intention of establishing permanent residency.

Incidence   The number of times a health issue occurs.

Indemnity plan   An insurance plan in which the beneficiary pays a premium to the health plan, which in turn reimburses the beneficiary when the individual uses covered service. The beneficiary then pays the provider.

Indemnity plans   Traditional fee-for-service insurance plans in which patients are reimbursed for medical expenses they incur after having met a specified deductible.

Independent practice association (IPA) model HMO   An HMO model in which the managed care organization contracts with individual physicians, who remain independent and care for plan members, as well as other patients.

Independent practice association HMO (IPA HMO) model   HMO model in which services are provided by medical groups and physicians who are independently contracted.

Individual providers   The professionals who offer private health care services such as physicians, dentists, chiropractors, and nurses.

Institutional providers   Include organizations that provide private health care services, such as physician's offices, medical groups, hospitals and nursing homes.

Insurance   Strictly speaking, protection against the risk of financial loss associated with an event among members of a group and is provided (underwritten) only when the potential loss is large (catastrophic) and beyond the ability of a group member to pay in the short run. In reality, health insurance plans in the United States are more akin to prepayment plans.

Involuntary commitment   A patient is committed against his or her wishes.

Legal immigrants   Immigrants who enter the United States after following the procedures outlined by the Bureau of U.S. Citizenship and Immigration Services.

licensed practical nurses (LPNs)   Provide basic, nonprofessional nursing care, such as observe patients, take vital signs, and keep records.

Long-term hospitals   Hospitals that treat individuals with chronic conditions requiring stays that can range from a month to several years; examples are psychiatric, chronic disease, and rehabilitation facilities.

Managed care model   Model in which health organizations manage care and cost by funneling all medical necessities through a primary care provider.

Managed care plans   The plan member still has access to health services, but to receive full plan benefits must relinquish some control regarding when to seek medical care, what type of medical care to seek, and which health care provider to use.

Managed care   A special type of service benefit plan that combines health insurance and provider functions.

Medicaid   A federal/state program that provides health care services to poor people. Although federally sponsored, Medicare is administered by the state.

Medical social services   Services provided by licensed social workers, who intervene on the patient's behalf.

Medicare Part A   A compulsory health plan that covers hospital-based services.

Medicare Part B   A voluntary, supplemental health plan that covers professional (primarily physician) services.

Medicare   A federally sponsored program that provides health insurance to eligible Americans who are elderly or disabled.

Mental disease   Term for an array of psychological, biological, chemical, neurological, and behavioral disorders that impair cognitive, affective, and social functioning.

Mission statement   The statement of purpose for an organization. It generally provides the context under which all decisions are made and the standard against which all strategies and outcomes are evaluated.

National Health Service Corps (NHSC)   A federal program administered by the Department of Health and Human Services, which recruits physicians to practice in underserved areas.

National Health Service Corps and Loan Repayment Program   Federal program providing scholarships to medical students and loan repayment to recent residency graduates in exchange for medical service in HPSAs.

National Institutes of Health (NIH)   Part of the U.S. Department of Health and Human Services. Conducts and supports medical research and is composed of twenty seven institutes and centers.

Nominating committee   Standing committee responsible for nominating new board members and officers.

Nonprofit hospitals   Hospitals that are organized as 501(c)(3) tax-exempt corporations. They are "owned" by the community in which they operate, or by other charitable organizations such as religious congregations, fraternal organizations, and associations.

Nurse anesthetist   Registered nurse who, after extensive training and national certification, provides services similar to those provided by anesthesiologists.

Nurse midwife   Registered nurse who, after additional training and certification, oversees pregnancies and births and, in some cases, deals with other gynecological issues.

Nurse practitioner   Registered nurse who, after additional training and certification, is licensed to perform physical exams and other medical services, including writing prescriptions, usually under a physician's supervision.

Nursing homes   Long-term-care facilities that provide a mix of intermediate-level nursing and personal services on a 24-hour basis to people who are either temporarily or permanently unable to care for themselves and require attention by a licensed nurse.

Open arrangement   A type of network in which independent physicians are admitted to the hospital's medical staff.

Optometrists   Medical professionals who diagnose and treat vision problems and some diseases of the eye.

Osteopathic physicians   Physicians who graduate from an osteopathic medical school and place greater emphasis on the neuromusculoskeletal system, preventive medicine, and holistic care. Known as DOs.

Palliative care   Care that eases the symptoms or discomfort of the condition but doesn't cure it.

Parent board   In a health system, the one centralized (or corporate) board comprised of representatives of the smaller boards. The parent board is responsible for ensuring that the health system's centralized mission, values, and philosophy are maintained and perpetuated across the various subsidiary institutions.

Personal care facilities   Facilities for people who can no longer perform the functions of daily living without help.

Personal care homes   Smaller, less institutional assisted living facilities.

Pharmacists   Medical professionals who provide consultation to, and dispense drugs ordered by, physicians and other practitioners, as well as counsel patients about the medications they've been prescribed and their appropriate use.

Physical therapists   Medical professionals who focus on the musculoskeletal system and provide services that restore functioning, improve mobility, and prevent or limit disabilities.

Physician assistants (PAs)   Non-physician medical professionals who provide a broad range of diagnostic and therapeutic services, and in all but a few states, prescribe medications. They work under the supervision of a physician.

Physician workshop stage   Evolutionary stage of hospital development in which hospitals sought better and more effective diagnostic tools and treatment strategies.

Planning or strategy committee   Standing committee responsible for long-range institutional planning and organizational strategic planning.

Podiatrists   Medical professionals who diagnose and treat diseases and injuries of the foot and lower leg, in addition to providing preventive care.

Point-of-service (POS) plan   A managed care plan that combines the characteristics of HMOs and PPOs. A POS plan offers both HMO and PPO services, and members choose which option they use at the time they seek health care.

Population-based medicine   A concept that requires PCPs to be concerned with every patient on their panel, not only those who actively seek health care.

Preclinical education   Also called academic education, the period during the first two years in medical school when students study basic sciences that are fundamental to medical practice (anatomy, physiology, biochemistry, pathology, microbiology, pharmacology) and learn how to take patient histories and conduct basic physical examinations.

Preferred provider organization (PPO)   A managed care plan that includes a provider network but doesn't use primary care physicians as gatekeepers.

Primary care   General preventive and curative care that is provided to a person over an extended period of time, including coordination of all primary, secondary, and tertiary care that the patient receives.

Primary care physician (PCP)   Physician who acts as the point of entry into the health care system, provides general medical care, and provides referrals for and coordinates specialty care.

Primary care team   A team approach to primary care in which division of labor is shared among a group of primary caregivers.

Private HCOs   Provide services that are consumed by, and affect, individuals. The goal of these organizations is to protect and enhance the health and well-being of individuals.

Private health care   Health care dealing with the provision of health services to individuals.

Professional and related occupations   Health care providers (such as physicians, nurses, pharmacists, and other direct caregivers) who work directly with the patients.

Proprietary health organizations   Private organizations that operate for a profit.

Proprietary hospitals   Hospitals operated for the purpose of producing a return for their investors.

Provider networks   Network of care providers, including physicians, hospitals, and so on, that have a contractual agreement with the managed care plan to provide services for a negotiated rate.

Providers   The health care organizations and individual professionals who deliver health care services.

Public HCOs   Provide services that targeted the health and well-being of populations or communities.

Public health agencies   Government agencies that promote health and prevent disease in populations, such as the Centers for Disease Control and Prevention.

Public health care   Health care dealing with preventing disease and promoting health in populations.

Purchasers   The primary payers (typically employers and federal, state, and local governments).

Quality credentialing committee   Standing committee that deals with ensuring that privileges, credentials, licensures, and certifications are appropriate, up-to-date, and in compliance.

Quality/performance/process improvement committee   This committee has ongoing responsibility in reviewing quality initiatives and performance regarding patient care, safety, and service delivery.

Refuge stage   Evolutionary stage of hospital development characterized by institution building.

Registered nurse (RN)   A graduate trained nurse who has been licensed by a state authority (as a board of nursing examiners) after successfully passing examinations for registration.

Regulators   Government agencies and private organizations that regulate health care institutions and professionals, such as state licensing boards, state insurance agencies, and federal agencies.

Rehabilitation centers   Facilities that help patients recover and/or manage specific conditions, addictions, or impairments. Also known as *rehab centers*.

Residency   A period of advanced medical training and education that normally follows graduation from medical school and completion of an internship. Residency programs include supervised practice of a specialty in a hospital and in its outpatient department, as well as instruction from specialists on the hospital staff.

Sarbanes-Oxley Act   Act, passed in 2002, intended to protect investors by improving the accuracy and reliability of financial statements and by establishing harsher penalties for those who violate the law.

Scientific method   A process of scientific testing that relies on the following five steps: observation, inquiry, hypothesis, experimentation, and theory.

Secondary care   Care that is typically provided in a hospital by medical specialists who generally don't have first contact with patients.

Self-funded plans   Insurance plans in which employers provide health care benefits without purchasing insurance from or paying premiums to a health plan.

Service benefit plan   An insurance plan in which a purchaser (employer) contracts with a health plan and pays it a premium for each beneficiary (employee and family members); beneficiaries, in turn, usually make contributions that cover a portion of the premium.

Service workers   Medical support staff (such as patient assistants, attendants, and aides; food preparation, maintenance, and housekeeping) who offer support services to the health care providers and maintain the facilities in which the providers work.

Services   Intangibles that are produced and used simultaneously.

Short-term hospitals   Hospitals that treat individuals with acute problems requiring inpatient stays that average about five days.

Solo practices   Physician practices consisting of an individual physician, generally assisted by several clinical and administrative personnel.

Specialist   A physician who completes a residency program (a period of advanced knowledge and supervised experience in a particular medical field) and passes a medical specialty exam, which qualifies him or her to specialize in a particular medical field.

Specialty care model   A health care model in which patients are not required to consult with a primary care provider before seeking general or specialty care; nor do patients have to have their care coordinated through a PCP.

Specialty hospitals   Hospitals that treat a narrow range of patients—children, women, or those with a specific condition such as cancer or orthopedic problems.

Sponsors   Family members or others who will cosign for any health care cost an immigrant incurs.

Staff model HMO   An HMO model in which the managed care organization hires physicians as employees.

Standing committees   Often permanent (but sometimes temporary) committees that address specific areas of needs.

State or local hospitals   Hospitals that are run by state and local governments and are paid for by tax dollars. They can be specialty hospitals, such as mental health facilities or community hospitals.

Subacute care   Care for conditions that fall between acute, or sudden onset, and chronic, conditions that are long lasting or never changing).

Subsidiary board   Functioning board for a health care organization that exists as part of a larger health system and that is accountable to the health system's parent board.

Suppliers   Organizations that provide products and services to the health care industry, such as pharmaceutical manufacturers, hospital supply and equipment companies, and medical consulting firms.

System stage   Evolutionary stage of hospital development characterized by a focus on forming and managing a diverse array of enterprises and relationships that allow hospitals to compete in current markets.

Tertiary care   Specialized consultative care, usually on referral from primary or secondary health care providers. Tertiary care, generally delivered in teaching institutions that have the personnel and facilities for special investigation and treatment, handles rare and complicated illnesses.

Theory   A judgment, concept, or formula that is considered true or accurate based on experimental evidence and generalizations of fact, but not yet accepted as a law.

Tiered health plans   Health plans in which hospitals, clinics, and doctors are placed in categories based on quality and cost, which plan members can choose and pay for accordingly.

Title VII programs   The major federal vehicle for generalist training.

Underinsured patient   Individual who has some insurance benefits but lacks the quality and scope of benefits that other insured groups enjoy.

Uninsured patient   Individual who lacks private health insurance coverage and who doesn't qualify for either Medicaid or Medicare.

Urgent care facility   A health care organization that evaluates and treats conditions that aren't severe enough to require an emergency room visit but that are serious enough to require treatment beyond normal physician office hours or before a physician appointment is available.

Utilization reviews   Managed care mandates requiring patients to get approval from the managed care organization for certain services before receiving treatment.

Vertical systems   Combine functionally different organizations, where patient outputs of one organization in the system are inputs of another. Vertical systems always combine organizations within a given market.

Veteran   A person who serves (or served) in the U.S. armed forces.

Veteran's Health Administration (VA)   U.S. governmental agency that provides hospitals and health care services for veterans.

Vital statistics   Statistics related to births, deaths, marriages, health, disease, and so on for a population.

Voluntary commitment   A person voluntarily commits to a care facility such as a psychiatric ward, hospital, institution, or treatment center. Generally the person is free to leave at will, with given notice.

Voluntary nonprofit health organizations   Private organizations that perform charitable functions or provide a community service.

World Health Organization (WHO)   United Nations agency whose function is to act as a coordinating authority on global health issues; established in 1948.

INDEX

X